M000280131

THE
NEUROFEEDBACK
SOLUTION

"Clearly written and exciting in scope. The contributors assembled here represent the 'who's who' in research-based neurofeedback. They pioneered the use of sophisticated technology and developed effective protocols to treat a variety of disorders."

LES FEHMI, PH.D., DIRECTOR OF THE
PRINCETON BIOFEEDBACK CENTRE, DEVELOPER OF OPEN
FOCUS TRAINING, AND AUTHOR OF *THE OPEN-FOCUS BRAIN*

"This book comes close to having it all: the past, present, and future of neurofeedback and neuroplasticity; the theories; and the stories of real people who, using neurofeedback and related technologies, discover and rediscover their true humanity and higher functioning. Here is the humanity with the technologies, and the technologies with the humanity."

LEN OCHS, PH.D., FOUNDER OF OCHSLABS
AND THE LENS TECHNIQUE

"The brain can do far more for itself than drugs or other invasions, and the possibilities and realities are brought forth herein. The wisdom to self-regulate is contained in every brain. Larsen introduces a host of pioneers who are forging the future in this important emerging discipline."

THOMAS COLLURA, PH.D., BIOMEDICAL ENGINEER,
NEUROPHYSIOLOGIST, AND FOUNDER AND PRESIDENT
OF BRAINMASTER TECHNOLOGIES

"Stephen Larsen has done an amazing job of pulling together state-of-the-art neurofeedback treatments into an easy-to-read book that will be useful to experts in the field as well as the general public. Those already doing neurofeedback as well as those with no background at all can learn from this book."

JEFFREY A. CARMEN, PH.D., LICENSED PSYCHOLOGIST
AND CREATOR OF THE EZPIR HEG NEUROFEEDBACK SYSTEM

The Neurofeedback Solution

HOW TO TREAT AUTISM, ADHD, ANXIETY, BRAIN INJURY, STROKE, PTSD, AND MORE

STEPHEN LARSEN, Ph.D.

Healing Arts Press
Rochester, Vermont • Toronto, Canada

Healing Arts Press
One Park Street
Rochester, Vermont 05767
www.HealingArtsPress.com

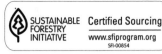

SUSTAINABLE Certified Sourcing
FORESTRY
INITIATIVE www.sfiprogram.org
SFI-00854

Text stock is SFI certified

Healing Arts Press is a division of Inner Traditions International

Note to the reader: This book is intended as an informational guide. The remedies, approaches, and techniques described herein are meant to supplement, and not to be a substitute for, professional medical care or treatment. They should not be used to treat a serious ailment without prior consultation with a qualified health care professional.

Library of Congress Cataloging-in-Publication Data
Larsen, Stephen.
  The neurofeedback solution : how to treat autism, ADHD, anxiety, brain injury, stroke, PTSD, and more / Stephen Larsen.
    p. cm.
  Includes bibliographical references and index.
  Summary: "A guide to neurofeedback for better physical and mental health as well as greater emotional balance, cognitive agility, and creativity"—Provided by publisher.
  ISBN 978-1-59477-366-2 (pbk.) — ISBN 978-1-59477-810-0 (e-book)
  1. Biofeedback training. 2. Affective disorders—Treatment. I. Title.
  RC489.B53L373 2012
  616.85'27—dc23

Printed and bound in the United States by Lake Book Manufacturing
The text stock is SFI certified. The Sustainable Forestry Initiative® program promotes sustainable forest management.

10 9 8 7 6 5 4 3 2 1

Text design and layout by Priscilla Baker
This book was typeset in Garamond Premier Pro with Trajan and Myriad Pro used as display typefaces

All images courtesy Stone Mountain Center, New Paltz, New York, except for the following: Fig 1.2 courtesy of Jasper and Penfield (1949); 3.2, 3.3 courtesy of R. Thatcher; 3.4 courtesy of OchsLabs and J&J Engineering; 9.1 courtesy of E. C. Hammond; 11.2, 11.3 courtesy of E. Baehr; 12.1–12.4, plate 12, plate 13 courtesy of V. Zelek, NCSC; 14.1 courtesy of E. Peper; 14.2–14.4 courtesy of J. Gunkelman, Q-Metrix; 14.5, 14.6, plate 1, plate 16 courtesy of J. Acosta-Urquidi; plate 4 courtesy of National Library of Medicine; plate 10, plate 11 courtesy of D. C. Hammond; plate 14 courtesy of M. P. van den Heuvel/ *Human Brain Mapping;* plate 15 courtesy of P. Hagmann/*PLoS Biology;* plate 17 courtesy of Rollin McCraty/Institute of HeartMath Research Center.

This book is dedicated to three of the great pioneers
and innovators—whose lives spanned the twentieth century
and who lived into the twenty-first—
who have made our field possible:

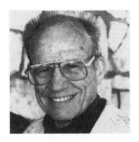

*Elmer Green, who first
hooked up yogis and
explored the boundaries of
science and mysticism.*

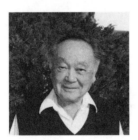

*Joe Kamiya, who discovered
brain wave discernment
and thus empowered a new
discipline for Psychology.*

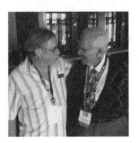

*Hershel Toomim (right),
who invented machines,
both practical and healing,
to bring new dimensions to
biofeedback therapy.*

CONTENTS

Foreword

Nancy White, Ph.D., and Leonard Richards, Th.D.

In his second book about neurofeedback, Stephen Larsen takes us further into the fascinating odyssey of this promising field: its birth, its adolescence, and now the dawn of its emergence into a mature treatment modality. The story the author tells us here is far from the final chapter in this rapidly developing discipline, and his current work chronicles significant aspects of neurofeedback's grown-up life: what it has become and what it can do today. Attention is duly given to the knowledge, understanding, and inventiveness that current practitioners have gained by "going to school" for a generation, under the tutelage of the field's original researchers—to whom this book is dedicated. Like Dad finally giving us the keys to our own car, today's practitioners are taking the results of their mentors' toil and driving more skillfully and safely into the future.

Important research findings in neural science regarding the physiology and functioning of our brains corroborate and support the findings of neurofeedback researchers—conducted for the most part without the extravagant funding available for more conventional projects—to provide an evidence-basis that gives the field greater acceptance than ever before. Stephen Larsen chronicles some of these developments, devoting an entire chapter (chapter 2) to the mainstream neuroscientific underpinnings of neurofeedback.

This field didn't always have the level of acceptance it does today. I (Nancy White) was one of the first professionals who brought neurofeedback from research into daily clinical practice; this began in the 1970s. Back then, many in the medical establishment treated neurofeedback with disdain, if not outright derision. On more than one occasion a parent reported to us that her child's pediatrician told her not to bother with neuro-feedback because she was "wasting her money." They found otherwise when they proceeded with neurofeedback therapy and their children improved markedly. At the end of an interview we gave to Houston's business newspa-per in the mid-1990s, a well-known local psychiatrist was asked to comment; he laid waste to the entire article with his own relatively uninformed negativ-ity. But today an entire section of his practice is devoted to neurofeedback.

On another occasion in the early 1990s we attended a dinner party in the elegant gardens of a friend's home. At our table sat a much older couple; the man introduced himself as a neurologist who remembered Houston's venerable Medical Center "when it was a corn field." At some point in the conversation he turned to me and asked, "And what is it you do, my dear?" I replied that we trained people's brains to improve neural function, at which point the old doctor pulled his glasses down on his nose and with a stern look said, "Poppycock, my dear, you can't train brains!"

Today, neurofeedback is conducted on a small scale at Baylor College of Medicine in Houston and at the University of Texas Medical Branch in Galveston. In our own clinic, we offer a variety of neurofeedback and related treatment modalities to improve brain function—in cases ranging from ADHD through traumatic brain injury to Asperger's and autism. How we use these modalities is guided by a wide range of testing and diagnostic tools, recently developed but increasingly accepted as reliable in the mental health professions.

We're a long way from the old-fashioned brown box with the 1970s blinking light, which signaled "feedback." Today's venues may be the simi-lar but the conversations are growing in sophistication and confidence. That's how far the field of neurofeedback has come and that's how much the rapidly growing body of research gives evidence of its efficacy.

And outcomes of this marvelous adventure are what Stephen Larsen gives us in this book.

More than a sequel to his earlier work, *The Healing Power of Neurofeedback,* this offering, *The Neurofeedback Solution,* takes us much further, much deeper, into this fascinating field. The distinguished professional contributors in this volume lay out salient aspects of today's neurofeedback in detail, but they do so in an accessible and conversational tone, despite the technical details included. We're introduced to a spectrum of areas in which neurofeedback has shown itself to be truly helpful. We believe neurofeedback can be life-changing, for ourselves, for loved ones, and for the many people so obviously helped by it, from difficult conditions otherwise unresponsive to conventional treatments.

At the very end of this book, we are given brand new perspectives on the mysterious field of consciousness itself—from a neurofeedback perspective—with Stephen interviewing some of the foremost brain wave experts in the world; they help us to understand the relationship between the brain and human behavior, at ever-deeper levels. This entire book gives both detailed science and warm and engaging human wisdom on how our minds work and how we can heal ourselves. You can trust that the science is sound, but you will not bog down in its details, because the overall message is so accessible and so universally human.

Enjoy!

NANCY WHITE AND LEONARD RICHARDS

NANCY WHITE, PH.D., QEEG, BCN Fellow, is cofounder and clinical director of *Unique MindCare* in Houston, Texas (formerly *The Enhancement Institute*). She is a past president and board member of the International Society for Research and Neurofeedback (ISNR), a consulting editor of the *Journal of Neurotherapy*, a member of the Quantitative EEG Certification Board, and a frequent presenter at professional conferences internationally. She has published a number of research articles and is a contributing author to the first and second editions of *Introduction to Quantitative EEG and Neurofeedback* (Academic Press 1999, 2009). She lives in Houston, Texas, with her professional and life partner, Leonard Richards.

LEONARD RICHARDS, M.B.A., TH.D., is a clinical associate at *Unique MindCare,* specializing in deep-state neurofeedback therapies for addiction, depression, anxiety, and post-traumatic stress disorder. In private practice he serves as a coach to senior executives and entrepreneurs. He has chaired or served on a number of charitable and educational boards. He has also written a number of magazine and journal articles, is a contributing coauthor to *Introduction to Quantitative EEG and Neurofeedback, Second Edition,* and coauthors research articles with Nancy White and others. He lives in Houston, Texas, with his professional and life partner, Nancy White.

WHY ANOTHER BOOK ON NEUROFEEDBACK?

W hy indeed? Simple answer: Neurofeedback is at the cutting edge of mental health care. Neurofeedback is one of the few evidence-based alternatives to pharmaceutical approaches. Neurofeedback helps people perform at the top of their game in an increasingly challenging world. Neurofeedback is about brain-computer interface—as in science fiction. In short, neurofeedback is a very "happening thing."

We are referring to the human biocomputer talking to a silicon chip–type computer, just like "Hal" in *2001: A Space Odyssey*. Much like Michael Knight's talking car on the old TV show *Knight Rider,* the human brain talks to the machine, and the machine extends the reach of the brain through information it couldn't quite get on its own—*about its own vital functioning!*

Miraculous as the capabilities of the machine are, without the "higher power," the *human* consciousness directing it, it is basically useless. The robot can both do much more and much less than the human being can do. In biofeedback, if we hook ourselves to a machine, it can tell us things about ourselves we don't know—about our temperature or blood pressure; and in *neurofeedback*—about our brain waves. Who out there knows when they are producing a certain brain wave? (But we know the *effects* of the shifting kaleidoscope of our brain energies—we are sleepy, we are alert, we are anxious, we are deeply engrossed in an inner fantasy.) We are also learning that we have to give our mechanical servant the right kind of instructions, skillful instructions, so it knows how to talk back to us politely and intelligibly, so we can learn from our own creation.

Some have likened the cyberrevolution to a genie that has not only gotten out of the bottle, but is now is *talking back to us,* in global surveillance systems and automated menus on telephones and computers that drive us crazy! We're supposed to be in charge, and the Frankenstein monster is abroad, in every mall, in our cars, on our cell phones, and in our e-mail. It is an open question whether our creature will ultimately help us or kill us.

There is an old Chinese curse: "May you live in interesting times!" *This is a very interesting time!* (In case you haven't noticed!) In biofeedback and neurofeedback, there is a focused attempt, by lots of very smart people, *to create healing robots.* We can learn about the brain from computers, and computers, after all, were built by—and are children of—the brain. If we expect our children to learn from us, can we learn from them? Can we form a healing partnership with our own creation?

I think we can.

My first book on this same subject, *The Healing Power of Neurofeedback,* was published by Healing Arts Press in 2006. I am told my book has played its own small part in helping the intelligent general public learn about neurofeedback and make their own better-informed decisions about whether to avail themselves of this gentle, noninvasive treatment method that can ameliorate many problems involving the nervous system—problems that lie in a zone not so well addressed either by the dominant medical paradigm or by traditional psychotherapy.

Healing Power concentrated on the LENS (Low Energy Neurofeedback System), the cutting-edge brain technology I have both learned from and contributed to over the last decade and a half. The LENS can sometimes provide breathtakingly short courses of treatment, sometimes even for intractable-seeming problems. I am told that thanks to the book and the wider visibility it afforded the LENS, there are now twice as many practitioners as there were, worldwide, and they bring to the field their own art and science; this book in part reflects their contribution.

In much the same way as *Healing Power* brought together clinicians and brain theorists, this book brings together a whole new colloquy—very much *not* the "same old, same old." There is not only new equipment but also new protocols for established equipment (as is described in later chapters), as well as whole new theories accounting for how this healing modality called "neurofeedback" actually works. Moreover, the clinicians, and the whole science itself, are in a state of development and transformation— as people realize its incredible healing potential. While in the earlier book I tried to honor the historically significant contributors who led up to the development of the LENS, as well as Dr. Len Ochs's own contribution to a whole new direction in neurofeedback, the LENS remains a small enclave within a field that itself is not that large, and the field itself has been involved its own complex evolution.

The good news is, you don't have to have read either book to understand the other, and I have deliberately written them so that each stands alone on its own merits. *Healing Power* examined neurofeedback up until 2005 (when the manuscript was turned in), and *The Neurofeedback Solution* details the developments from that point onward. Also, while *Healing Power* focused on the LENS as the culmination of neurofeedback to that time, as I believed it to have been, *The Neurofeedback Solution* focuses on what has happened since that time, as more people than the founder see the possibility of the method and write their own protocols, or use the LENS in combination with other methods.

In effect, since the turn of the millennium, there has been a kind of quantum explosion in this exciting field of brain-healing technology. As I prepared to write this book—attending conferences and talking to the innovators, who are both clinicians and innovative computer geniuses who are making it happen—I was "blown away" again and again by the rapidity with which our knowledge base is expanding. There is a whole new breed of scientist whose purview reaches beyond solid-state circuitry into mathematics, physics, probability theory, neuroscience, and healing. Talk about new "Rennaissance men" (and women)! As knowledge expands, the humans trying to *grok* it (Robert Heinlein's word in *Stranger in a Strange Land*) are able to master unique and useful ways of deploying that knowledge—for healing and consciousness exploration. The age of specialization has yielded to the age of dialogue—and synergy; it is nothing short of what teenagers call "awesome!"

I am humbled by the vastness of the evolving knowledge base about the brain that I have explored to write this book. I *gassho* to the many brilliant thinkers I have interviewed and taken seminars with, and I recognize how many people there are who know much more than I do. Understanding this, I had to identify my own role and find my own voice, as it were, as a (hopefully useful) expositor of a quantum technology. Only your *feedback* after reading this book will tell me if I have been successful. (I have only been willing to try because of some very nice feedback I have gotten in the past.) In fact, the magical utility of feedback is the theme that runs throughout this approach to healing the brain and the mind. Below you will find some basic terms that are used throughout this book; I also want to add that there is a list of acronyms in the back of the book, which you should refer to, as well as a compilation of neurofeedback resources for the interested reader. Please also know that the "Conclusions" at the end of the various chapters are my own.

A Definition of Basic Terms

Biofeedback: Any machine-mediated, often electronic device that feeds back to an organism information or a signal that helps the organism learn or change something.

Neurofeedback: A brain-based form of biofeedback, usually using brain waves. There are many schools of neurofeedback, each with its own protocols.

The LENS: The Low Energy Neurofeedback System developed by Dr. Len Ochs, which uses subliminal (radio frequency) signals to produce dramatically rapid results. Can be used to treat small children and animals, as well as adults.

Operant conditioning: A reward-based system of learning, in which an organism must discriminate between stimuli in order to obtain the "reinforcement."

Classical conditioning: A type of learning based on the innate, nervous system–based responses of the organism.

ONE

WHAT IS NEUROFEEDBACK?

The Helpful Little Robot

A biofeedback machine is a type of helpful little robot. First thing, it doesn't lie.

Any psychotherapist knows how beautifully defended most people's psyches can be—in the service of preserving the status quo—even if their way of being in the world is making them sick and crazy. They may fiercely hang on to what seems to everyone around them a "neurotic" set of compensations—some would call them "symptoms." That is why some psychotherapists have to use really sneaky techniques to effect therapeutic change—hypnosis, Neuro-Linguistic Programming, even years of (expensive) psychoanalysis. (That's why some therapeutic environments count on group therapy, because really well-defended people, like alcoholics or sociopaths, can defeat the attempts of even the most skillful therapist, and it takes a "whole group" to bring about positive change.)

But now imagine that the therapist has "a little helper," *who everyone knows tells nothing but the truth.* In fact, he is a robot—so you can't argue with him or deny what he says. Years ago a patient who was herself a psychotherapist came to me for a consultation. After years of therapy, including some of the most cathartic and expressive approaches, which were very popular at the time—such as bioenergetics, psychodrama, and even "primal scream" therapy—she was possibly worse, but certainly no better. Some of the most skillful veterans in our therapeutic community had tried with her—and failed.

In our first psychotherapy session, she readily got in touch, once more, with her primordial angst—the "emotional self" she called her "inner child." Just think, a few skillful questions, and this patient was in touch with her primal pain. (That's the point at which, off guard, you could say to yourself, "What a good therapist I must be—to have gotten to the problem so quickly!")

But I did my own usual kind of "proprioceptive" biofeedback. How did I, the therapist, really feel inside as my client was having her dramatic catharsis? Was I feeling empathic, vindicated in my approach, and as if I had really accomplished something?

No, I actually felt bored, and maybe a little bemused at the spectacle (which is not my usual response to a patient in distress). Then I remembered my little helper I had just brought over from the college biofeedback lab.

"Would you mind if I just hooked you up to a little robot?" I asked. Astonished, she stopped the emotional pyrotechnics for a moment, and agreed. I hooked her to a GSR or skin galvanometer (at the heart of the classic "lie detector" test).

I then invited her to resume, and she willingly obliged—it was a very familiar therapeutic MO for her, and she jumped back in.

But the little robot was absolutely unimpressed. According to the GSR machine, she was flatlined, as if there were no genuine (physically arousing) emotion at all.

I gently confronted her with the disparity. I hinted that the "abreaction," the emotional discharge, instead of being therapeutically useful, might be a learned response to the environment (the privilege of working with psychotherapists who embrace the emotional-discharge school of therapy).

Instead of the kind of shrill doubling of the emotional output, as had happened in the past when discerning psychodynamic therapists had accused her of "secondary gain"—that is, "getting something" out of the emotional display (like attention)—she sighed, shrugged her shoulders, and said, "Oh, well." (How do you argue with a "little robot" who always tells the truth?)

We were able to begin some far more useful and insight-yielding therapy from that point onward, with a far more appropriate affect that fluctuated within normal bounds.

Biofeedback and neurofeedback skate elegantly between the paradigms of psychopharmacology and psychiatry on the one hand and psychodynamic or behavioral psychotherapy on the other. Relying neither on medicines nor on lengthy talking analyses and interventions, it does a third thing. It hooks someone up to a machine, which is neutral. The machine puts no one on drugs, nor does it analyze one's Oedipal dilemmas or "flawed reinforcement history."* Instead it says, "You have a lot of muscle tension" (EMG) or, "Your hands are freezing and your head is on fire—which is fueling that migraine!" (temperature biofeedback). Or, "Your brain waves are similar to those we have seen before with head-injury patients" (EEG or neurofeedback). "Can you think of any traumatic brain injury you forgot to tell me about?"

It is a different form of communication, and invitation to response, that the little robot offers. It does not say: "Improve your attitude" or "Think positively," things one can fail at; it simply says: "Turn on this tone, or that animation, or play that movie with sound—and some good things might happen." Succeeding or failing is not limited to whether you are a good responder to this or that drug, nor whether you are a compliant or insightful psychotherapy client. Instead, success is predicated on how much you can produce this result, or play this little computer game (say Pac-Man).

What a wonderful alternative to the *terrifying obligation to get better* by having to change oneself in all kinds of ways (reform programs often doomed to fail, psychoanalysis, where one "doesn't get it," or a behavior modification program in which one is lax or inconsistent). The biofeedback is more immediate and less cluttered with sociocultural baggage.

Change this light, make this music or video play, and in effect learn to trust the thing inside you that can do that; making it happen *like a miracle*

---

*Flawed reinforcement history refers to operant conditioning theory, whereby one has inadvertently received "reinforcement" for inappropriate or dysfunctional behaviors— getting lots of attention for a tantrum, for example.

of which you don't understand the agency, but which is real nonetheless. The implicit value system of biofeedback agrees with the fundamental tenets of psychoanalysis *or* behaviorism. It says, "Yes, you are capable of affecting *the unconscious mind"*—even "classically conditioned" reflexes you felt totally helpless to control. Try this little piece of self-influence, and see if anything changes in the relationship with your unconscious mind—on which you depend for nine-tenths of everything you do anyway. Without the vaguest idea of how to produce what you would like to happen, you do it anyway—and thus are in sync, and in a pretty good rapport with the *terra incognita* inside. Biofeedback opens avenues to dialogue with the unconscious in which you are not simply "fighting yourself" but are open to influencing not just the unconscious but your relationship to it. There will be more discussion on this in the clinical examples that follow.

The Existence of Brain Waves

The very existence of brain waves was not really described systematically till the end of the 1920s, by Dr. Hans Berger. During World War I, Berger was almost killed in a military operation by a runaway piece of military equipment. His sister, many hundreds of miles away, showed an inexplicable knowledge of the fact that her brother had almost died—at the very time of the near-accident. Berger, of a scientific mind, set out to probe the inexplicable. Using an extremely primitive string galvanometer, he measured the oscillatory waves that could be recorded through the skull and scalp. These are measured not in thousandths but millionths of a volt—called "microvolts."

Berger gave the first waves he found, all over the scalp, the name *alpha,* after the first letter in the Greek alphabet. In turn, the other brain wave ranges were discovered. *Beta* is a faster frequency associated with mental effort and thinking (also anxiety). *Delta,* the slowest frequency, is found in abundance in deep sleep, and it also indicates injury or deep kinds of depression. *Theta* is the gateway frequency that seems to connect the conscious and the unconscious mind. It appears in the hypnagogic and hypnopompic states that lead into and out of sleep and is also found in hypnosis, mystical experience, and deep reverie—as well as attentional problems.

All this is covered in basic neurofeedback books and in *The Healing Power of Neurofeedback,* which also shows how different schools of thought applied different training procedures up till the discovery of the LENS. This is fascinating, because the LENS does not reward or signal out a specific range for training; it stimulates the *dominant frequency* at an *offset* (a frequency measure in Hertz or cycles per second), thus allowing the brain to self-regulate.

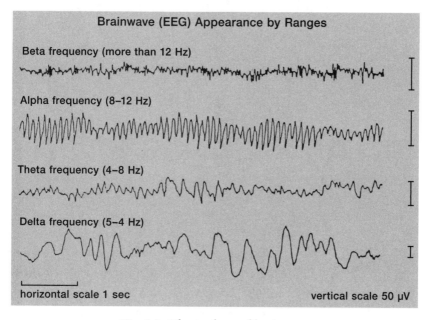

Fig. 1.1. Classic chart of brain waves

This book includes many wonderful stories and cases from the LENS as the treatment modality I know best, but it also takes a second look at traditional neurofeedback and the amazing things we can learn from going right to the *source,* in our biofeedback command-central, the brain itself. Later in this book we will look at how basic neurofeedback can be used in multiple ways: to supplement or follow the LENS; to work with traditional—or, as it is called, "peripheral"—biofeedback (such as heart rate variability or muscle tension); and to work with new technologies that use something other than "waves" to talk to the brain (such as "slow cortical potentials") and the simple dynamic of blood flow to the brain (HEG, or hemoencephalography). In short, since the publication of my first book on this topic in 2006, this field has not been idle; instead it is growing with the technology, particularly the brain-computer interface technology.

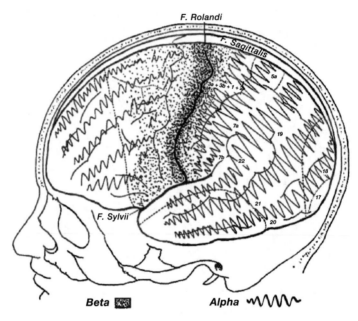

Fig. 1.2. Electric fields of the brain. Cortical surface regions where alpha rhythms were recorded in a large population of epilepsy surgery patients are indicated by wavy lines. The dotted region near the central motor strip indicates beta activity. EcoG activity was characterized by counting zero crossings before Fourier transforms were used in EEG. Reproduced from Jasper and Penfield (1949).

Surfing the Waves

I'm working on this book on my brand new Apple computer. I wasn't sure I wanted to learn a new computer technology; after all, I've been with Windows for years, and it's all ploddingly familiar. But I wanted a different tool to work on this book: zingy, versatile, with good graphics capabilities. Besides, I wanted a rugged little machine with a good battery that I can carry anywhere, on the Trailways bus, or at the airport, for when inspiration comes calling.

Great idea, but can old dogs learn new tricks? I'm in my late sixties, and here I am, standing in front of this kid who can't be more than
twenty, a third my age, and he's an Apple "genius." Now he's showing me
all kinds of things I never saw before: unfamiliar icons, little guitars and
palm trees and stamps in a strip at the bottom of my computer. My mind
is racing to take it all in.

I recognize the state: just short of anxiety, but with a unique acquisitive
energy to multiprocess information, a little like surfing on a big gnarly wave
of information; it's *beta waves* I need to produce now, right around 15–18
Hz. I first learned to really identify this range on one of Siegfried Othmer's
classic EEG Spectrum machines back in the 1990s. After an intensive ten-
hour day in Summit, New Jersey, all on EEG neurofeedback, with Siegfried
and his wife, Sue, I was tired and mentally wiped out. In the middle of a
three-day intensive training, I was looking forward to crashing on a relative's
couch, next town over, and starting the same regimen again the next day.

On the way out the door, there was a vacant machine sitting there,
and I ogled it uneasily. (*Too much brain on the brain!*) What the heck! I
attached the single electrode to my scalp and told the machine: *Reward
beta, inhibit theta,* and listened for the signals. Soon I wasn't tired any
more; instead, I was *wired.*

Driving home after the seminar, the state rose up suddenly again on
the New Jersey Turnpike; suddenly traffic was zooming all around me
in three tightly channeled lanes and all well over the speed limit. A low,
malicious chuckle broke out of me, and I stepped on the gas, weaving in
and out of traffic, giddily relishing the speed, like Mr. Toad in *The Wind
in the Willows.* It's the sensation of a brain on overdrive, but it sure gets
things done, and it gets you where you're going, in the fast lane. (After
years of experience, I'm convinced it's the safest way to drive in aggressive
New York traffic. Daydream, and you're doomed!) Arriving at my relatives' house, I chatted wildly, a ball of fire. I didn't realize EEG biofeedback could actually *do something* like this! After all, I was physiologically
as well as mentally exhausted. Could it galvanize the body via the mind?

Arriving home after the seminar, I realized I was thinking faster than
my family members; maybe I was even a little hard on them, talking too
fast, impatient.

"Oh, oh. Down, boy!"

Time to slow down. How about a glass of wine and a dunk in the hot tub? Ah . . . That's better; I'm back to a mindless, content "alpha" (8–12 Hz). I'm not looking at the clock any more, and I'm not expecting anything unusual of anyone.

As I write this first chapter, I'm looking for a way to communicate to my reader how exciting are the possibilities that neurofeedback can open for us, a technology that puts the mind and the computer together and lets them talk to each other. It's a healing technology that expands our options for mental control—and it's also an an optimal performance technology.

The advantage of having done years of neurofeedback is that I have developed a different kind of cognition, call it a *metacognition* even, that allows me to identify the state, or the dominant brain wave range, I am in and thus exert some kind of control, either directly or indirectly, over what's happening inside my head.

Back to the Apple store, where I started, and the present: By the time I'm done processing everything the brainy kid has told me, and daring to imagine I can remember anything, I sort of go limp. By the time I'm home I just want to relax, close my eyes, and sink into reverie. Hovering close to the borders of sleep, colorful images swarm around, and I hear themes from classical music in my mind, as clearly as if I were in a concert hall—a unique faculty I have often enjoyed. It's very restful, and it goes on for some time, because here time doesn't matter at all . . .

As I slide back to normal waking consciousness, that is, the "place of thinking," I marvel at the richness of the theta state that I just passed through (about 4–8 Hz). I was swimming in mental imagery, seeing and hearing things. But not to worry, theta's just as important in the daily cycle of things as beta or alpha. In fact, theta helps me recover my wits and delivers some unexpected inspiration. (And by the way, theta is deeply involved in forming long-term, meaningful memories via a little brain organ called the "hippocampus.")

"That's great for personal experiences and narrative consciousness," some scientifically oriented readers might be saying, "good storytelling, but how do you know these beta and theta states correspond to anything in the real world?"

An inspiration has just come to me. I think I'll tell them about John Gruzelier's heavenly musicians and the dance, the *pas de deux* between beta and theta experiences.

Gruzelier's Heavenly Musicians

British researcher John Gruzelier* is a cultured, soft-spoken scientist, a professor of Psychology at Goldsmith's College, University of London, who has designed some of the most highly regarded experiments in neurofeedback, real studies with experimental and control groups, statistics, and a blinded panel of experts. Gruzelier's list of 250 scientific publications includes work on the immune system, schizophrenia, and hypnosis, but for our purposes, let's look at a paper I heard him give at a major international conference (Gruzelier 2009).

His theoretical question, now to be put to the experimental test? *Could neurofeedback offer anything whatever to music students in a highly competitive music conservatory environment?* Judges are routinely used to evaluate students' accuracy and musicality, so it was relatively easy in this study to *blind the judges*—that was their job; they simply did not know anything about the students they were evaluating beyond their performance. The students who had received neurofeedback training to strengthen their beta brain waves performed discriminably (and significantly according to the judges) better than the control group, especially on tasks requiring sight reading and musical accuracy. Teaching the students' brains to speed up made it easier for them to master the complex processes of reading and playing a musical score.

This was finding number one, which Gruzelier documented indisputably. It is not impossible that Ritalin or amphetamines could produce similar improvements in score, but these drugs have a narrow window of efficacy (no effect before the drug begins to work, and afterward the musician may become "buzzed" or "wasted"). ("Speed freaks" do not usually last that long in the realm of professional musicians; they are rather like meteors that streak through the sky, casting a great trail as they burn themselves to oblivion.)

---

*For more on John Gruzelier, please visit www.gold.ac.uk/psychology/staff/gruzelier.

But the next finding of Gruzelier leaves crude pharmaceutical influence in the dust. He wondered what would happen if the musicians were now led to explore theta, at the other, slower end of the brain wave spectrum. Theta brings in the flavor of emotionality, reverie, opening the portals of the "deep unconscious." When the students were exposed to theta training and then went before the judges yet again, the judges felt that there was more than mere accuracy in their music (the higher frequency beta): there was *soul,* there was expression, there was deep rapport and communication of the musician with the listener, from theta.

Try that one with pharmaceuticals: Dexamyl perhaps, the stimulant Dexedrine with amobarbital, a barbiturate derivative. Frankly, I have never heard that great musicians are produced by such a druggy combo. The outcomes of this type of neurofeedback further illustrate the principle that in this realm, monolithic approaches are counterproductive, whereas flexible approaches, tentatively and pragmatically applied, seem to produce the richest and the best outcomes. The neurofeedback has the delicacy to mobilize endogenous systems within the person, whereas the pharmaceutical approach simply floods the brain with chemicals, and the brain now has the additional task of sorting out how to function normally while under an alien (nonendogenous) occupation. No wonder it gets exhausted, especially when the chemical invasion is repeated day after day, and it must try to mobilize itself as best it can under these circumstances (think of life in Baghdad trying to return to normal while an occupying army is still present).

Morphogenesis and Neurofeedback

A colleague, Jeremy Narby, a professor of Psychology at Ohio University, cued me to a very subtle application of the principle of pedagogical influence. He noticed that over years of teaching the same course in transpersonal psychology, the class seemed to "deepen" both intellectually and experientially each semester. It is not unexpected that this should happen when students acquire a new vocabulary and become familiar with the subject matter; their questions would be better, and the discussions would become really interesting, drawing forth new dimensions of the psychological problem that was before them. The surprising part, though, Narby told me, was that semester to semester, even with brand-new students, *they would seem to start at a higher level of discourse* and then take it to still higher and more sophisticated levels.

A skeptic might say that it was just due to his own development as a professor and educator, and indeed, that variable can't be discounted. Because he was the professor, naturally he was the only observer with the continuity to form a judgment. As science, such an idea must remain speculation, though an interesting and perhaps testable hypothesis could come out of it. I thought I had already observed some version of the same thing in a college course I taught called "The Psychology of Consciousness." Admittedly, the course tried to empower students and encourage them to be their own "field study" in consciousness, tracking dreams, daydreams, and reveries, the effects of prolonged concentration, the effects of meditation or sensory isolation. I had to agree with Narby after about ten more years of teaching. The students seemed almost to take up where their predecessors had left off.

I believe something like this has taken place in biofeedback and neurofeedback as fields. Yes, they are fields in which "consciousness is studying itself," so you can guarantee that there are going to be surprise "field effects." Not everyone always gets along by any means, and people have different paradigms for studying the phenomena in which they are interested. But major breathroughs ripple through the field like chemical reactions. For example, there are now about three hundred LENS practitioners worldwide. The subject is on the agenda at major neurofeedback conferences, and the articles appear in professional journals such as the *Journal of Neurotherapy*.

Another example: About ten years ago, I felt I must be a maverick neurofeedback clinician and researcher for being so interested in heart-rate variability (HRV), a measure of cardiac health. I finally went to Boulder Creek, California, got trained and licensed at HeartMath as a provider, and went on to study the work of Rutgers professor Paul Lehrer and his detailed analyses of the HRV.

But I should really be concentrating on brain waves, the EEG, shouldn't I? They are demanding enough as a subject, after all. But now, HRV has swept the self-regulation field, and there are many, many

Defining Emerging Brain-Changing Technologies

HEG or **hemoencephalography** (a term coined by Toomim and Carmen to define the clinical diagnostic tool they developed; see chapter 13) uses simple blood-flow biofeedback to change brain waves (neurofeedback).

HRV or **heart-rate variability** (Doc Childre's HeartMath and/ or Eliot's Coherent Breathing, as well as other approaches) uses breathing (about 5–6 breaths per minute) and concentration on a positive emotion to change the brain.

The NeuroField, developed by Nicholas Dogris, uses pulsed electromagnetic fields to stimulate and balance the entire nervous system.

Slow cortical potentials (SCP), developed and used in Europe by Nils Birbaumer, are more DC than AC.* Infra-low frequency (ILF) training (developed by Othmer and Smith) is AC so slow that it seems like DC. Both SCP and ILF can be trained with operant conditioning techniques; they affect the entire AC spectrum of brain waves.

Z-score training (developed by Smith and Collura, using Thatcher's NeuroGuide database) is based on qEEG (quantitative electroencephalographic) databases that do moment-by-moment comparison of the subject being trained to normative metrics such as *coherence, connectivity,* and *phase.*

---

*Electrical energies in the brain can be measured by AC (or alternating current—the familiar frequencies of alpha, delta, etc.) or DC (direct current, slow carrier waves), similar to the "currents" of acupuncture.

---

approaches, although Doc Childre and HeartMath were right there at the beginning. It turns out HRV training is a major physiological marker for what the rest of the nervous system, including the brain, is doing.

Independent researchers such as Stephen Eliot have brought new ways of thinking about systemic resonance and coherence to the process. Almost everyone that comes to our office gets training in coherent breathing and HRV. It didn't take long for all our staff to be trained and to use it along-side of neurofeedback sessions to help keep patients in balance as we work.

Minds and hearts at work means integrative healing methods that involve the best our minds can do, but also with the human emotional life taken into account or included: "a path with heart."

Infra-Low Frequencies, or ILF, HEG, and Z-Score Training

Because these terms will be found in the text and in interviews with professionals, I'm going to give the reader the briefest of introductions to these things, just as I did with biofeedback, neurofeedback, and the LENS. They will be covered in greater depth in chapter 13. Here are three unusual forms of neurofeedback, which are very salient in the professional community these days:

Infra-low frequencies (ILF) seem to lie in the DC realm instead of the AC realm of "brain waves" (and hence are often confused with slow cortical potentials, which are "true" DC). ILF fluctuations are slower than delta (.5–4 Hz by most reckoning). They lie below a frequency so low that many EEG machines cannot register it; it is called "the corner frequency." Against the vivid up-and-down frequencies of the conventional EEG spectrum (with rhythmical, frequent sine-wave excursions above and below the Y axis), this inexorable energy probably corresponds to the same energy that moves through the acupuncture meridians and points. More on this will be discussed later, but this energy may correspond to something seldom spoken of in Psychology these days: *the will.* Amazingly, training this energy has been said to reduce negative symptomatology and help in recovery from trauma and emotional injury.

The training of hemoencephalography (HEG) begins with the work of Drs. Marjorie and Hershel Toomim, venerable pioneers in the realm of biofeedback (nirHEG), and Dr. Jeffrey Carmen, a New York clinical psychologist, each working independently (pirHEG). Rather than train-ing the brain waves themselves, the Toomims and Carmen focused on the circulatory system that nourishes the brain. We know that if you deliver more oxygen and glucose to areas of the brain, they suddenly begin to work better. A way of verifying this is that the EEG frequencies speed up. Different biofeedback modalities actually offer a scientific and objective way to measure modalities that affect completely different parameters. So I have people practice deep muscle relaxation measurable on an EMG, and I see that their EEG also actually changes—there is a statistically noticeable increase in alpha (8–12 Hz). The Toomims used simple operant conditioning to increase blood flow to people's frontal areas. Not surprisingly, even though this may seem like an indirect way of getting there, the brains of these individuals began to work better.

Z-score training is a brilliant, dizzyingly complex "brainchild" of Mark Smith and Thomas Collura, and it is based on the NeuroGuide database of Robert Thatcher. The first thing required is a qEEG, or quantitative electroencephalogram of nineteen "sites" (according to the International 10–20 system) acquired through a "cap" on the scalp. What is the difference between this and the EEG you get in a neurologist's office? Almost nothing except the manner of interpretation. The neurologist counts on his specialized training—up to two years—and his expert eye to scan the raw EEG for anomalies, mostly relating to epilepsy or some form of TBI.

The "q," on the other hand, uses computer parameters to analyze the data in the blindingly rapid calculations of the microprocessor. Not only can the computer do fast Fourier transforms (FFTs) to turn the raw data into a "power spectrum" that compares the amount of the different brain wave ranges—alpha, beta, delta, and so on—but, in a feat worthy of an interstellar navigator on a spacecraft, compares the metrics that instantly appear in the EEG to a "cohort," a representative group of people matched as to age and gender to the subject being measured. This is the "Z-score." Your brain is instantaneously compared to a "normative database" (people who are "normal" because they are like lots of other people).

The qEEG is examined and used as a basis for the Z-score "training." Where does the brain listen or fail to listen to *itself*? The FFT is used to compare the qEEG (done with the nineteen-site "cap" that measures sites simultaneously) for *phase* lag or advance between the sites. (I will explain this in greater detail a bit later in the book, as well as provide more information on Dr. Robert Thatcher and his NeuroGuide database as we learn how this space-age hybrid came to be.)

The NeuroField is the brainchild of Dr. Nicholas Dogris. At first I was reluctant to consider this machine "biofeedback" at all. Rather, it seemed more akin to "energy medicine," because the NeuroField does its work through pulsed electromagnetic fields that are preprogrammed and selected by the operator.

But Dr. Dogris, on the threshold of FDA approval, has made his device use both biofeedback and neurofeedback after all, by an ingenious method that will be described in more detail later. (He built in both an HRV monitoring device and an EEG monitoring device that show the results of the energy field "sweep" or treatment that is given. This is real science: administer your wisp of a radio frequency that you hope will help someone's arthritis, or depression, or TBI, and then see how it affects the cardiac environment and the brain itself.) Dogris thought there might be value in the widely applied practice of muscle testing—done by many bodyworkers to determine whether a substance or a situation is good or bad for you—but he thought the procedure was far too subjective, so he got a couple of little robots, who couldn't lie, to help him. There will be an in-depth analysis of these systems in chapter 13.

We are left with the fact that with almost any kind of feedback system—whether the unconscious, subliminal operation of the LENS; the time-honored techniques such as alpha-theta that helped Eugene Peniston's war veterans with drug and alcohol dependence; the SMR (sensorimotor rhythm) that helped Barry Sterman's cats be seizure-free even when exposed to seizure-inducing chemicals; the beta, explored by Joel Lubar and the Othmers for intellectual activity and problem solving; or the very high frequency gamma believed by Davidson and others to accompany states of near-"enlightenment" or optimal performance—we have the single, simple underlying dynamic of the brain exercising itself by changing its functioning. If physical exercise relates to improved functioning of both body and mind (as it does), then the same principle holds "in spades" for the brain.

We look next to movements in a mainstream, university-based science—neurobiology, or neuroscience—which comment poignantly on the change in thinking we are talking about!

TWO

THE CHANGING BRAIN

NEUROPLASTICITY AND THE
PARADIGM SHIFT

The entire rest of this book is believable and comprehensible only if you have an open neurological paradigm. Or, as one bumper sticker from the nineties said: *Minds are like parachutes, they work best when they are open.*

I believe neurofeedback makes sense only if you see it in the broader context of *neural plasticity,* a concept now sweeping the entire field of neuroscience, with implications so broad for humanity that they are staggering. We now know that the brain is able not only to change its functioning—we all seem to have accepted that—but its very physiological substrata: the neurons, their synapses, and the entire biochemical environment dwelling there, on which modern psychopharmacology has based its enterprise (and it is a vast and lucrative one indeed).

Old assumptions, so fundamental to our consumer culture that professions and economies are based on them, are in the process of being replaced. Something needs to die so that something new, something healthier, more flexible, and more alive can take its place.

The Death of the Old Paradigm

Thomas Kuhn, who gave the term *paradigm* its modern meaning and then popularized it so that everyone in the intellectual community knew what it meant, once quipped: "The old paradigm indeed will change, one funeral at a time!"

I came to learn more about what he meant as I did the background research for my recent book, *The Fundamentalist Mind*. People are extraordinary, versatile, creative geniuses, but we are also capable of getting stuck in our own habitual ways of thinking. Age and experience may not help; rather, they may consolidate or petrify what we already know till we *know* we know! (A genteel friend of mine, instead of saying someone was rigid or closed, would say, "Well, he's just had a hardening of the categories"—or, "He suffers from *logosclerosis!*") And this same condition afflicts *the scientist* no less than the rigid, fanatic world of the religious right.

Underneath what the Germans call *die Weltanschauung,* the "worldview," lie fundamental assumptions about the way reality is put together. To examine an early dilemma from Psychology: Is the science of the human psyche to be examined *structurally* or *functionally*?

Not surprisingly, researchers pursuing both paradigms learned important things. For example, Walter Cannon learned that a major part of emotion in organisms is mediated through a central little organ called the *hypothalamus* (a structural analysis). He was right. But William James and Carl G. Lange, a Danish physiologist, at the same time came up with the idea that when an emotion is felt, it ricochets all around the body, so that the stomach and the heart become involved along with the brain (a functional analysis). Also right, especially with new sophisticated physiological measuring devices. Partisans of each perspective claimed they knew the answer.

In this book we seek to cultivate new ways of looking at old problems and to examine new technologies that did not exist during most of the last century. In this way we learn to open our paradigms, parachuting into the new and fantastic worlds of microbiology, microelectronics (as in the EEG), and previously unimaginable things like gene expression and neural plasticity.

The No-New-Neurons Orthodoxy

No less an authority than the venerable Santiago Ramón y Cajal had stated, not long after the turn of the twentieth century: *Neurons do not regenerate.* For ninety years that remained the dictum and the orthodoxy; lacking evidence to the contrary, neuroscientists passed the lore along like a piece of indisputable Bible-based theology (call it a type of neuroscientific *fundamentalism*).

Joseph Altman knew what political and social fundamentalism could do to the human mind from surviving the *Wehrmacht* in Hungary, where, as a Jew, and highly vulnerable, he invented for himself a kind of "aparanoia," in which he held his head high and "refused to cower" (like the mouse hero in *Despereaux*). Surviving the Nazis, he "could not tolerate the rising Communist dictatorship," thus becoming a "stateless displaced person" in West Germany for some years. He then emigrated, first to Australia and then the United States. After completing his graduate studies as a neuroscientist, he found a job at MIT (Gross 2009).

By the 1960s, now in his late thirties, Altman published the findings of his studies of rodent brains using *thymidine autoradiographic* techniques, which described the proliferation of new neurons in the *dentate gyrus* of the hippocampus, the *olfactory bulb,* and the *neocortex* of both rats and cats. The implications were revolutionary for the scientific community, demonstrating the physiological underpinnings of learning and opening whole new avenues of exploration for medicine and neurotherapies. It also offered to turn a shibboleth of modern neurophysiology on its head: the "no new neurons" orthodoxy, on which not a few experts had staked their professional reputations.

Though Altman published his findings in prestigious journals such as *Nature* and *Science,* for decades the old belief system, congruent with the scientific paradigms of the time, prevailed over the evidence. As late as 1970 an authoritative textbook of developmental neuroscience stated: "There is no convincing evidence of neuron production in the brains of adult mammals" (Gross 2009, 230). In effect, the field was held to a dogma by "minds that couldn't change themselves."

Then, fifteen years after Altman's first publications, Michael Kaplan and his associates at the University of New Mexico reported evidence from electron microscopy (the only technique fine enough to show details in the neuronal environment) supporting neurogenesis in adult rats and adult macaque monkeys. (The "adult" part is important, because everyone knows juvenile brains are plastic; once matured, the brain was not believed to exhibit physiological changes.)

The traditional authority in the field of neuroscience had emanated from Yale's prestigious neuroscientist Pasko Rakic, who said of Kaplan's findings, "These may look like [new] neurons in New Mexico, but they do not look like neurons in New Haven!" Both Altman and Kaplan were to suffer professionally because their research was aligned with an unpopular paradigm.

But there was additional evidence of plasticity from another source. During the same period, Fernando Nottebohm and his associates at Rockefeller University had been studying the amazing ability of songbirds to alter their songs year by year, even season by season. The same thymidine labeling process that had been used on the rodents showed the growth in birds of new neurons with long axonal processes and the formation of new synapses. (People all over the country were hearing blue jays and magpies that had learned how to sound like their cell phones—clearly a learned rather than a genetic response.) Still, the bird research was dismissed as an exotic abberation of flying creatures, whose ultralight brains need to learn new things over and over.

And as for rodents? Well, rodents were perpetually immature. Mice, as Disney shows us so plainly, never grow up! Rakic and his associates would publish research in 1985 that categorically denied neurogenesis in any adult organism.

Proving Neural Plasticity

Only four years later, in 1989, a young neuropsychologist named Elizabeth Gould was doing research on the lethal effects of stress and impoverished environments on neurons, particularly in the *hippocampus* (a limbic organ intimately associated with memory). While counting cells in stained, ultrathin slices of rat hippocampus, she unexpectedly found evidence of *neurogenesis* (cell growth) in addition to the *apoptosis* (cell death) from the effects of environmental impoverishment that she was studying. This was not supposed to happen. She kept on carefully counting. "There were too many cells," she said.

Going back into the Rockefeller Institute's archives on neurological research, she found Altman's twenty-seven-year-old research, which announced that neurogenesis existed in the brains of rats, cats, and guinea pigs. His work should have occasioned decades of neurobiological research, if not founded a whole new field with implications for education, neurotherapy, degenerative diseases such as Parkinsonism, and implications about the roles of stem cells and *neuroglia* in neuronal damage repair. But the budding field of neurogenesis had withered on the vine. The old paradigm had announced the truth: *there is no neurogenesis in adult organisms.* Without acceptance in academic circles and professional journals, funding sources dried up too.

Curiosity, and maybe an indignant awareness that injustice had been done both to Altman and to the truth itself, led Gould to pursue eight years of feverish neurobiological research. Not unexpectedly, Gould's work was soundly criticized. Finally she decided to confront Rakic's findings directly by documenting neurogenesis in brains of primates: *adult* marmosets. She found new neurons in the olfactory cortex and hippocampus. (Now a Princeton professor, she had taken Yale to the mat.) By 1999 Rakic recanted his earlier position and admitted in print that he himself had seen new neurons in the hippocampi of macaques. To Rakic's credit as a scientist (not a scientific fundamentalist) this is not an easy thing to do.

Gould's work was to have other social—and even, perhaps, political—implications. She was to show how stress and deprived environments kill brain cells, whereas well-being and enriched environments grow them. The enlivening principle, of course, is stimulation, as well as the friendliness and diversity of the environment. Gould's research was to lead to some major conclusions, all of which are important for their neuroscientific, as well as clinical and social, implications:

1. Hormonal regulation of cell production. This has led to research, spearheaded by Emory University scientists, showing that estrogen and progesterone therapies, administered in a timely manner to those with recent head injuries, can have major impact on healing and cell regeneration.

2. Experience-dependent changes in neurogenesis, particularly the ability of stress-related factors to inhibit neuron growth.

3. The importance of complex environments, particularly those resembling the natural living conditions of the animal. "Natural" burrows for adult rats or natural foraging environments for macaques affect the animals' ability to regenerate neurons.

The functional role of new neurons, particularly those that mediate the stress response, and learning how to cope with the stress.

Stress, which causes the secretion of glucorticoid hormones, inhibits neuronal growth and shrinks and depletes the brain and central nervous system (CNS)—especially over time. (Implication: War and international stress zones generate less-than-optimally intelligent human beings, who in turn may be easily exploited for extreme political agendas. The old paradigm holds in concentration camps and for caged animals.)

A recent *Seed Magazine* article says: "The social implications of this research are staggering!" If boring environments, stressful noises, and the primate's particular slot in the dominance hierarchy all shape the architecture of the brain—and Gould's team has shown that they do—then the playing field isn't level. Poverty and stress aren't just an idea, "they are an anatomy. Some brains never even have a chance" (Lehrer 2008, 2010).

For those of us who, as psychologists, were raised on behaviorism so to speak, it is an interesting idea that a rat in the impoverished environment of a Skinner box follows those Skinnerian operant conditioning paradigms so well because they're the only game in town. But give rats, or monkeys, enriched or more naturalistic environments, and their behavior changes. Thus Gould's contemporary research has these more stimulating types of environments for her experimental animals. If bare Skinner boxes wither neurons, enriched environments can restore them and help grow new ones. Gould believes the proliferating new neurons in the hippocampus have two major roles: learning and modulation of the stress response.

Eric Kandel Loves Snails (in a Different Way Than the Rest of Us)

But maybe that's because they helped him win the Nobel Prize in 2000! Much of the modern work on the functioning of neurons was done on marine creatures, which (are lucky enough to) possess giant neurons. (Another advantage is that you can poke microelectrodes into the cell to see how its electrodynamics work in living action. My colleague Juan Acosta-Urquidi—see chapter 14—who worked at Woods Hole Marine Biological Lab, has described how this is done with the squid neurons, with glass micropipettes inserted into the pulsing, living cell to sample its internal chemical dynamics.)

Discovering how snails protect themselves by withdrawing their siphon, easily observed in the giant neurons, Kandel and associates showed, at the molecular biological level, how what Donald Hebb called "consolidation," the transmutation of short-term into long-term memory, took place. Snails could be "aversively" conditioned by pairing a neutral stimulus with a noxious one. When the researchers repeated the noxious conditioning over a short period up to forty times, the snail retained the memory for several hours. When the aversive learning trials were reduced in frequency, not intensity, and spread out over several hours, long-term memory was potentiated for up to three weeks.

From this and other experiments, a new science was developed, now being studied in microbiology labs all over the world: *gene expression*. While all our cells contain all our genes, the majority of them are not expressed, or activated, unless special conditions supervene. Mostly genes just replicate themselves (the template function). What was being discovered by Kandel, and replicated in many other labs, was the "transcription function" that switches genes on and off. It was this factor that was causing the neurogenesis, which is also called *neural plasticity*. Sprouting was going on, to the extent that in neurons with 1,300 connections there were now 2,700, more than twice as many (Doidge 2007, 220).

The old neurobiological orthodoxy had not dreamed of, nor anticipated, "gene switching" nor "transcription factors." Everything was conceived of in a much more simplistic, mechanical way.

Neural Plasticity Everywhere: The Plot Thickens

Alvaro Pascual-Leone, the distinguished Harvard neuroscientist, considers Ramón y Cajal his spiritual preceptor, and ultimately he would become involved in disproving his master's century-old dictum, *no new neurons!*

During the 1990s, as Elizabeth Gould was doing the meticulous electron-microscope neuron-counting in rat and marmoset brains, Pascual-Leone was using a kind of energy-medicine procedure: transcranial magnetic stimulation (TMS). Eventually he came to the same conclusion she did. In 1999 he published a paper with his associates called "Transcranial magnetic stimulation and neuroplasticity" (Pascual-Leone et al. 1999).

Pascual-Leone would more gently replicate some of the legendary Wilder Penfield experiments that Wilder had done during open-brain surgery, using a copper wire and low voltages to touch a part of the brain, suddenly evoking concrete memories or experiences from the person's past. (It is out of this work that much of the modern brain mapping that stresses *localization* has come, and we will return to that topic a little later.) We have all seen the grotesque little guys made out of cortical gray matter that are called *homunculi,* with the big mouths and lips and thumbs, that show either sensory or motor reception or control of the body from regions in the brain.

Pascual Leone felt that the new TMS stimulation was far less invasive (than copper wires on recently opened brains, for example). In doing so, he pioneered work that was to have profound clinical implications in what is called rTMS, "repetitive" transcranial magnetic stimulations, used as therapy for depression and other problems.

Faraday had shown that any electrical current through a conductor produces a magnetic field. Likewise, magnetic fields can affect conductive wires—or neurons, for that matter. TMS could be used alternatively to turn neuronal groups, fairly tightly localized, either on or off.

Working in Spain with teachers of the blind, who, as part of their training, agreed to wear light-impermeable blindfolds for a week, he discovered astonishing changes in very brief periods of time. Not only, as folk wisdom everywhere seems to know, did the other senses of the blinded become more acute so that they could visualize space better than previously and hear echoes from objects (all signs of neuronal plasticity), but as they undertook the daunting process of learning Braille, within days their brains began to reorganize. Instead of learning just with the areas of their brains associated with touch, the visual cortex showed activity. (They were learning how to "see" with their fingertips.) Confirmation was provided in totally unexpected subjective reports: when subjects were touched, or heard sounds, they reported "hallucinations of beautiful, complex scenes of cities, skies, sunsets, Lilliputian figures, cartoon figures" (Doidge 2007, 210).

Thus the *synesthesias* reported by people in altered states of consciousness or after ingesting psychedelics: sounds can become colors, colors qualities of touch or emotion; the usual boundaries of the five senses are blurred. Reading Pascual-Leone's experiments, I thought of the Kogi, a "lost tribe" of Colombia, in which children who are deemed to possess psychic or visionary abilities are isolated in darkness for nine years and only gradually introduced to the light, whereupon they become a specialized type of shaman, a seer, who is said to be able see in *both* the physical and the spiritual worlds.

Although Pascual-Leone has become a great advocate of neural plasticity, that doesn't stop him from contemplating its opposite: neurological rigidity, the very subject I take on in *The Fundamentalist Mind*. I propose in that book that primate attention is sensitized to dominance hierarchies and the tendency to be subservient to others of superior rank. Mirror neurons then help us imitate such "authority figures" (the ultimate symbolic form of which is "God"). In the presence of fear, the amygdala becomes involved, and we have rigid attitudes favoring dichotomous choices: "Are you a believer or an infidel?" Clearly, violent and discriminatory behavior can be a consequence.

Ritual also helps cement what was originally plastic into firm behavioral patterns that will now be resistant to change. Religions know and understand this and hence are made up of rituals and "credos," saying the things in which one is supposed to believe over and over until they are second nature. What "fires together, wires together," said neuropsychologist Donald Hebb in the 1950s.

It is not so far from Hebb to Pascual-Leone. Behaviors repeated again and again not only affect synapses, they probably foster new neurons and dendrites. The neurological "traffic" gets directed down these routes, and they become the highways and superhighways of our functioning. Eventually the behaviors slip from habits into behavioral rituals (and all the things "old dogs" are said to acquire so you can't teach them "new tricks" any more). There are thus not only ritualized behavior patterns, but beliefs, attitudes, and values that go along with them.

Even when a behavior or attitude clearly does not serve a person—in fact is downright dysfunctional or embarrassing, as in the rituals of obsessive-compulsive disorder (OCD), for example—it may persist. Psychotherapists often make their living attempting to change the secret mainsprings of these problems. But, as often as not, verbal understanding doesn't affect the behavior or the emotions. However, neurofeedback may have better tools. In the EEG domain, these fixations can be associated with a frozen dominant frequency, a rhythm that seems stuck in the brain, or problems in coherence, connectivity, and/or synchronization or the lack of it.

Later in this volume I will take on the controversy that exists in neuroscience between the importance of *locations* in the brain and their complex interconnecting energy networks. These are the factors measured in qEEG work called "coherence," "comodulation," and "phase synchrony."

There can no longer be any question that single locations are not responsible for everything having to do with a particular brain function. The Nobel Prize–winning work of Gerald Edelman suggests that rather than any simple isomorphic representation of perception or function, there is a kind of *competition between patterns,* which he calls "operators," found with representations throughout the brain, in which, for example, the visual and the tactile ideas of space and dimension are involved in someone's ability to perform an action like reaching for an object on a shelf. Functions are clearly shared between operators such as the visual and tactile-spatial assemblies. Information flows fluidly around in our brains from one neural assembly, or operator, to another. In Edelman's version of human maturation, there is a kind of Darwinian competition between assemblies to see which ones can fit the bill or serve the need best.

In "higher order processes, maps can be combined to form concepts," which he calls "primary."

Edelman attaches great importance to *higher order* processes— concepts are *maps of maps,* and arise from the brain's recategorising its own activity. Concepts by themselves only constitute primary (first-order) consciousness: human consciousness also features secondary consciousness (concepts about concepts), language, and a concept of the self, all built on the foundation of first-order concepts.*

I remember a colleague, an earnest history professor, who came to me in genuine consternation. He said, "Steve, I'm trying to find some way to justify the liberal education to my kids—and to some kind of conservative adults who are arguing with me! I know it does something for people, something that makes them people of breadth and substance, who contribute something, who, er, you want to hang around with! Is there any neuroscience to prove it?"

I replied that I totally agreed with him and his viewpoint, but that I didn't know any hard science that supported what he was saying. (It was the 1980s.) I wish I had known then what I know now. There is substantial evidence now that abilities acquired in one domain can overlap to others. That is to say, an art form is more than a learned virtuosity; everything that artists do and have done that makes them human affects their performance. We, in effect, borrow from ourselves all the time. The ability to read or play music affects your ability to write literature. Your ability to do hard science improves your philosophical reasoning. Your ability to self-regulate in one area seeps over into an adjacent area. Joseph Campbell's ability to read in several languages extended his grasp of myths and their symbolic grammars and syntaxes.

Pascual-Leone's caveat is well taken: Neural plasticity is good news and bad news. It helps us see how society and culture, the very company we keep, shapes our brains—and thus our behavior.

Learning Neurogenesis from Prozac

Listening to Prozac is the title of an interesting book by Peter Kramer, a psychiatrist who looks at both the dismal failures and the unexpected contributions of a popular antidepressant: Prozac (fluoxetine), first released

---

*For more on this, please visit www.consciousentities.com/edelman.htm.

in 1986 and widely prescribed since then. Its manufacturer, Eli Lilly, touted the drug as one of the first "selective serotonin reuptake inhibitors" (SSRIs); this was believed to be the cause of efficacy. (The "feel-good" neurohormone *serotonin,* manufactured by one's own body, is kept active in the synapses longer than usual without the drug, and people, well, "feel good.") The criticisms of the drug claim that when it wears off, people can become irritable and depressed, even explosively angry and suicidal. (*Talking Back to Prozac* is another book, authored by Peter Breggin, on the cons as well as the pros of Prozac!)

Yale researcher Ronald Duman, professor of psychiatry and pharmacology, has furthered the enterprise of "listening to Prozac" but in an unexpected way. Duman was as confused as the rest of us in the mental health field about the "Prozac lag," the first three weeks the person is taking the drug, during which the SSRI is supposed to be operating, and yet the person feels not one whit less depressed—until gradually, it is supposed, like a great ship turning around, the chemistry of the brain changes, and the person begins to feel better.

The secret, Duman's research shows, is actually a *deus absconditus,* a "hidden god"—or a "causal agency" no one suspected (Lehrer 2008, 2010). Prozac triggers a cascade of what are called "trophic factors." While stress decimates neurons, trophic factors (the best-known of which is "brain-derived neurotrophic factor") cause them to grow and proliferate. Perhaps the "Prozac delay" was simply the time that Prozac took *to actually effect neurogenesis,* and the result had *little or nothing to do with the reuptake of serotonin.* Could it be that it was actually (the forbidden) growth of new neurons that helped the sufferer's depression, not what the manufacturers believed and promulgated for the last forty years? (*Myth,* or *mistaken paradigm?*)

This could indeed have some relevance to the $12-billion-a-year search for the next generation of antidepressants, for example, *because the exact mechanism of pharmaceutical efficacy actually matters.*

"Our working hypothesis hasn't been right," says Duman. The brain-derived neurotrophic factors may matter much more than anything involving serotonin. Acknowledging inspiration from Gould in his own work, Duman published a paper in the *Journal of Neuroscience* that set out his observation that SSRIs increase neurogenesis. "It was just an accident," he says of fluoxetine, the chemical name for the compound marketed as Prozac, "that it stimulated neurogenesis." And the work of René Hen at Columbia gave a further observation to Duman's work. When brain growth and neurotrophic factors were neutralized by doses of radiation, the antidepressant effect was also canceled (Lehrer 2008, 2010).

Though "a howl of criticism" has greeted Duman's work, the combination of Duman's and Gould's research has intensified interest in the stimulation of neurotrophic factors. The *Seed* article concludes: "Depression is not simply the antagonist of Happiness. Instead despair might be caused by loss of the brain's essential plasticity. *A person's inability to change herself is what drags her down.*"

Could Neurofeedback Affect Neural Plasticity?

In my first draft of this chapter, I was being scientifically conservative and cagey. I wrote, "Though there is no scientific evidence, *yet,* that neurofeedback directly affects neural plasticity, almost everyone who practices it suspects that it does."

In 2010 an article from the *European Journal of Neuroscience* entitled "Endogenous Control of Waking Brain Rhythms Induces Neuroplasticity in Humans" came to me on my BrainMaster e-mail list. The study was a team effort headed by Tomas Ros, M. A. M. Munneke, Diana Ruge, John Gruzelier, and John Rothwell. The list of authors is impressive, with major institutional affiliations and long lists of scientific publications. The study basically shows that brain wave neurofeedback (the "endogenous control" of the title) produces physiologically measurable responses to transcranial magnetic stimulation, "producing durable and correlated changes in neurotransmission."

Basically, alpha *suppression,* achieved through a "noninvasive" neurofeedback procedure, increased cortical excitability that was measurable for up to twenty minutes. The magnetic stimulation was used to produce motoric evoked potentials (brain responses to stimulation, usually measured as spikes in the EEG). The changes in the EEG were robust, and the frequency range examined stretched from very slow potentials, a cycle or less per second (slow delta), to those over a hundred Hz (a range much broader than usually measured in EEG studies, or neurofeedback scans, for that matter). The study takes on added significance because *cortical excitability* is a perennially interesting topic for neuroscience, affecting everything from kindling (brain excitatory activity, which is often preliminary to seizures) and seizure activity to anxiety and panic attacks. (Psychiatrists and neurologists utilize anticonvulsants, tranquilizers, or inhibitory neurotransmitter agonists such as Neurontin [gabapentin] to try to achieve the same effect.)

We know that the neurofeedback asks the brain to do something that it doesn't normally do, so it exercises our "neurological muscles," so to speak. As I have written in *The Healing Power of Neurofeedback*, almost any kind of neurofeedback seems to be good for the brain. The effects aren't always what one expects or is "trying" to do, as in the case I have written about in the book where a woman practicing alpha (unexpectedly) acquired the ability to concentrate, while (expectedly) gaining some control over emotional volatility. It's a little along the lines of the way stretching a muscle can make it more elastic and actually stronger.

In the LENS technique, this principle is brought to a fine edge, because the very idea is to "bump the person out of his or her parking place"—or habitual neurological state—again and again with small bumps. The desideratum for the LENS, as I explain, is not to try for either faster or slower brain waves but to let the brain itself do the choosing. In the early days of the LENS, our "USE-2" (an early version of the software) had an exciting bar graph that showed the dominant frequency as a white bar (the highest one) that was free to move up and down the entire EEG spectrum. If a person was "stuck" somehow, the dominant frequency bar would remain frozen. But sometimes, after a treatment, we would see the previously frozen bar suddenly scurry up and down the spectrum like a pianist playing arpeggios. Subsequently people would report improvements in their emotional and cognitive flexibility. Emotionally, they would be less likely to get stuck in the doldrums or an OCD loop. Cognitively they would become more creative, inventive, and playful. ("Ah, freedom at last!") This seems to me very close to the principle informing neural plasticity.

Neural plasticity, denied for so long, now looms as the single most important issue in the neuroscience of the future. Along with it, I submit, comes neurofeedback as the clinical methodology most able to help the nervous system overcome its deficits and impairments, moving toward full functionality.

How could it do this? In the middle of the last century McGill University's Donald Hebb proposed the "reverberating circuit" idea of learning. It made intuitive sense, and it turned out to be applicable to learning theory in a variety of ways. After you've had an experience, it is captured in a kind of temporary way by neuronal circuits; "what fires together wires together," as mentioned above. The neurons fire around and around in a kind of loop. Short-term memory is a transient neuronal dynamic of this kind. Frequent rehearsal gradually *consolidates* the memory into long term. And Eric Kandel has identified the precise neurobiological mechanism and thus vindicated Hebb.

We learned in General Psychology that the best thing to do after learning was to sleep or rest, to allow for the consolidation. Something chemical is being changed, so it needs peace and quiet to complete its work. This is why Ramón y Cajal's discovery of the synapse, and hence the neurotransmitter environment, won him the Nobel Prize. Your first college Psychology course taught you about synapses, the places where nature has arranged *for neurons not to touch each other.*

If neurons touched, the circuit would be sealed. The loop would be like an electronic (mechanical) reverberating circuit. This is hardly the wiring for a creature of advanced capabilities. (No, thank you, I am not your dial tone or alarm system!)

With the synapse, the sodium-calcium exchange that powers the neurons down the long axons suddenly meets a different kind of environment, in which far more complex chemicals are involved. True, this slows down our conditioned reflexes, compared, say, to those of a fly. But it is also what makes us far more flexible and better able to learn from experience.

It was Ramón y Cajal's work that revealed how important the synapse was and provided the physiological underpinnings for Hebb's theory. The organic chemistry of the nervous system, where complex indoles, amino acids, and an incredible variety of other substances ply their trades, introduces a whole new dimension into our functionality. Hebb's theory suggested that the repeated use of synapses compelled the complex molecules that migrate the gap between neurons to change. All organisms need to change and be adaptable, but for the first time in nature, with human beings, *change is the name of the game*. We live by learning. Being able to modify our neurological response to external environments becomes crucial and decisive. And indeed this is where modern psychopharmacology has decided to invest its whole portfolio. We have the technical ability to change the *chemical* action of the interneuronal synapses—the wonders of modern chemistry!

We do not or will not (says profit-driven psychopharmacology) look at the *action* of the neurons, the software or the programs that are put into the circuit, the exercising or utilization of the circuit. We will look at the *chemistry*. On a certain level, it does work splendidly, and I would like to affirm that I believe psychotropic drugs can save lives, intervene in desperate situations such as psychosis or clinical depression, and ameliorate suffering. (And those of us in the mental health professions know that there are problems too deeply grounded in our physiology for talk therapy even to touch.) But by definition, chemicals miss the exquisite specifics and refinements of psychological and cognitive growth, and, painting with way too broad a chemical brush, cause wholesale—hence crude and unintelligent—things to happen.

Neurofeedback is in a unique position, right between *physiology and psychology*. It avoids the "bipolar" fundamentalism that says, "If talk (or even behavior modification) therapy can't help you, then I must reach for the prescription pad."

If long-term change is predicated on change at the synapses, then neurofeedback has to show that it can produce those changes. Hard-science physiological studies (such as the one cited above) are saying it can. And evidence has been accumulating for some time in the biofeedback and neurofeedback communities (for example, that HRV training actually modifies the balance of glucocorticoids such as cortisol, DHEA (dehydroepiandosterone), and salivary IgA, or immunoglobulin A; and that EEG training helps control muscle tension or panic attacks—that *cortical excitability* evidence). It can also accomplish the same kind of up-regulation and down-regulation of the CNS that pharmacology prides itself on being the only agent of—and it does this without flooding the entire CNS with chemical agents, which remain in the body long after the intended effect has been accomplished.*

True, biofeedback is not "natural" in that it uses machines, but the machines are becoming more sophisticated by the day; the more sensitive the machine, the more likely it is to become part of the "learning loop" that Hebb described. The same principle of rest or sleep following learning experiences that ensures maximum consolidation of the learning process also seems to apply in neurofeedback.

In effect, the little machine, with its transistors and silicon chips, is integrated into the exquisite circuitry of the nervous system, and even when it is withdrawn, the nervous system retains the memory of its (hopefully benign) presence. It is "benign" if its major function is *to enable the brain or nervous system access to something (information) that it needs,* something heretofore unavailable, something useful. Changing the nervous system on a relatively permanent basis does in fact change neurochemistry and physiology, and it requires recuperation time.

The skill of the biofeedback programmer comes in regulating the usability of the new information available. For example, the clinician in Z-score training sets the "reward threshold" on the processor so that the attained behavioral targets—say establishing a new connectivity circuit in the brain, or dissolving a pathological old one—is rewarded at the optimal level for learning and consolidating, or incorporating the new learning into the allostatic state† of the organism.

Now it's time for a little more on the paradigm idea with which we began this chapter: Is the brain a boring old Newtonian organ of cause and effect, push coming to shove, reeling between reward and punishment, pleasure and pain? Or has it not something of a paradoxical *quantum* nature, where light behaves as particle and wave, where positrons and charmed quarks do not obey conventional rules like mass and gravity at all but insist on paradoxicality, popping up in new ways in unexpected places, finding new possibilities? Can we learn to see the CNS as a *self-*

---

*For more on this, please visit www.HeartMath.org, a research website.
†An "allostatic state" refers to the dynamic self-regulation of the entire organism.

regulating dynamical system, with its own *emergent properties,* rather than something that merely responds to influences from the outside environment? Mechanistic neurobiology is a tired runner now and must yield the baton to an emergent quantum world including neural plasticity and metacognition!

The possibilities of the human brain were underappreciated before computers—that is to say, before we had a more closely appropriate machine analogy. In the early days of Psychology, hydrological and gas dynamics were used to explain things like *repression, sublimation,* and *reaction-formation.* Pavlov showed us the analogy of conditioning and reflexes to electrical circuits, Skinner expanded the paradigm through the use of reward and punishment contingencies, imagining simple equations based on discrimination, generalization, reward contingencies, and so forth, and pushing in the direction of *instrumental behaviors* (that is to say, the opportunistic actions of goal-oriented captive creatures in their artificial environment).

We now find that when the brain is put in touch with itself (the elemental principle of biofeedback), miraculous things begin to happen. Among other things, it is eminently capable of modifying itself without chemicals or other mechanical help. Abberations such as depression and anxiety are not "things" (symptoms) to be "eliminated" but suboptimal *conditions* of the nervous system when it isn't working so well. When functionality is restored, and the system begins intelligently to self-regulate, the "symptoms" drop away by themselves.

Illusionist Magic: Neurofeedback That Doesn't Look Like Neurofeedback

In 2010 I was privileged to meet the illustrious neuroscientist V. R. Ramachandran. He was an invited plenary speaker at the Association for Applied Psychophysiology and Biofeedback (AAPB) annual meeting in San Diego, and I, and the sizable audience, hung on every word.

Of Ramachandran's unique background and preparation to be one of the world's top neuroscientists, Norman Doidge has written:

In India, Ramachandran grew up in a world where many things that seem fantastic to Westerners were commonplace. He knew about yogis who relieved suffering with meditation and walked barefoot across hot coals or lay down on nails. He saw religious people in trances putting needles through their chins. The idea that living things change their forms was widely accepted; the power of the mind to influence the body was taken for granted and illusion was seen as so fundamental a force that it was represented in the deity Maya, the goddess of illusion. He has transposed a sense of wonder from the streets of India to Western neurology, and his work inspires questions that mingle the two. What is a trance but a closing down of the gates of pain within us? Why should we think phantom pain any less real than ordinary pain? And he has reminded us that great science can still be done with elegant simplicity (Doidge 2007, 195).

We are used to thinking that neurofeedback must be mediated by complex electronic circuitry and computers, but it was indeed "illusionist neurofeedback" that Ramachandran spoke of at that conference. Ramachandran described how he used a simple mirror-box to help people with the painful "phantom limb" affliction.

First described by battlefield surgeon Silas Weir Mitchell, the phantom limb phenomenon occurs after the amputation of a limb, when the patient feels the missing part is not only there, but that it has sensation, including, not infrequently, intolerable pain. No amount of logical reasoning or persuasion seems to help, and the problems may persist for years. Ramachandran came to believe there were complex neurological circuits involved, and because of the intensity and immediacy of the pain, it must be a problem of rewiring along the sensorimotor strip of the brain, and thus involving our ugly little friend, *the homunculus*.

Believing the brain is a kind of "virtual reality" machine, he sought to reprogram it. But when he went to Hollywood technicians to create a virtual-reality hand or arm, he learned it would cost a million dollars or so. So he set out to design something that would accomplish the same thing for about fifty dollars. He calls it "the mirror box."

Let's say the missing limb is a hand or part of the arm and hand.

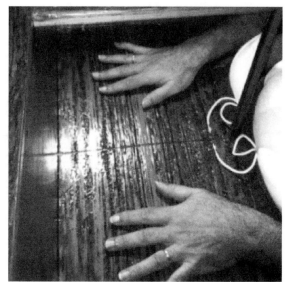

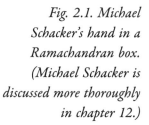

Fig. 2.1. Michael Schacker's hand in a Ramachandran box. (Michael Schacker is discussed more thoroughly in chapter 12.)

The patient's good hand is inserted into a hole in the mirror box, and he or she leans over slightly, and presto, it looks like the hand is its opposite counterpart. The patient is instructed to move the good hand, which appears to be the missing one that is actually moving; the movement are simple and subtle at first. Eventually, with repeated trials and more complex movements, the brain begins to reprogram itself. The patient can, for example, "unclench" a fist that no longer exists but feels "clenched." With this, some patients experienced considerable relief and loss of pain.

The part I have become more interested in (as shown in the photo of Michael Schacker's hand in the mirror box) is the restoration of feeling to a hand paralyzed by stroke. The results are preliminary, but promising.

This, my friends, is neurofeedback.

I don't care whether the feedback is invisible LENS, a tone or a light, along with the quantum-flickering numbers of the Z-score training, or the illusion that reprograms the brain that its missing limb exists again and can relax. If it talks to the brain in a language it can understand, it is neurofeedback.

Our next chapter moves to how neurofeedback can be used to help in diagnosis and for clinical purposes in the amelioration of problems. How does neurofeedback know what it knows, and how can it be used to help people?

THREE

THE EVOLUTION OF NEUROFEEDBACK

BRAIN MAPPING AND SCOPE OF TREATMENT

With Joel Lubar, Ph.D., BCIA-EEG

Mapping the Brain

There is something magical about any device that lets us see into the brain. The MRI has awesome capabilities of identifying structural anomalies, and the fMRI evokes gasps of wonder and awe as we see different areas of the brain light up while doing a task and realize that we are seeing more than structure—we are seeing function, the brain in action.

Most modern brain-scanning devices are in the hands of medical doctors and radiologists; they're used in hospitals and diagnostic facilities. This is as it should be, because the technologies—from the X-ray to the MRI—are powerful and, if not used skillfully, potentially harmful. They are also very expensive, costing hundreds of thousands of dollars for computed axial tomography (CAT) scanners, up to a couple of million for the more powerful (3Tesla)* MRIs. They must be run by specially trained and

---

*A Tesla, an SI unit named after pioneer Nicola Tesla, is a unit used to measure a magnet's strength. One Tesla is equal to one Weber per square meter.

licensed technicians and interpreted by medical specialists such as neurologists and radiologists.

The MRI is touted as less "invasive" than machines such as the X-ray and CAT scan because they use ionizing radiation, which may have a role in cancer. But the MRI is so powerful it causes any ferric or ferromagnetic material to become a potentially lethal projectile. Positron-emission tomography (PET) and single-photon emission computed tomography (SPECT) scans require the ingestion or injection of radiotracing or radiopharmaceutical substances.

X-rays, first used in 1895, revolutionized medicine. They allowed doctors to see inside the body and thus identify hard-tissue anomalies, especially bone fractures. They became invaluable for diagnosing sports injuries, broken pelvises, and shrapnel in the body. Unfortunately, some of the early researchers did not understand the consequences of repeated exposure to ionizing radiation. (The energy carried by X-rays is so powerful that it strips electrons out of the material through which it passes, creating *ions*.) I can remember looking at my own feet in a shoe-store "fluoroscope," a little uneasily, as a ten-year-old, and seeing my own fragile bones inside the shadowy shoes. (You could wiggle your toes and the bones moved.) Later, it was commonplace to see what was going on in one's jaw at the dentist via X-rays. By now, the effects of ionizing radiation are better known, and so the patient is draped with a lead-lined apron to protect certain vulnerable areas from the radiation, and the technician retreats behind a lead shield as the picture is taken.

CAT scans, or computer-assisted tomography, which uses the same basic principle, did not appear until the 1970s. A ring of scanned images allowed for the presentation of "slices" (the *tomos* of "tomography," which means "slices") through the medium being surveyed. CAT scans, like X-rays, though, use ionizing radiation and, because they hold the subject being scanned in the apparatus for much longer, expose him or her to much more radiation than an X-ray. Recent breakthroughs in computer technology make possible the combination of CAT with PET or SPECT scans.

The appearance of PET and SPECT scans increased the sophistication and resolution of soft-tissue imaging and made it much easier to identify cancer or other tissue pathologies. With SPECT, a radioisotope is injected into the bloodstream. The *radioligand* forms bonds with tissues, and then the suspect area is photographed with a gamma wave–recording camera, revealing abnormalities.

As noted, when the MRI first appeared, it was touted as noninvasive because it does not use ionizing radiation. The MRI uses very powerful magnetic fields, rated in the 1.5–3 Tesla range, accompanied by radio frequencies (millions of times stronger than the LENS, for example) to spin molecules. (Free water spins differently than bonded water, adipose tissues show up entirely differently in the scan than muscle or circulatory tissue.) The MRI is a specialist in picking out pathological features such as tumors and demyelinating disorders such as multiple sclerosis (in which the insulating "myelin sheath" around the neuron is slowly destroyed). Diffusion tensor imaging, based on MRI, is used to detect whether bundled neuronal pathways are intact or have deteriorated. (Please see plate 4 of the color insert.)

Functional magnetic resonance imaging, or fMRI, allows for precise anatomical locations of behaviors or mental events *as they are happening*.

While MRI is touted as noninvasive, it does often use dyes to increase the contrast between tissues, and not everyone responds well to these. But

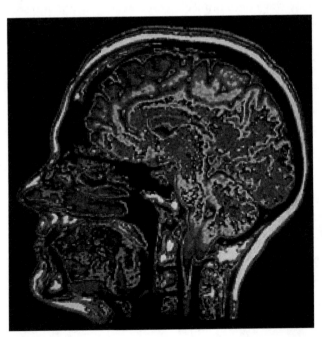

Fig. 3.1. MRI, or magnetic resonance imaging

due to the power of the magnet, "missile-effect accidents, where ferromagnetic objects are attracted to the center of the magnet, have resulted in injury and death" (www.mrisafety.com). Think about implants and artificial joints that involve stainless steel. Think about cardiac pacemakers (no, don't think about them!). Shrapnel acquired in battle, or metal fragments from industrial accidents, long forgotten but still in the body, can become missiles, as can wired-together joints.

There is one additional factor that introduces a lot of unknowns into the use of magnets this powerful on the human body and brain. There is indeed ferromagnetic material, called magnetite, present in the brain. Its greatest concentrations are in the pineal gland and in the hippocampus. Biologists believe this material enables some animals (loggerhead turtles and geese among them) to navigate geomagnetically—that is, by Earth's magnetic pole. There is no proof, but papers have proposed this as the "antenna" that responds to LENS and NeuroField treatments. Some of the famous or infamous "overdoses" have happened to people from energies as minuscule as 10^{-18} (ten to the minus-eighteenth power) watts per square centimeter. What happens on these same levels when people are put into extremely powerful magnets, millions of times stronger than the neurostimulation? We simply don't know. I have sometimes heard TBI patients say they "didn't feel right" for days after an MRI. Others are just fine.

On the positive side, the scanning and imaging methods mentioned above have enormously expanded our ability to look into the body without opening it surgically. In fact, they have made it possible to identify and localize tumors, strokes, and ischemias, so that precise surgical intervention becomes possible. The fMRI has made it possible to identify areas of the brain that are indisputably involved in certain key behaviors and even mental processes. This is all to the good for humanity. One more fact, however, deserves mention. Except for the X-ray and CAT scan, which directly reveal structural anomalies, all these methods rely on *indirect* imaging: blood flow, oxygen, glucose, metabolites, radioligands.

Now we move to a brain-mapping technology *that is truly noninvasive,* because it only measures AC microcurrents that make it through the *pia mater, dura mater* (the brain's covering layers), skull, and scalp, to be read at the skin of the patient. This does not keep the measurements from being very precise in terms of what may be revealed; nor does it limit them to merely surface details as can be revealed by individual component analysis of the EEG or the astonishing technology derived from it by Roberto Pasqual-Marquis, starting in the 1990s, called LORETA (Low Resolution EEG Tomographic Analysis). The LORETA uses mathematical formulae called "the inverse solution" to picture structures beneath the cortex. Later developments with even higher resolution in voxels are called s-LORETA, and still higher, the zero error, "exact" or e-LORETA (there is more on LORETA below, and in chapter 13).

Furthermore, the anomalies and imbalances in the brain detected in the qEEG suggest treatment strategies and locations. We will even discuss studies where EEG analysis directly suggests which medications might be the most advantageous, and further down the treatment decision tree, how well the patient's brain is responding to psychopharmaceutical assays already attempted. This latter fact alone is already making this "people's technology" of interest to "big pharma." (See Gunkelman et al. 2008, on pharmaceutical phenotypes as revealed through the EEG.)

The Modern qEEG Is Born

To explain what a qEEG is, we first have to differentiate it from the kind of EEG you might get at a neurologist's office or a hospital. And what kinds of things can you learn from an qEEG that make it different from all the other kinds of diagnostic instruments? First, a little history.

While brain waves were discovered by Hans Berger in 1924, and his research was published in 1929, the neurology field made very little of it, and Berger died in 1941 feeling his discovery was never really recognized.

It was during the 1940s in America, though, that Gibbs and Knott identified EEG changes throughout the life cycle of the organism. Children's waves on the whole are much slower (delta and theta), gradually yielding to alpha and above, the betas being the high frequencies that characterize working adult cognition. In the 1960s the "alpha craze" was born, and it was realized that people could actually identify what range of brain waves they were producing (Kamiya 1979; Brown 1977).

In 1989 David Joffe and Michael Hickey founded Lexicor Medical

Technologies. A Denver-based fund, Columbine Ventures, financed development and manufacture. Their machine, the Neuro-Search 24, which at that time cost under $20,000, considerably lowered the cost of medical EEGs. Two thousand Lexicors of different vintages and generations would be built and sold over the next decade. Early researchers and innovators—Joe Kamiya, Barry Sterman, and Joel Lubar, as well as E. Roy John and Robert Thatcher—immediately saw the potential of the machine and were brought aboard to work with the Lexicor and develop the databases of which you will hear much more shortly.

Up until this point, roughly 1990, the primary use of the EEG was the detection of seizures, seizure-proneness, traumatic brain injury (TBI), and clinical death. There was no systematic work that tied certain patterns in the brain waves to clinical syndromes such as anxiety or depression. Most of these researchers were psychologists—Ph.D.s, not M.D.s. Their thinking was statistical and probabilistic. They wanted to do large numbers of maps on large numbers of people, so they could find the *normative*.

Fortunately, the rapid development of computers paralleled what the researchers wished to accomplish, and so over two decades, qEEGs decreased in size and increased in portability, while also requiring computers with more sophisticated internal architecture (16-bit machines yielding to 32- and finally 64-bit machines). The computers would have to be powerful enough to crunch the numbers and make sense of them. More powerful processors would allow these early researchers not only to detect epilepsy but to localize and determine the severity of TBIs, assess what *kind* of ADD or ADHD a child might exhibit, allow the analysis of the autistic spectrum of disorders, and many other things. The age of the full-cap qEEG* was born.

Most modern EEG processors utilize nineteen points on a prearranged grid that covers the parts of the head and scalp that have brain beneath. It is called the International 10–20 system. For the most part, these metrics are based on extrapolating from these points to the spaces between, and that is how they create the "area rugs" in some of the maps you will see. Some brain researchers use 32 or 64 or even 128 points, in a much denser

---

*A full-cap EEG uses a cloth or mesh "cap" with nineteen "sensors" or electrodes built in to measure nineteen sites simultaneously.

The Full-Cap Nineteen-Channel qEEG Processors

Lexicor, USA, David Joffe

DeyMed, Czech Republic

Mitsar, Saint Petersburg, Russia, Yuri Kropotov

Nexus 32, Mind Media BV (simultaneous EEG and other BF modalities such as EMG, GSRO), The Netherlands

Discovery 24 (BrainMaster), USA, Tom Collura

The Databases

Neuro-Navigator: Barry Sterman

Skill Database: William Hudspeth

Nx Link ER: E. Roy John and colleagues at the NYU Brain Research Lab

NeuroGuide: Robert Thatcher

---

array, for more precise calibrations. But most diagnosticians and clinicians feel the nineteen-point map or cap is sufficient for their purposes. Most caps, resembling elastic bathing caps, can fit a range of head sizes and allow the clinician without exact knowledge of the International 10–20 system to simply put a cap on the patient's head and be fairly confident that the points on the cap are accurate to the standardized mapping system within several millimeters.

Add powerful statistical sampling procedures to the mix, and you have something totally unavailable in orthodox medical circles—in fact, they can't touch this mix of cybergenius with neuroscience. It is a "people's science" that grew up alongside formal medicine and the powerful scanning techniques made possible by modern physics.

That may be why the trained neurologist, possibly with two years of postdoctoral study and board certification behind his reading of the EEG, may resent the qEEG folks. "A computer couldn't possibly do what I do!" he says, petulantly. And we answer, "Of course not; the human biocomputer is infinitely more capable of discernment and interpretation; and your postdoctoral internship in EEG is nothing to sneeze at."

However, what the computer can do that no human can (or would want to) do is to make hundreds of numerical calculations a minute, or even in a few seconds, and compare the results to normative databases. Nor can human beings store or remember millions of bits of demographic data and statistics. But a board-certified neurologist, such as Jonathan Walker, M.D. (www.neurotherapydallas.com), who also uses and interprets qEEG data (possibly from several databases), can provide an extraordinary wealth of data from a qEEG, things ordinary neurologists never even guess at: whether depression is endogenous or anxiety-driven; or whether there are layers of TBI or metabolic disturbances showing in the EEG. (Please see plate 1 of the color insert.)

In fifteen years as a neurofeedback professional, reading neurologists' reports, I have almost never seen textured or nuanced interpretations of executive functioning problems, affect regulation or impulse-control difficulties, aphasia, agnosia, or even, for that matter, ADD or ADHD, or poor emotional intelligence. But these interpretations—often accurate, and pointing to therapeutic strategies—are found in the reports of qEEG diagnosticians. These guys are willing to listen to the little robot.

The qEEG offers a wealth of data. The data may be in "raw" form for the discerning eye of the expert. The power spectra graphing shows FFT graphing of the different sites in different colors. The topographic maps are derived from the raw data and compared by color to normative data; the LORETA maps show the extraordinary images that can be extrapolated using mathematical formulas called the "inverse solution" from the data that actually reaches the electrodes pasted to the skull.

LORETA is remarkable because it is not only noninvasive, it is a transformation of *data already aquired in the qEEG,* and yet it gives a picture of problems and potential pathology much deeper in the brain than the outer layer of the cortex (which is measured in EEG and neurofeedback). According to Robert Thatcher, LORETA is a "smeared resolution" like a "probability cloud" (Thatcher 2010, 135). (Please see plates 2 and 3 of the color insert.)

Joel Lubar, Robert Thatcher, Marty Wuttke, and Tom Collura are working to develop neurofeedback protocols based on LORETA, that is, what is going on deeper in the brain. Someone with a brainstem TBI or a thalamic stroke (very serious kinds of deep injury) could engage in neurofeedback training at the very site of the problem. (LORETA-based biofeedback is a work very much "in progress," but with promising results already—see chapter 13.) To show the versatility and information richness of qEEG, please refer to plate 3 of the color insert in which we see views of the same patient showing *asymmetry* between specific sites in the left and right hemispheres. The asymmetry is extreme in this case because most of the left hemisphere is missing or badly damaged.

Maps of this type could be used to help design a treatment protocol in Z-score training, using complex computer-mediated algorithms to reward the patient when he or she is strengthening or weakening abnormal connections. This provides a good example of how the diagnostic and imaging modalities used in neurofeedback can provide a direct link to treatment modalities.

Why Is qEEG Reliable, or Valid?

As I prepared to answer this query about why the qEEG is valid, I was taken back in time forty to fifty years or so into the 1960s and '70s, while I was still in graduate school at Columbia, to an early "turf war" between psychiatrists and psychologists. At stake was congressional legislation pertaining to mental health law. The American Psychiatric Association claimed that as medical doctors, with all rights and privileges pertaining thereto, and better educations, psychiatrists should occupy the high ground in the mental health field. Not only was their knowledge of brain physiology and pharmacology greater, their evidence basis was better or more scientifically proven (and they should generally enjoy administrative privileges and draw commensurate salaries in a higher bracket than the psychologists).

I had already worked for a year as a psychiatric social worker in the State Department of Mental Hygiene, a public agency, where the M.D.s usually lorded it over Ph.D.s and M.S.W.s, not to mention Psychology bachelor's-level counselors, like I was. Now I was back in graduate school preparing myself as a career psychologist, while many of my friends were in medical school, so I was interested in the issue, to say the least.

One immediate controversy involved the revision of the *DSM*, or *Diagnostic and Statistical Manual of Mental Disorders*, the basic manual for all mental health providers of every professional category. The psychologists were determined not to let this one go. After all, *they had their own guild*, the American Psychological Association, with more members, in fact, than "that *other* APA" (the American Psychiatric Association). Congress became a proving ground (even a "jousting field") between champions representing both professional moieties. Each side would have to demonstrate its evidence basis.

Since the professional area of both groups falls into human services or social sciences, the playing field would be defined by the terms *reliability* and *validity*. Reliability means, basically, would two (or potentially many) psychiatrists give the same patient the same diagnosis?—important because a reliable *diagnosis* (supposedly) leads to an effective *treatment*. It is easier to see the *validity* aspect in relation to treatment rather than diagnosis. Does the therapy or treatment bring about results in the real world? (Spitzer and Fleiss 1974, 341).

The rest is mental health history. The two *guilds* (and perhaps the medieval term pertains more than we would like to think, at least in mental health!) presented their evidence. The rules of the playing field are an annoying something called *statistics*—or, how much more than the *null hypothesis*, results due to chance, can be demonstrated? The outcome actually led to the revision of the *DSM*, with much more probity given than heretofore to the methods used by psychologists. For example, in diagnosis (a reliability test), when the psychiatrists, with their somewhat archaic Latin and Greek terminologies for human conditions, came up with poor reliability scores, it was questioned whether anything with poor reliability could even be valid (Kirk and Kutchins 1994).

Why?

The psychologists used instruments more objective than off-the-cuff clinical diagnosis. (No matter how astute the psychiatrists may have been in those days, they are much more sophisticated today.) Standardized tests, such as the MMPI, the Minnesota Multiphasic Personality Inventory, which usually consists of 566 questions, has a much higher reliability and validity (70 plus percent) than the clinical-interview method (Spitzer and Fleiss 1974; Spitzer, Endicott, and Robins 1978; Grove 1987).

In the last decade or two, computer-mediated and scored tests such as the TOVA (Test of the Variables of Attention), used for assessing ADD, also demonstrate high reliability and validity rates. Way back when, Congress decided to grant some probity to statistical evidence basis and granted psychologists their seat at the table. The latest version of the Diagnostic and Statistical Manual of Mental Disorders, *DSM IV-r* has had much input from psychologists. (Maybe there is increased legal parity between Ph.D.s and M.D.s, but physicians still usually draw much higher salaries—and it is true, their education probably costs more. Don't get me wrong, psychiatrists are usually highly professional and helpful to people with diagnoses or conditions that warrant medication. Some of my best friends are psychiatrists!)

In the current controversy involving the probity of the qEEG in court, its admissibility as evidence in court, or even its reimbursability by third-party payers, I am having déjà vu (and the year is 2010, not 1960). Traditionally the EEG has been the bailiwick of the neurologist, an M.D., who might do as much as a two-year postdoctoral residency and/or become board-certified in reading the EEG. Unfortunately, despite the awesome abilities of the human biocomputer, that means a physician eye-balling an EEG for anomalies and making a comment on the kinds of anomalies noted. For the most brilliant EEG-literate neurologists, it is a field day. No one else can do what they do.

The qEEG is a different animal. It has been mostly developed and used by Ph.D.s, research psychologists in graduate departments, such as Harvard's Frank Duffy, E. Roy John at New York University, or Robert Thatcher, formerly of NYU (more on Thatcher in chapter 13).

I have evoked the mythos of "the little robot who doesn't lie." This is the truth of the qEEG. It samples gigantic amounts of data and compares individual people to the normative database. John and Thatcher, while gathering EEG evidence for studies on ADD and ADHD, put together the database that is used not only in creating qEEG and LORETA (diagnostic tools), but also in live Z-score training, a biofeedback treatment

	Standards	Yes	No
1	Peer reviewed publications		
2	Amplifier matching		
3	Artifact rejection		
4	Test/retest reliability		
5	Inclusion/exclusion reliability		
6	Adequate sample size per age group		
7	Approximation to a Gaussian		
8	Cross-validation		
9	Clinical correlation		
10	FDA registered		

Fig. 3.2. Standards for evaluating qEEG databases

modality that is suddenly a realistic option because of great advances in computer processing abilities and speed.

Dr. Robert Thatcher says in his 2010 article "Validity and Reliability in Quantitative Electroencephalography," published in the *Journal of Neurotherapy* (vol. 14, no. 2, April–June 2010), that qEEG is better than visual EEG inspection "because qEEG has high resolution in the millsecond time domain and approximately 1 cm in the spatial domain, which gives qEEG the ability to measure network dynamics that are simply 'invisible' to the naked eye. Over the last 40 years, the accuracy, sensitivity, reliability, validity, and resolution of qEEG has steadily increased because of the efforts of hundreds of dedicated scientists and clinicians that have produced approximately 90,000 qEEG studies cited in the National Library of Medicine's database."

He goes on to say, "Since approximately 1975, it is very difficult to publish a non-qEEG study in a peer-reviewed journal because of the subjective nature of different visual readers agreeing or disagreeing in their opinions about the squiggles of the EEG."

Thatcher clearly favors the "q" approach, not just because he is a Ph.D., but because he appreciate human limitations. *Computers cannot do what we can do, and we cannot do what they can do.* Thatcher goes on to talk about how qEEG has given superior results in three kinds of validity: criterion, or predictive, validity; content, or face, validity; and construct validity. The basic issue in all three is how well the hypothesis compares to other measuring or imaging techniques, such as the MRI, or another way of gauging the method's relation to the real world. Thatcher also mentions that unless a measure is reliable, it can't be valid; that is to say, until you see that something is reproducible in a variety of conditions, you cannot judge its relationship to reality.

Correlation between qEEG data and IQ (content validity) is high, for example; or how well does qEEG data correlate with the Glasgow Coma Scale in severe TBI (predictive validity)?

In studying TBI, there is a good correlation of qEEG data with MRI pictures. This is construct validity, integrating theoretical constructs and empirical measures.

There are also comparisons of LORETA images derived from the qEEG with fMRI data, with PET and SPECT scans. There is test-retest

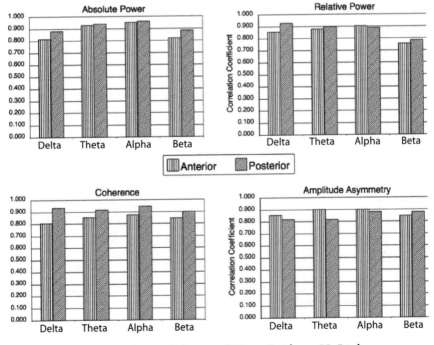

Fig. 3.3. Cross-validation of NeuroGuide vs. NxLink

reliability, also called "stability reliability." The reliability of qEEG data can be further examined at the National Library of Medicine's database.*

The Neurofeedback Museum and Hall of Fame at the BrainMaster Home Office, Bedford, Ohio

During the 1970s, my biofeedback lab at the State University of New York–Ulster had two EEG units: an Autogenics 70 and a big, powerful Autogenics 120 processor. They could measure both frequency and amplitude ranges, and you could set reward thresholds in whatever brain wave range you wished: theta, alpha-theta, alpha, or beta. My lab had Toomim EMGs and American Biotech GSRs and temperature trainers. The devices were stand-alone, and, at the time, "state of the art," each in its handsome wooden case.

I have written elsewhere of how people practicing the voluntary control of inner states relaxed tense muscles, abated headaches, and lowered blood pressure. There was, however, no combined-modality screen, such as I now have on my BrainMaster Atlantis, for monitoring several biofeedback modalities at once and seeing how they relate to each other, so we can form a complex picture of the interaction of psychophysiological variables. Nor was there any kind of report generator, where you could look at a recapitulation of the session to examine the progression of training. (These important results of the session would have to be gleaned from subjective reports by the trainee or the trainer-clinician.)

The importance of these machines is that they were pioneering prototypes, using the best solid-state technology at the time, to give people information back about their bodies and brains. The designer-engineers were often clinicians as well. The machines would be made in home shops or nearby electronics manufacturers where there could be continual interface with the designers. Adam Crane, founder of American Biotech, was my first neurofeedback mentor, and I can still remember the hundreds of hours Adam spent devising and calibrating the reward

---

*Please reference this at www.ncbi.nlm.nih.gov/sites/entrez?db=pubmed. (If you enter "EEG and reliability" there are 368 citations, and the majority of these pertain to qEEG.)

tones for his training machines. When you succeeded in, say, producing alpha and inhibiting theta, and your muscles also were relaxed, the auditory feedback would produce a beautiful three-part tonic chord, which was pleasant to hear. Thus the feedback really was reinforcing. People performed well and got good improvements on those American Biotech machines.

The Neurofeedback Hall of Fame (also at BrainMaster's home office) honors people who have contributed to the development of biofeedback.

I will list below the 2009 recipients honored on BrainMaster's website, with the briefest description of their contribution:

Adam Crane: Founder of American Biotech

Tom Budzynski: Early researcher in EEG and EMG

Hans Berger: For the development of the original EEG in the 1920s

Joe Kamiya: For the first controlled experiment during the 1960s that showed subjects could discern what brain wave state they were in

Barry Sterman: For the 1970s development of the first antiseizure protocols using the sensorimotor rhythm (12–15 Hz)

Joel Lubar: For adapting the adaptation of the sensorimotor rhythm to attention-deficit problems (1970s to the present) (more on Lubar and his importance below)

Lester Fehmi: For developing the whole brain synchrony protocols and the Open Focus technique (1970s to the present)

I have often emphasized how much biofeedback and neurofeedback are a "people's technology." Yet some of the most important inventions in our modern world have come from clinicians with small labs and modest incomes—with nonetheless great and shining motives and tireless energy to realize the goals.

I wanted to interview some of the awardees for this book, and then the following description from Joel Lubar arrived on my BrainMaster user e-mail list. It contains the essence of his contribution in his own words, and a thorough inventory of "conditions treatable by neurofeedback."

Dr. Lubar's Involvement
with Neurofeedback
JOEL LUBAR, PH.D., BCIA-EEG

My work with seizure patients using neurofeedback actually began in my laboratory at the University of Tennessee in 1973. We published our first paper on this in 1975. (I became interested in the seizure work following Barry Sterman's first publication in 1971 of a single case using neurofeedback to reduce seizures.) In our work in 1973 and 1974 with about eight patients who had significant and severe seizures that were uncontrolled by medication, I observed that as they acquired the ability to increase *sensorimotor* rhythm (12–15 Hz) and at the same time reduce slow wave paroxysmal activity, they became more attentive and alert.

Since scientific discoveries are often based on observation, I extrapolated that this treatment might be helpful in dealing with what was known at that time as "the hyperkinetic disorder" of childhood. Now it is known as ADHD. Starting in 1974, and continuing from that date, I began a project along with Margaret Shouse, which in fact became her dissertation. She then continued the work after she graduated. What we found in our early work was that if we trained children to *increase SMR* over central sites while *inhibiting theta,* their hyperkinetic behavior often decreased markedly, but they still had problems with focus, concentration, and attention.

Even at that time, there was considerable literature that indicated that *beta activity* was associated with a more alert and focused state, so, following that lead, I instituted a second type of training in which I *reinforced beta activity* along central sites Cz in children and at Fz in adolescents and adults, again inhibiting slow activity either in the theta or sometimes even in *thalpha* (6–10 Hz).

This second paradigm was particularly effective in improving attention, focus, and concentration. Currently, I often do this training in the left frontal region or in locations that are indicated by the qEEG to show excessive slow activity and insufficient fast activity.

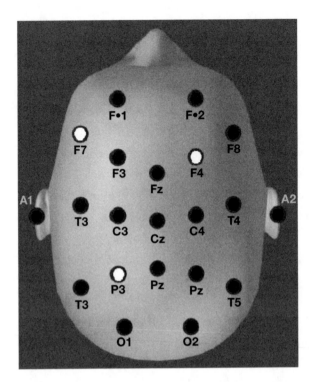

Fig. 3.4. A basic map of the brain

Thus, my early work with ADD and ADHD was based upon observations developed working with seizure patients. Over the years, but particularly starting from 1991, there was considerable publicity about our early work with ADD and ADHD using neurofeedback, both in *Woman's Day* magazine and in *Reader's Digest*. Today neurofeedback treatment of attention deficit is the largest single application of neurofeedback and also the best documented, and it is considered to be both efficacious and specific, according to our recent review in the *Journal of Neurotherapy*.

However, the seizure work still stands as highly effective for many patients who do not have adequate control with medication. It is most unfortunate that this area has not shown the degree of interest that the work with attention deficit has. Back in the 1970s it was often stated in the neurology literature that only 75 percent of epileptics respond well to anticonvulsant medications. This number has only changed from 75 to 80 percent in the current time—even though a number of new medications have been introduced.

Then there other areas of neurofeedback that deserve considerable recognition as being highly effective, for example the use of the Peniston protocol* for treatment of alcoholism and certain types of drug addictions.

There is equally promising work with severe depressive disorders employing protocols that were developed by Peter Rosenfeld at Northwestern University and also by Elsa and Rufus Baehr in Illinois. Some of their patients, who would have been on multiple medications and psychotherapy for years with little progress, showed considerable progress when they were presented with neurofeedback involving the alpha asymmetry protocol.† Some of these patients have now been followed for more than ten years posttreatment and still show significant improvement of their depressive symptoms. There are many other applications of neurofeedback that have been shown to be highly effective.

While it is true that often the ideal double-blind, randomized controlled study with multiple control groups has not been done, the clinical data is overwhelmingly supportive. It may be years before these perfectly designed control studies are completed, and there is no question that therapist variables are very important. There are very few neurofeedback applications that stand completely alone, in the sense that the patient is connected to the machine and no therapist needs to be present. In my own practice with my wife, Judith, we were always in the room with the patients during every session of neurofeedback. In the laboratory studies that I have published, some of which were double-blind, the therapist was not present, and still positive results were obtained, both for ADHD and for seizure disorders, but this is not good clinical practice. The therapist clearly has to be part of the feedback loop, providing encouragement, especially since feedback can be long and tedious in some cases.

However, the basic model for all forms of neurofeedback is operant conditioning, based on nearly a hundred years of solid learning theory and

---

*During the 1970s and 1980s Eugene Peniston applied his protocol to alcoholic and addicted Vietnam War vets, with such a high degree of reported success that it was regarded as controversial in the field—surely no one could get such good results with such a difficult population.

†Davidson shows that many depressed people have an overactive right frontal cortex associated with pessimistic thinking and an underactive left frontal cortex associated with optimism.

thousands of journal articles, involving both animal and human models, that show which schedules of reinforcement are most effective, and in dealing with the problems of extinction reacquisition* and maintenance of gains acquired during learning.

Let me return to one other aspect of treatment, the integration of neurofeedback with medications. We all know that medications are not "magic bullets" and that the side effects sometimes outweigh the main problems they were designed for. Many medications have been removed from the market because of these effects. Nevertheless, when we begin treatment using neurofeedback, we leave the patients on whatever medications they are on, without changing the dosages. As the neurofeedback progresses, if the patient's symptoms are decreased and they feel that they have made significant progress, we work with the referring physician in trying to slowly and in a stepwise manner reduce those medications that have the most deleterious side effects, until the patient is stabilized with neurofeedback, and hopefully on a much lower dose of medications, which is less dangerous and more helpful. There are many cases in which medications have been eliminated entirely—for example, in treating chronic anxiety disorders, depression, ADD, and ADHD. In the case of epilepsy, patients usually have to remain on lower doses of their anticonvulsant medications. When we work with seizure patients, we run blood levels on a regular basis to make sure they're in the therapeutic range. In rare cases where the seizures disappear entirely, it may be possible to remove patients from all medications, but they have to be very carefully followed.

In all my work, regardless of the disorder being treated, we obtain pretraining, during training, and posttraining qEEGs. I started working with qEEGs back in the mid-1980s when I was associated with the pain disorders center at St. Mary's Hospital in Knoxville, Tennessee, where we had a very active biofeedback program. At that time the main interest in qEEGs was to see if they correlated with different psychiatric disorders, and of course the equipment at that time was very primitive compared with today's. I strongly recommend in all my workshops and consulta-

---

*Extinction reacqusition is the "unlearning" of already learned behaviors, according to Watson and Skinner's operant conditioning theory.

tions with professionals that they use qEEG extensively. More recently, they have the qEEG instrumentation and NeuroGuide (the Thatcher database), so that they can do connectivity training for coherence and phase, as well as amplitude and frequency training.

Some Terms Pertaining to the qEEG

Coherence: Refers to shared activity in the frequency domain, which can look like areas or "rugs." One definition of coherence is the degree to which there is a constant or variable phase relationship between pairs of sites for a particular frequency or frequency band.

Comodulation: The rate at which shared activity varies together over time. Most neurologists refer to a similar measure as "spectral correlation" (Sterman and Friar 1971).

Connectivity: To what extent are two sites connected? That is, do they share activity in frequency, amplitude, or phase? Connectivity is indicated on the maps by lines between sites. Thicker lines are more unusual or distant from the norm, thinner are more weakly connected.

Phase synchrony or separation: In what way do the troughs and peaks of waveforms coincide, or are they 180 percent of some other measure, out of phase? Includes angular relationship between waves. This is the specialty of Fehmi's approach.

Conditions That May Benefit from Neurofeedback

The same disclaimer with which we began this book pertains here. *Neurofeedback does not pretend to cure any illness or diagnosed problem.* Through relaxation and attunement, it simply makes the symptom easier to live with, or it may facilitate a self-healing response from within the patient.

What defines conditions that are likely to benefit from treatment by neurofeedback? Think of anything affected by the central nervous system (especially our brains): anxiety, depression, insomnia, hypervigilance (for whatever reason); but also the more severe mental problems such as obsessive-compulsive disorder, attention deficit and hyperactivity, especially in childhood; and explosive or anger disorders based a chronic irritability. Neurofeedback may facilitate pharmaceutical treatment or combined approaches such as psychotherapy or autogenic training, and so forth.

Then there are disorders not expected to be more than minimally treatable, if at all, such as autism and Asperger's syndrome. By simply calming and balancing the nervous system, and by increasing the patient's own sensitivity to internal cues or problems, neurofeedback may make things a little easier, and more graceful, for them.

Moreover, neurofeedback can help ameliorate the sequelae of disorders normally regarded as problems only treatable by medicines: Parkinson's disease, notably, and multiple sclerosis. Again, no cure is offered, only more ease with side effects such as tremor, anxiety, sleep disturbance, and nightmares.

An area in which conventional medicine offers very little is TBI, traumatic brain injury, in all its many inflections: automobile accidents and falls, impact and blast injuries in the military, sports injuries, anoxias and ischemias, strokes and aneurysms. While some neurologists remain stuck in the old paradigm of "no neuronal regeneration," neurofeedback, as we have discussed, promotes neural plasticity, glial repair, and dendritic proliferation through injured areas, as well as the reassignment of lost functions to new areas.

Neurofeedback has shown special promise in helping to resolve PTSD (post-traumatic stress disorder). Some clinicians believe neurofeedback can provide therapeutic relief from flashbacks, nightmares, and explosive or seizure disorders subsequent to traumatic exposure. It can soften the difficulties of "soldier return" syndrome of damaged warriors attempting to integrate into civilian life.

Seizures and seizure disorder have a special appropriateness to neurofeedback because they occur in the brain and involve the same brain waves that neurofeedback measures. We have mentioned the early work of Dr. Barry Sterman, first with cats and then human epileptics. Then there is the theory of Dr. Len Ochs, that subclinical seizures—and the brain's own attempt to control them—may be implicated in many kinds of other disorders, such as paroxysmal anger or depersonalization. He believes that as seizure disorders resolve, neuropsychological energy is released for other activities and functions.

Neurofeedback prides itself on being included in "complementary and alternative medicine." That is to say, the best neurofeedback clinicians work integratively with physicians, nurses, and physical and occupational therapists as well as psychotherapists to achieve more complete outcomes than single modalities alone can usually achieve. Neurofeedback may facilitate or free up the brain to make much more profitable use of many kinds of therapeutic and rehabilitative techniques.

Neurofeedback can also, by making patients more sensitive to all forms of stimulation or input, help with the side effects of prescription medications, to the point that the doctor may be able to lower the dosage. Neurofeedback has also helped with the aftereffects of chemotherapy or radiation (instead of using other medicines and further compromising an already overburdened system).

Some neurofeedback clinicians have also had experience with trying to restore brains compromised by multiple ECT (electroconvulsive therapy) treatments. The gentler treatment may help restore damaged memory, or fine-tune cognitive clarity lost in the overwhelming impact of the ECT.

In conclusion of this section, we should mention one more important application: the use of neurofeedback in *optimal performance*. Many neurofeedback researchers, as well as clinicians, have focused on helping athletes and performing artists such as dancers and musicians to get out of their own way and let creativity shine through. We have mentioned John Gruzelier's study of the effect of neurofeedback on conservatory-level musicians, where it helped improve accuracy and virtuosity, but also helped the musicians enhance their emotional communication. We know of no comparable studies for writers and poets, but the author has seen neurofeedback be very helpful to people with "writer's block" and the inability to finish plays, novels, or doctoral dissertations.

FOUR

THE COMPASSIONATE HEALER

OR, HOW DOES A PERSON BECOME A NEUROFEEDBACK PROVIDER?

With Nicholas Dogris, Ph.D., Mike Beasley, L.M.T., and Richard M. Smith, Ph.D.

The Healing Gate

The theme on which this chapter is based takes us into the heart of compassion, and into healing. Those of us who work in the field and attend professional conferences know that a large number of our company (neurofeedback professionals) have arrived through the same gate: the urgent need to help a loved one in distress. It is a testament to the effectiveness of our method not only that the help brought relief to the afflicted person but that it then enabled the practitioner, through the skills learned, to establish a profession.

The first narrative is from Nick Dogris, a California psychologist whose son almost didn't make it but now is fully here. Nick has not only written innovative protocols for the LENS treatment; he also designed and mobilized his own healing technology, the NeuroField, about which we learn more later in this book.

The second case is also about saving a child, in this case the daughter of corporation CEO Mike Beasley; she was shot by an overmedicated convict and has had a long, slow, and painful road back to normalcy (now happily married). The third story is how the self-healing of a healer helps others: Richard Smith is a North-Country (Plattsburg, New York) professional psychologist in his seventies, on the threshold of retirement. In his own professional training (by the author), not only was he healed himself but new life was brought to his practice.

In the following essays, with minimal editing, I have let these three practitioners tell their own stories.

AJ All the Way: Bringing My Child Fully into Himself
NICHOLAS DOGRIS, PH.D.

It was Monday, July 22, 2002, and I had just finished working a twelve-hour day. People who know me know that I have a lot of energy. I was born with it, and in the years that followed this day I would use all of it to develop a way to heal my son. This is my story about how I developed protocols for the LENS and would eventually come to develop my own technology, known as NeuroField. It's a story about how a father and mother came face-to-face with some of the best and worst medical providers. A story about the American medical system and how thinking outside the box changes lives. A story about my experience as a neurofeedback professional and a father. A story about my quest to help my son and what I went through to get there.

This is a story that needs to be told over and over again because it represents the spirit of exploration and the need to look at different methods of healing to help people. There is more out there than you know, and it is my hope that the telling of this story will encourage you to look further than the physician that you visit. To look outside the box and to ask the hard questions. To challenge the status quo of using suppressive medical techniques to treat problems that are much more complicated and pervasive than anyone knows. To walk side by side with a competent and adequately trained health care provider in an effort to achieve the highest quality of care that you possibly can. Here is my story about someone I value and love deeply: my son, AJ. He is the light of my life and the inspiration that fuels my intention, my will, my desire. Here is his story.

My wife, Julie, was pregnant and had been on bed rest for several months. She was staying at her parents' house in La Crescenta, California, because hers was a high-risk pregnancy. We had gone to hell and back trying to have a child. She was determined beyond belief and had retained a very good physician who worked out of Huntington Memorial Hospital in Pasadena, California. This facility had the number-one neonatal intensive care unit in the country, and we did not want to take any chances with our baby, so Julie moved 275 miles from our home and was ten minutes away from the hospital.

We had lost twins in 2001, a month before the tragedy of 9/11, after Julie had gone into sudden premature labor at five months. She came within an inch of dying losing those babies, and we were determined not to relive that nightmare again. So this time she obtained a cerclage after being pregnant for twelve weeks and began a very difficult stint of bed rest. Regardless of these measures, she went into premature labor during the thirty-first week, roughly two months early, and drove herself to the hospital at two o'clock in the morning. The doctors did their best and tried to stop the labor by giving her magnesium and terbutaline. The measures worked for a couple of days but then failed, and Julie ended up back in the hospital with the doctor saying that she would spend the remainder of the pregnancy there.

I had driven back to my home in Bishop, California, the night before. I felt assured that Julie was in good hands at the hospital and left to resume the responsibilities of my neurotherapy practice. At the time I was transitioning into a full-time private practice while maintaining employment as the program chief for Mono County Mental Health. I would work a full eight-hour day at the clinic and then drive to my private practice and log in another four hours. Looking back, I wonder how I did it, but then again I wonder how I do a lot of things. Anyway, I drove home and had just walked through the door when the call came. Julie was calling me from her cell phone and said, "You need to get down here, he's coming." She had broken through the intravenous magnesium they were giving her, and she knew it.

I hung up the phone, quickly threw some clothes in a bag, and fed the animals. While I was doing this, Julie called back and said, "He's coming now; they are taking me to the delivery room. You're not going to make it. Don't rush." I was four hours away by car, and Bishop does not offer air service to Los Angeles unless you are critically injured. I took a deep breath and gathered my strength. I was exhausted after working all day and had a 275-mile drive ahead of me, but the notion of being a father was exciting and terrifying all at the same time. Soon I was ready to leave, but just as I was about to walk out the door Julie called again, and this time I could hear the sound of my son, AJ, crying. Because of the magnesium, his nervous system was depressed and he had trouble breathing, and so then the doctor intubated him immediately. Julie barely had a moment to see her newborn son before they rushed him into the neonatal intensive care unit. He had been born two months before his due date.

By the time I arrived at the hospital, it was around 3:00 a.m. I was guided to the intensive care unit and met my son for the first time.

As I stood there taking him in, I was informed by the doctor that he was breathing "room air" and that the intubation was just a precaution. His lungs were working fine, and his prognosis was good. I was consumed with emotion but became almost immediately aware that AJ had been born anoxic. The magnesium had depressed his nervous system enough to warrant intubation. The doctor said that had they not intubated him, he would have been blue within minutes after being born. The doctor in me turned on at that moment, and I asked to see the chart that they allowed me to review. They had saved my son's life by taking the measures they did after his birth, but they had also caused a low-level anoxia that caused brain damage. I knew I would have to treat him, but the neurotherapy measures I was using at the time could not be used on children until they were roughly four to five years of age. I would have to find another way to help him.

I began my search by scouring the Internet. I was astounded by the amount of "energy" modalities being offered by people who had little to no qualifications for offering these types of treatment. However, there they were, and I began the process of studying each of them. Over the period of two years I invested over $100,000 purchasing devices and trying them out. I found some items that I felt had merit and others that were pure garbage. Many people claimed to be professionals but had no formal training in any health care modality and claimed to have certifications that afforded them the ability to work with people. Many of them simply wanted to "do good" and had the intention to help. However, I found many of the "do-gooders" did more harm than good and ended up giving alternative therapies a bad name. As I sought help for my son, it became very apparent to me that I would have to be mindful of what I chose, but the clock was ticking, and I needed help.

My son was almost two and was showing significant cognitive deficits. He was behind in milestones and had severe sensory integration problems. He had severe hypotonia and could not sit up without assistance, was late to walk, talk, dress himself, and maintain his bowel. He was extremely sound- and light-sensitive and would get overstimulated easily. Since AJ was born two months premature, he was automatically enrolled in an early start program and began physical therapy. This program was helpful, as the physical therapist was able to model movement for AJ and helped him become stronger with increased movement. However, his sensory issues were difficult to treat, which led the physical therapist to request further medical consultation. So we were referred to a traveling pediatric physician who worked for the early start program. My wife and I were willing to allow the examination, as we recognized that AJ was progressing but was falling behind in his development. As a parent, I remember feeling fearful of what life would be like for my son if he could not be helped.

We went to the appointment. The physician looked at him and said, "He has a big head!" The physician then took out a measuring tape and measured my son's head, saying that he believed he had "hydrocephalus." I was stunned and glanced at my wife, who had a perplexed look on her face. So I said, "I have a big head too. Maybe he just takes after his parents." The good doctor measured our heads and then said, "He needs an MRI and should get one immediately."

I had seen cases of hydrocephalus in my career, and my son did not show symptoms that I thought would warrant that diagnosis. My own head was reeling, and I began to question if I was becoming defensive or was in denial about my son's problems. Was I refusing to accept reality, or was I asking appropriate questions? I remember numbly nodding and leaving the office with my family. As Julie and I talked about our experience, it became clear that we had just been seen by a physician who shot from the hip, did no formal workup, and made a snap diagnosis within seconds of meeting our son.

To say I was angry is an understatement. As I became aware of what this physician had done, I became incensed, because he did this not only to my family, but many others. In my humble opinion, doctors like this one need to have their licenses revoked and face disciplinary actions for unethical, harmful behavior. Why? Because they end up misdiagnosing their patients, placing labels on them that will affect their entire lives, and sending their families on a wild goose chase seeking treatment for a diagnosis that is incorrect. The impact can be life-changing and can lead to a horrible outcome if you simply follow the suggestions of the doctor. As Julie and I discussed what had happened, we arrived at the decision to seek a second opinion and to check our own defensive responses over time.

Eventually, the doctor sent his written report, in which he suggested encephalitis and the MRI. We took our son and the report to his pediatrician, who shook her head and refuted what was written in the report. It was a real eye-opener that caused Julie and me to approach physicians with caution and to ask questions that would make them responsible for the opinion they generated.

When AJ was roughly two years of age, after being given the MMR (measles/mumps/rubella) vaccination, he developed a serious blood disorder. This blood disorder, called idiopathic thrombocytopenic purpura (ITP), prevented him from creating the platelets he needed to keep from bleeding to death. This just added insult to injury, as AJ had an anoxic head injury and could have another simply by getting a bruise on his head. We were terrified, to say the least, and had to be on guard 24/7 to protect our son. At its worst, his platelet count dropped below 5,000, which is extremely dangerous. Should he have hit his head, it could have resulted in a potentially lethal internal bleed.

We began taking him to doctors in an effort to obtain help and guidance. AJ's problems were complicated and multilayered. This is when Julie and I experienced many of the limitations of Western medicine. AJ was diagnosed with many different things because he did not cleanly fit into any one box. The doctors scratched their heads and shot out diagnoses left and right, missing the mark on most of them. This was difficult to handle because our son was suffering, and we wanted answers. We obtained the services of a veteran hematologist from Children's Hospital in Los Angeles who did nothing short of saying he would grow out of the problem and should be given steroids.

The use of steroids depressed AJ's immune system and prevented his body from destroying its own blood cells. The treatment was brutal but effective in slowing down the progression of the disease. However, it also had serious side effects, including agitation and significant weight gain. AJ shot up to forty-two pounds and was in the ninety-ninth percentile for his age range. After giving him steroids for six months, the doctor announced that the problem was "chronic" and that AJ would be dealing with this issue for the rest of his life. He said that we should get ready to remove AJ's spleen, because that was the culprit.

I remember sitting there restraining the urge to punch this idiot in the nose as I attempted to ask questions about the proposed splenectomy. The diagnosis was such that there is no identified reason for the disease. The doctor was clueless about how it happened, but he was ready to cut my son open and remove one of his organs. When questioned about it, he became defensive and hostile, refusing to consider other ideas or alternatives. He never presented ideas outside of what was available to him. He remained in the box even though his patient could die as a result. I lost faith in him and Western medicine's ability to cure my son. Julie and I fired the good doctor and never went back.

We decided to search for another means to help AJ, and we scoured our resources. I guess when you put something into motion in that way it happens, because one of our friends told us about a doctor who practiced plant medicine. She told us a story of success using natural means. It was intriguing enough to place some calls and arrange for a consultation.

We took AJ off of the steroids and obtained help from a naturopathic physician. This doctor examined AJ and informed us that his liver was toxic. She suggested that this problem could have started in utero with the magnesium and terbutaline exposure. It made sense, because the doctor was trying to stop Julie from going into labor and assist her in carrying AJ as long as possible. However, the medications used to stop her contractions were theorized to have an impact on AJ's liver and digestive system. If his liver was toxic, then it would not be able to do the job of cleaning the blood. Liver toxicity can also lead to bone marrow depletion, as the liver pulls energy from the bones in an effort to stabilize itself.

The bones are responsible for blood cell development and create the platelets that AJ was deficient in at the time. As the liver pulls energy from the bones, they begin creating what are called "dirty" platelets. The spleen has the job of identifying "dirty" blood cells and will destroy them, because that is its job. Lastly, AJ's gut was toxic as well, and his ability to absorb vitamins and minerals was compromised. As a result his blood could not carry the fuel to various parts of his body, including his brain, so that it could repair itself.

The puzzle pieces came together, and we began giving AJ supplements to address these problems. Within thirty days, his platelets increased to safe levels, and his brain began to heal itself. This new doctor was willing to discuss what she did not know. She was willing to be open minded and to examine options and alternatives. She worked with us to create a workable plan. She empowered us and walked side by side with us. She was competent in her ability and shared information without hesitation. She was a real doctor, unlike the twenty-five-year veteran hematologist who wanted to cut out AJ's spleen, who would talk down to us, never once assessing my or Julie's abilities. Not once did he ask about our son's diet or take into consideration that the MMR vaccination may have impacted our son's immune system negatively. Never once did he engage us in a discussion about theory so that we could, together, try to formulate a workable plan to heal our son.

The memories of Los Angeles Children's Hospital haunt me to this day. The look of desperation and fatigue on the faces of parents who were seeking a cure for their children is burned into my soul, as are the vacant eyes of children who suffered from cancer and various diseases being treated by people who would not deviate from Western thinking even if it meant their young patients would die. I felt death there, and I knew I had to get my son out of there before this limited form of thinking claimed his life as well. Thank God we did, because removing AJ's spleen would have only worsened his condition and could have led to his death. As a health care professional with over twenty years of experience, I found myself humbled. I had a new respect for people and had been taught a valuable lesson about compassion, ethics, and competency. I also learned about my own feelings of love and compassion, and how my four academic degrees meant nothing if they were not linked with those feelings. I swore to myself that I would change the way I did things in my life and in my practice. The old saw "When the student is ready, the teacher will appear" applies to me. I was ready, and the teacher appeared.

It was during this time that my search led me to Len Ochs, Ph.D., the man who invented the Low Energy Neurofeedback System (LENS). Here was a legitimate professional, who had created this interesting system that he claimed had the ability to disrupt EEG activity by using a very small radio frequency pulse. It did not take me long to get into contact with Dr. Ochs. I ordered a system and hounded him for two months, as he was out of stock and was waiting for the next batch of EEG hardware to be shipped from J & J Engineering.

Len would take my calls and discuss his technology with me. I asked all sorts of questions and began to feel hope that I could engage my son in a meaningful early intervention, before he reached three years of age. Dr. Ochs was willing to answer my questions and would openly admit when he did not know something. He was genuine and sincere, even though his sense of humor was such that I found myself feeling light and happy when speaking with him about intense issues. My talks with Len seemed to occur effortlessly. I was ready to learn, and he was (and still is) ready to teach. I am reminded of an old proverb, "A teacher for a day is like a parent for life." I am extremely fortunate to have met Dr. Ochs, as he helped me and my family in ways that I am still trying to understand and will, more than likely, spend the remainder of my days examining. I feel an enormous amount of gratitude toward him that I simply cannot express in words.

In time my LENS system shipped, and I was off and running. My recent experiences with the medical world gave me plenty of motivation to learn about the LENS. Before I knew it, I was using it in my practice. I took to the LENS like a fish to water. I had been using traditional EEG biofeedback techniques for years and knew a great deal about brain wave entrainment,* but now I had to learn things about EEG and brain that were, in many ways, opposite to what I had previously learned. The LENS worked to *disentrain* the brain and would assist it in becoming unstuck. *It did not attempt to train the brain to function in a different way.* The LENS was based on the premise that the brain could heal itself.

It made sense to me almost from the word go. The fit was good, and I found myself pondering this technology in most of my waking moments. I had learned how to create brain maps and administer the basic LENS protocol. The people I worked with in my practice began to report changes, and I was still skeptical. It seemed too fast. In my experience with EEG biofeedback, it could take forty to sixty sessions to evoke a therapeutic clinical response, and when people began reporting changes after the first mapping session, I felt that this was placebo.

However, I could not deny that the EEG waveforms looked different. The data from the report generator would show dramatic decreases in delta and theta wave amplitudes that could not be denied. I had been trained by Margaret Ayers and had learned how to watch the EEG and recognize waveforms on the fly. Slow delta and theta waveforms are easy to pick out in the EEG and are predominant in people who suffer from brain damage. So, naturally, I checked my equipment to make sure it was working correctly. No problems found there, so

---

*Brain wave entrainment generally uses a rhythmical stimulus to cause the brain waves to follow the stimulus.

I thought it must be the computer system. No problems there. So I bought another LENS and built another computer system just to make sure. Same observations, with slow delta and theta amplitude reductions that went beyond anything I had observed in years of traditional EEG biofeedback training.

How could this be? It was simple yet complicated. The brain is a massive energetic system that can tune itself much like a person tunes a musical instrument. However, because of the billions of dendritic connections, it tunes itself in a chaotic fashion. The LENS tracks the dominant frequency in the EEG and then emits a small radio frequency that disrupts the brain for roughly one second. I would eventually tell people that I am very good at disrupting the brain and that the brain is very good at reorganizing itself. It knows how to repair itself, and the trick is knowing how much energy to give the system.

The LENS community has learned over the years that a simple whisper of energy is needed to nudge the system and evoke change in a positive direction. As simple as that statement sounds, it is a very challenging and daunting task. Just ask any experienced LENS practitioner, and they will confirm that this is the case. What I would eventually come to learn is that once disrupted, the system would engage in an energetic reorganization that would allow the brain to rewire itself energetically. As a result, the person is able to learn and become more functional in multidimensional ways. People get better because the system makes the correction, not the doctor.

It's an amazing thing to observe when you see it for the first time. Something as small and gentle as a LENS treatment can move a person in ways that are hard to believe. After all, I am a trained Western psychologist. I have worked in mainstream settings, including a psychiatric hospital, for seven years. My training as a health psychologist was part medical and positioned me to become a prescribing professional.

After working with the LENS for around three months, I felt ready to begin working with my son. I began by taking a brain map and looking at the raw EEG waveforms. What I saw made me take a deep breath and exhale slowly. AJ's delta and theta amplitudes were very high in several different regions of his brain. (Please refer to plates 6 and 7 of the color insert.) They display a topographic brain map with high amplitudes, and a histogram of EEG amplitudes in delta respectively.) AJ's high delta and theta amplitudes meant that there was significant damage to his brain and that he required a great deal of treatment. After his mapping, AJ was given four one-second sites per session with the LENS. He was comfortable and did not show any signs of overstimulation or potential side effects.

Within four weeks, Julie and I observed big changes. I remember sitting on the couch when AJ walked over to me and climbed up on the couch. He stood up, smiled, and then jumped on me. AJ's speech began to improve on a consistent basis, and his developmental process appeared to be accelerating. AJ's sensory issues began to decrease in severity. He became more tolerant of light and sounds, with an increasing ability to be around crowds and loud noises. His sense of humor emerged, and we began to see our child as a person. It was, and remains, a cherished memory. This was all I needed to see, and I jumped into the LENS headfirst.

After I had treated my son for roughly six to eight months, his improvement leveled off, and I was not seeing so many changes. It was then that I started professional consultations with Dr. D. Corydon Hammond. Dr. Hammond and I would talk twice a week, and I would bounce ideas and cases off of him and get his opinion along with mentoring to help improve my abilities. In our talks, we discussed Margaret Ayer's protocols to decrease the amplitude of delta and theta wave activity. It was then that I came up with the idea to modify the LENS. At that time, the standard LENS protocol would search to a dominant frequency in the 1–48 Hz range and then deliver feedback to the person.

I wondered what would happen if we focused the LENS on the slower delta and theta ranges between 1 and 8 Hz. In the dark of the night, I found a way to modify the LENS software to do just that. Nick's 1–8 protocol was born. I went to bed, awoke early, and called Dr. Hammond for my supervision. I remember confessing that I had changed the LENS software and that I was really excited about it. Dr. Hammond asked me if I had told Dr. Ochs, and I said that I had not but would in time.

Eventually, with a little trepidation, I did call Dr. Ochs. I breathed a sigh of relief because his response was so encouraging. (It was then that my neighbors reported seeing green lights and arcing electricity flickering from the windows of my house during the late hours of the night.) I had a flood of ideas based on traditional neurofeedback methods, some based on rocking a truck out of the snow and others based on a single strum of my *bouzouki,* or even a single note. It was a magical, intense time that I will never forget. Over the next two months I would develop a whole suite of protocols for the LENS that did a variety of things. People started calling them "Nick's Protocols," and they were used almost everywhere there was a LENS user.

My son began improving again and was progressing. We observed improved speech and more comprehension. His little personality emerged, and it turned out that AJ was a funny kid. His sensory issues began to decrease again, and I found myself forgetting that he had had the issue in the first place. However, it was not gone, and sometimes AJ would get overstimulated, which would remind us to be sensitive and mindful of his needs while at the same time celebrating his improvement. It was at this time that I conceived of NeuroField, to be discussed in more detail in another chapter.

As AJ went through preschool and kindergarten, his abilities jumped, and his testing showed great improvement academically. He began to show more compassion toward his parents and others. He would express feelings of love and was moved emotionally by the things that he observed. By kindergarten he had begun to demonstrate an amazing imagination. He loved to play pretend games with the kids and would organize them by assigning different characters to each of them. AJ's growth and improvement was apparent to his parents, his teachers, his friends, and his family.

AJ still has his challenges, but his ability to meet those issues head on is now a reality. Speech, sensory integration, and muscle-tone issues continue to be a problem for AJ. He is in speech therapy, occupational therapy, and physical therapy as of the writing of this book. He continues to see me for neurotherapy services and continues to respond to treatment. One issue that is turning my hair a steady shade of gray is the level of defiance that AJ can demonstrate. At first this appeared to be an expression of his personality, but then Julie and I discovered that AJ's sensory integration issues had evolved and matured over time. We would come to learn that his defiance was a way to control the amount of stimulation that he could tolerate. If AJ was getting overstimulated, he would either break off from the current event that was overstimulating or attempt to control it so that he could remain part of the event. This might involve his telling adults "No" when asked to engage in a task. In the old days he would lie on the floor face down and scream. Now AJ communicates and is becoming aware of the issue, and Julie and I can tell when things are "too much" or if he needs space.

We had come a long way from those days, and it appeared that AJ's sensory issues continued to change and become more manageable for him over time. AJ's speech continues to improve, and he is able to engage us in conversation that reflects thoughtful insight and a very sweet little boy who loves to be dramatic (like his mother). Lastly, AJ's muscle tone continues to improve through the concerted effort of his mother, who became a nutritional consultant. Julie focused on diet and has given AJ a very good, nutritious, healthy diet. As a result he has become stronger, which appears to have offset the hypotonia to some degree.

The LENS and NeuroField treatments changed AJ's life and improved it in ways that I doubt he would have achieved had he not received treatment. I shudder to think what would have happened had AJ not been treated. I feel so fortunate to be part of the LENS community, as these are intelligent, thoughtful, compassionate, and professional people. As I sought out help, I was given tips and guidance from many individuals who gladly shared ideas and insight into the use of the LENS and EEG neurofeedback techniques. The feeling of support was invaluable, and knowing that I could simply pick up the phone and call any one of the many LENS users allowed me to breathe much easier. I am honored to be part of your world, Dr. Ochs. A teacher for a day is like a parent for life. Thank you, Len.

How Healers Emerge from Adversity
MIKE BEASLEY, L.M.T.

Scientists are curious by nature. This, coupled with the ancient Chinese curse "May you live in interesting times," pretty much sums up how I got into the "new frontier" of healing. The transition from a career as a research chemist working with semiconductors to one in the healing arts focused on subtle energies and how they interact has been, well, "interesting."

The driving force for change occurred on March 13, 2001, at 5:30 p.m. This was when our daughter, Julie, was attacked while doing field research on a remote Texas ranch by a deranged stranger who had had an adverse reaction to prescription drugs. The stranger shot her twice with a high-powered rifle and then walked over to ascertain that she was dead. (She, wisely, pretended to be just that.)

The man then drove off in her car. Julie crawled two thirds the length of a football field, out of the rough, cactus-covered Texas ranch-land, dragging her nearly severed arm and destroyed hip, by pulling with her good hand and pushing with her one good leg. Then she came to the next obstacle, a barbed-wire fence. She pushed her way through the fence, tearing her side open, only to get stuck, totally exhausted, in the ditch of the dirt road.

There was an ongoing thirty-three-hour manhunt with a force of over 100 personnel searching for the perpetrator, because he had attacked four other people before he shot Julie. The manhunt included officers, support personnel, a helicopter, and a canine unit. A nearby rancher heard shots and called the police, which helped an officer locate her in this remote location. She was eventually flown by helicopter to the San Antonio's University of Texas Health Science Center trauma center, where she was given a 5 percent chance to live.

An AirLife pilot called the house and said that Julie had made it to the emergency room alive. My stunned response was, "I think you have the wrong number." The pilot asked if I was the father of Julie Beasley and gave me the details. In minutes, my wife and I were speeding toward San Antonio.

Dr. Animesh Agarwal, chief of surgery, gave us the news; our daughter's injuries were so severe that there was a 95 percent chance that she would not make it. Nearly all of her blood was lost; the damage was so extensive that they left her abdomen open that evening and packed it with ice in an attempt to find all the bleeding sources. They kept packing her abdomen with ice bags for nearly a week, while every other day would be another lengthy surgery. This began an "interesting time" in our lives. Months later, thanks to his team's efforts, the "Miracle Girl" crossed the university stage to a standing ovation to receive her summa cum laude degree in Biology.

The newspaper and local and national TV headlines read: "Shot Twice, Left to Die, 5 Percent Chance to Live, Graduates with Honors."

To date Julie has had about fifty-five surgeries to repair the impact from the two .270-caliber bullets. Due to the initial trauma, multiple hospitalizations and surgeries, and lengthy recoveries, Julie developed reflex sympathetic dystrophy (now referred to as chronic regional pain syndrome, or CRPS). Julie experienced CRPS types I and II. These conditions reduce vascularization and cause the affected limbs to become cold, grayish, and swollen. This was coupled with an unexplained tissue breakdown in the right elbow region that required more extensive surgery; more muscle grafts, tissue grafts, bone removal. No one really knew how to solve the problem.

One thought to explain the tissue breakdown was that it could the result of an allergic response, because no bacteria would culture out as positive. The most probable cause therefore seemed to be an allergy to the implanted materials—the titanium, steel, or plastic parts composing the prosthetic. There was no way to test for this type of allergy. I learned from Rush University that skin-patch test results were meaningless in this instance, and blood tests would not work because the blood had to be so highly acidified to keep titanium ions in solution that it destroyed the blood sample. I searched out two doctors to help me develop a new technique. From several locations in my body, we removed a core of tissue large enough to place a 2 × 8 mm titanium rod perpendicular to the skin's surface, then sutured the skin to enclose the rod. The rods were left in for weeks, and then they were extracted by removing larger cores of tissue that also contained the test rods. The tissue next to the rods was examined under a microscope for an allergic response. There was none. The technique worked on me, so now we would try it on Julie. The result of the test was that she was not allergic to the implanted parts. Another answer and possible cause was crossed off my list of seventeen reasons that might explain the tissue failures. More research was indicated.

Eventually, while reading research papers, a treatise on staph-adherent biofilms seemed to exactly fit what we were seeing. I called the Center for Biofilm Research at Montana State University. It turns out there were two doctors in the United States looking into bacteria-laden biofilms, and one was in Texas, Dr. Gerhard E. Maale. One phone call, and the data fit exactly; Dr. Maale even finished the sentences correctly before I could! My motto has always been, "Follow the data." The data led directly to Dr. Maale's office. We changed surgical approaches, against the advice of the world expert and many other doctors. It worked; tissue breakdown stopped.

The tissue breakdown problem was controlled, but the chronic pain was not. Chronic and burning pain was getting worse. Julie was on maximum opiate medication levels and had two spinal blocks on a weekly regime. She asked for more frequent blocks, even though the relief was down to about a day postinjection. The pain relief barely outlasted the surgical anesthesia effects. Her pain clinic issued her a transcutaneous electrical nerve stimulator (TENS), which she used four times per day for forty-five minutes per session, and the pain subsided somewhat during the device's use but returned immediately after the TENS was turned off. There was no long-term relief from pain. Once reflex sympathetic dystrophy (RSD) was identified, the medical prediction was that RSD would worsen; she would move into a wheelchair, deteriorate further, and expire. I told the medical world this was unacceptable and started researching chronic pain and RSD.

Serendipity intervened when Julie's orthopedic surgeon had knee surgery and experienced postsurgical pain. The doctor could bend his knee only 40 degrees, and it was very painful. This orthopedic surgeon remembered there was a company that wanted to show him a Russian device that was supposed to alleviate pain. He told the company that they could use the device on him, and if it worked, he would talk to them further. After a thirty-minute session with Dr. Zulia Valeyeva-Frost, his pain was essentially eliminated. He was shocked. He fully bent his knee, even crossed his legs, with very little discomfort. He said, "This is the real thing, isn't it?" and set up a pilot study that included twenty-three of his patients who were experiencing severe orthopedic pain from known causes.

In the pilot study, twenty-three patients were treated with a Russian device called a SCENAR for thirty minutes per day for three days in a row. Each day, data was recorded from pre- and postpain levels. Julie was the first patient on his list. Her pain went from 8/10 (the top of the pain rating scale) to zero inside of thirty minutes; her leg changed color back to pink, and the pain stayed away totally for sixteen hours. We were all stunned. This level of relief and/or color change had not occurred in over a year, much less from a thirty-minute non-drug, noninvasive therapy session. I got involved with the trial and asked the CEO, "How do we get one of these devices?" The CEO said, "Well, they are not approved by the FDA . . . they are experimental devices . . . and . . ."

I stopped him and politely said, "Excuse me, but that was not my question. My question was, specifically, how do we get one of these?" He smiled, having understood completely; we left with an "experimental device," the first of many to come.

Upon our return to Austin, Julie eliminated all her scheduled spinal blocks and requested that her pain medication level be dropped. There was no more mention of a wheelchair and/or death. Her pain doctor was perplexed and asked, "What are you guys doing?" "Experiments," we answered. "We'll let you know exactly when we have more data."

Julie was receiving some biofeedback treatments with Austin practitioner Lynda Kirk, which seemed to be helping. Lynda was involved in the national conference of the Association for Applied Psychophysiology and Biofeedback (AAPB) in Las Vegas that year and presented something about her work with Julie. Julie and I accompanied her to the conference. There Julie was also worked on by a rather famous Japanese healer named Kawakami, who had given an impressive demonstration in front of the psychologists that involved putting skewers through his face and throat. At that conference, Julie met many practitioners, including Eric Peper, who presented Kawakami, and Stephen Larsen, who, with his wife, Robin, was there when the healer worked on her. Afterward they had a very warm exchange. (See also chapter 14.)

A year passed, and now synchronicity was to strike again, because the AAPB conference was held in Austin. Stephen and Robin, once again attending the conference, met Julie in the lobby of the hotel where the conference was being held. Stephen, seeing how much pain Julie was in (the Scenar had given temporary relief but only for a period after application), asked her if she would like to try a LENS treatment. She said, "Please, anything." Since Stephen had his equipment with him, a LENS session was done right in the lobby of the hotel. During the "offset" treatment, lasting about ten minutes, Julie flinched visibly. When the session was concluded and she was unhooked, she said she had relived the shooting and flinched when she felt the bullets hit her.

Dr. Len Ochs himself was at the conference, scheduled to conduct a professional training at its conclusion, which Stephen had set up at Lynda Kirk's office in town. Dr. Ochs asked Julie if she would like to be the patient. Naturally, Julie, the researcher, jumped at the chance.

Julie sat comfortably in a chair while Dr. Ochs attached three small sensors, one to each earlobe and the third to her scalp. This began the LENS map process. LENS mapping involves moving one small dime-sized sensor to each of twenty-one sites located around the head. At each location the sensor is adhered with a small amount of conductive paste and left on the scalp for four seconds as the LENS measures brain wave activity. Then for 1/100 of a second, the LENS feeds back an extremely weak signal, so low that it can barely be measured, about 1/10,000th of the strength of the signal emitted from a quartz watch. However, low energy should not be confused with low efficiency; it is quite the opposite. LENS is extremely effective precisely because it uses low energy.

The body accepts low energy and polarizes against higher energies as a protection mechanism.

It was during this initial mapping process that at one site Julie physically reacted with a jerking motion of her right arm, torso, and left hip. She thought for a moment and said, "Wow, those were the exact motions . . . in the same sequence that I was shot." She described this while suddenly talking animatedly using both arms, not just one arm as she had done for the last four years. *She was back to her old self,* I thought. I laughed and told Dr. Ochs that I had noticed a curious side effect of LENS: the capability of turning people into Italians, a nationality we all love for "talking" enthusiastically with their entire bodies! Dr. Ochs shared that the brain tends to store traumatic memories as physical events that get released as the mind and body processes these informational memories, something I would learn to appreciate more as I studied somatoemotional release techniques.

The other curious phenomenon was that immediately after the LENS session, her burning RSD leg pain simply vanished for an entire week. She also possessed a new clarity; she recognized forms that appeared in her nightmares and understood what they were. They were not so troublesome any longer, and post-traumatic stress levels diminished. For example, in her nightmares, the cross was the "X" of the helicopter hospital landing pad and X-ray targeting light; the half-moon she often dreamed of was the mark her boots left in the dirt as she pushed her way toward the road after she was shot. It was a distant observation of these facts occurring within a relaxed but focused, almost meditative, state. This clarity shifted her; colors were brighter, details were sharper, and the nightmares subsided. She had obviously entered into a more parasympathetic, relaxed, and healing state. It seemed to me that LENS had somehow facilitated the body's healing response.

"Len, how do I get one of these?" I asked. This question had evidently developed into something of a pattern. When a technology worked, no matter how far out it seemed, we adopted it, used it, and tried to understand how it worked later. We were adding to the "Julie Toy Chest." Julie's life had changed. Things were greatly improving on all fronts because of these technologies.

When in doubt, follow the data.

Russian SCENARs were researched further, back to the original patents, which led to inventor Alexander Karasev's company, LET Medical in Russia. While working with Dr. Irina Kossovakia, a colleague of Dr. Karasev's, I came to appreciate that the devices made by the original inventor worked better than the clones. I owned eight different SCENARs from various manufacturers, and we had "Julie Tested" them all. The fact that devices associated with LET Medical performed the best was really not a big surprise. Dr. Karasev was several generations ahead of anyone else. The clones, while they did work, had not successfully copied everything. Plus, he was deep into newer, more regenerative models. We acquired the latest versions, and these worked faster and better for Julie. It was during this time that we also ran into a Soft (also called the low-level or cold LASER) 42mW multiple wavelength LASER and observed an increased healing rate of postsurgical wounds—another toy added.

Julie's results began to surprise more of her doctors, and they would ask me from time to time if we could do what we did with Julie for another of their patients. We were always glad to help. Julie would explain things, and my wife or I would use the devices. This small activity and constant pushing by a few friends and caring doctors moved us toward a new avocation called NeuroPaths in Austin, Texas.

My old career had ended because I chose to focus entirely on our daughter, Julie. As things got better and better, we no longer had to spend all day changing bandages, checking IV drugs, and maintaining peripherally inserted central catheter (PICC) lines. Julie was using the SCENAR and LASER on herself. She even had her own LENS system. With all her spare time, she met a really nice man, and they got married in 2009. She doesn't own a wheelchair but does have a JPS (Julie Positioning System!), used to locate great buys in shopping malls.

The healing arts represented a radically new vocation and passion that oddly enough grew out of desperation. The future now involved work that had encompassed days, nights, and years of learning, researching and doing noninvasive, nondrug therapies. The new goal became to use nondrug, noninvasive therapies in a responsible way. My wife had her

M.Ed. and LPCI (licensed professional counselor intern) in counseling, so she was in an associated area, but I was a nerd.

The question became, how does a chemist "change horses" and go into the healing arts? The suggestion was made to me that I become a massage therapist. I proceeded to get my Texas, Florida, and national massage licenses and attended more LENS, LASER, and SCENAR trainings, eventually teaching many of these same modalities to others. This included the military, which asked me on several occasions to explain how these devices work and/or to hold workshops with their complementary medical teams. This was an honor for two reasons: first, it was an Army surgeon, Dr. Lyons, who was very instrumental in saving our daughter's arm; and second, there was the chance to help our returning soldiers by alleviating their chronic pain and post-traumatic stress disorder (PTSD).

Within the massage curriculum, craniosacral therapy and somato-emotional release caught my attention because they use low force and subtle energies. A very low force of less than 5 grams, the weight of a nickel resting on your fingertip, is used over an extended time to affect large shifts in a person. As the practitioner's and client's subtle energy fields blend, the person relaxes. It made sense. Low energies from devices and/or a person's subtle energy could make tremendous changes in a person. I began to look into the chemistry and physics that would explain how these effects were possible. Soon it was evident that biophysics was leading the effort to understand these weak field interactions. One memory clearly surfaced. It was during my more linear life when I saw *Reiki* for the first time as a very strange ritual . . . until I recalled its effect on Julie, who was a much happier person after each Reiki session. Resonant frequencies and low energy began to attract my attention. What I needed was a very precise frequency generator.

During an advanced LENS training, Nick Dogris, who developed some advanced LENS protocols, mentioned that he had run into a former SETI engineer and was now making a precise frequency generator, which he called the NeuroField. "How do I get one of these?" I asked. After experimenting on myself with the NeuroField, I immediately began writing programs for the device. Julie, always the researcher, volunteered for duty as a lab rat, with the result that she reduced her medications even more sharply. The problem was how to get off the meds safely and titrate down.

The more I learned and thought about subtle energies and/or energy/ vibrational medicine, the clearer things became. Perhaps this was partly due to a scientific background. It occurred to me that the spirit/mind/ body connection is a remarkable system driven by almost imperceptible forces. Quantum fields and subatomic particles cluster together vibrationally to make atoms; atoms have electrons whizzing around their exterior space, signaling and even combining into neighboring atomic shells to form molecules; one or more molecules clump together to form structures.

Molecules and their structures move according to songs of resonance that result from moving electrical charges that in turn induce magnetic fields capable of changing the shapes of the molecules to facilitate joining with other atoms or molecules. Eventually, enough of the right molecules congregate to form specific cells that combine to form tissues according to cellular DNA songs that allow communication via electromagnetic and vibrational waves. The atoms and molecules make up instruments that join into a larger set of cells and tissues that form an orchestra of life. Tissues join and construct specific organs. Combine enough of the right organs, and systems develop. Put enough systems together, and there is a person or entity projecting its internally driven songs outward to interact with other myriad fields and songs resonating in the universe. We are part of a larger whole.

To further comprehend these phenomena at a basic level, consider that as muscles move/contract/extend, electricity is generated. This is accomplished by a piezoelectric effect whereby pressure change on a semiconductor's surface generates an electrical discharge. The electrical charge travels along connective tissue and fascia of the body because of the body's properties as a semiconductor. Even the blood supply is designed as a highly conductive saline solution that allows electrical charges to flow throughout the body. The body communicates constantly with itself, passing information instantly via biophotons, electrical current, and magnetic and vibrational energy fields. Humans are an electrochemical system that produces magnetic fields as molecules vibrate and electrons move throughout the body. A moving charge produces a magnetic field perpendicular to the electrical field, and any moving magnetic field will generate electricity.

The body has one very strong muscle that is constantly pulsing from contractions, the heart. These muscle contractions produce an electrical signal used for diagnosis of the heart's overall health. As the heart produces this electrical signature, a magnetic field is also generated. The heart's field energy, or force, can now be easily detected up to fifteen feet from the person. So "getting a vibe" from someone is literally picking up on a person's informational field energetics. Some but not all fields and vibrational waves may diminish as their source gets farther away, but in any case they never equal zero. Fields and waves of information are constantly interacting from every part of the universe. There are those who can tap into this. Consider healers who "focus with intent" to affect a positive change in another person. These "healers" have been measured and shown to tremendously increase output fields in their hands as they focus their intent. This ability to use and manipulate very low, subtle, but measurable energy opens fascinating possibilities. Many people are working on refining these possibilities.

The International LENS Conference focuses on such low-energy work. This meeting brings together caring and highly creative out-of-the box thinkers who range from acupuncturists, biophysicists, counselors, chemists, and chiropractors to massage therapists, nurses, professors, psychologists, psychiatrists, and conventional medical doctors. Such an environment is highly conducive to brainstorming and development. It is a natural consequence that most everyone gets lost in thinking how to improve, refine, and/or develop protocols and procedures.

The new LENS platform allows one to write programs easily, so I became interested in developing new protocols and helped a group of very creative people—Dr. Sara Hunt Harper, Dr. D. Corydon Hammond, Jill O'Brien O.M.D., and Dr. Nick Dogris. These protocols were all added to Ochs's original protocols, strengthening the tool set. While certain tools may work well for certain applications, even better results may be obtained if multiple techniques are combined into a mixed-modality approach to respond to a problem.

One tool set or multimodality "toy chest" that is very effective combines LASER/photonic stimulator, SCENAR/COSMODIC, LENS, NeuroField, and subtle energy techniques (craniosacral therapy, acupuncture, Reiki, etc.). It is important to consider how these modalities combine to facilitate positive changes. The Soft LASER/photonic stimulator (Light Systems) helps increase energy (speeds up the Krebs cycle*) and tends to promote tissue healing. SCENAR/COSMODIC devices tend to up-regulate changes from the skin's surface to the peripheral nervous system/central nervous system (PNS/CNS) to the cortex. The LENS tends to down-regulate information from the cortex to the CNS/PNS. NeuroField bathes the system in vibrational notes. Acupuncture, Reiki, and craniosacral therapy tend to rebalance and redirect our subtle energies. These modalities, in combination or in a standalone fashion, tend to reduce swelling, promote improved vascularization, release regulatory peptides, and produce relaxation affects.

Combining these modalities often results in a shift away from the anxious, sympathetically driven "fight-or-flight" state toward the more relaxed parasympathetic "rest-and-digest"/healing state. This is accomplished by "nudging" the dysfunctional stuck state. Once the dysfunctional state is interrupted, the body automatically rebalances to a more adaptive and healthier homeodynamic (actively self-regulating) point. The more the process is repeated, the better the body gets at returning to its truly adaptive nature, and the healthier it becomes. It is when the body stops adapting that "dis-ease" occurs. What is great about this process is that the mind/body does this automatically as it rebalances, irrespective of any diagnosis.

After Julie's mechanical systems were stabilized by groups of very talented surgeons, conventional approaches to help with alleviating chronic pain, PTSD, and RSD failed. "Interesting times" redirected my energies to understand and conquer what was diminishing my daughter's quality

---

*The Krebs cycle refers to the generation of ATP or adenosine triphosphate by the mitochondria of the cells.

of life. It was essential to keep an open mind, use the tools that serendipity and/or research supplied, and to always follow the data. This was the approach I used during my years of internship at "Julie University," a term of endearment that describes both the adventure and the steep learning curve that led me into the alternative/complementary world of energetic and vibrational medicine.

As the healing journey pulled one way and then the other, ultimately the path led to further considerations of subtle energy, spirit/mind/body connections, and interactions of the surrounding universe. Sometimes these connections and interactions combined to make a person feel better. Sometimes the intersections led to new protocols and/or new modalities. The entire adventure certainly brought about a new direction and focus to my efforts, focused efforts that merged knowledge from the scientific arena with a new appreciation of the human spirit and how we are all connected to each other and the universe.

One result is that I more easily "tune in" to others and feel subtle vibrations that yield informational messages. Perhaps, as difficult as this adventure was, it forged me into a much more empathetic and caring human being, and in the process produced a practitioner with a strange but highly effectively tool set. Perhaps it takes "interesting times" to produce "interesting results."

Restoring a Psychotherapist
RICHARD M. SMITH, PH.D.

My thirty-six years of clinical practice began with a strong interest in the biology of the brain and consciousness. A year after I graduated from high school, Neal Miller demonstrated that instrumental learning could influence the autonomic nervous system. He succeeded in rewarding rats to gorge one ear with blood and blanch the other. During my graduate studies, Joe Kamiya showed that verbal feedback when the alpha rhythm is present could increase this brain wave. This pivotal research revealed a new way to experience animal nature, and biofeedback was initiated.

As the years went on, I developed a busy psychology practice in a small town by paying attention to the needs of people throughout the intense seasons in the Champlain Valley of New York. I came to use methods like meditation, rhythmic light and sound, and other psycho-therapies beyond my initial training in behavior therapy. Establishing therapeutic relationships with patients was most important. When a new method of interest distracted from the therapeutic relationship, my clinical work would falter. Carl Rogers was my guide to get the optimal balance back. Then a synergy with the application of appropriate thera-peutic technique and the client-centered relationship would reemerge, and the world would seem right.

At what ordinarily would be the end of my career (I am in my seven-ties), a promising method "happened along." It had an intriguing quality that struck me as humility with power. I learned of its existence on the Internet when Dr. Siegfried Othmer made favorable comments regard-ing Dr. Stephen Larsen's first book about Dr. Och's LENS method. This book turned my curiosity into an imperative. I had to learn more, I had to get experience with LENS. After reading Stephen's book in March 2007, I sought some LENS treatments from him. These worked well enough that I enrolled in professional training and finally in the necessary sophis-ticated hardware and software.

I began to treat myself and my younger son in August of 2007. Soon I was applying LENS in my practice. It was easy to stay humble with LENS, because the gentle feedback came from and was directed back to the brain. The brain, not me, orchestrated the changes. The therapeutic change process is largely hidden from the awareness of the patient and therapist. The positive changes "spontaneously" appear, usually hours or days later, but rarely at treatment time. Thereafter, the symptomatic his-tory seems mostly irrelevant. There is great respect for the specialization of conscious and unconscious processes.

For several months it was hard for me to have a heartfelt or gut accep-tance that the extremely low-energy feedback could possibly be having the graceful but powerful effects that typically occur. Difficult biological tem-peraments would "spontaneously" give way to more socialized behaviors. Compared to my pre-LENS clinical experience, the improvements were more easily won, and they seemed ideally suited for each patient. At times

I remind people that it is their brain that produces the lively energy that is recorded in the feedback process and that their own brain is assimilating and using this feedback. It seemed appropriate to be the joyful servant and cheerleader who guides and shares his relevant experience when appropriate and maintains proper boundaries. Most interesting, the mechanism of change takes place outside the awareness of patient and therapist.

Clearly, it is gratifying to participate in the paradigm shift to the energy health and energy psychology that LENS enables. I am a lucky man who experiences a renewed sense of fulfillment.

Yes, retirement will have to ensue eventually, but for now there is a need to carry on and eventually train someone to continue this satisfying practice. Then there will be the flexibility and opportunity to gradually slip into a more relaxed practice, which would have its own sense of satisfaction, transition, and grace. There is also the security to know that members of the LENS practitioner community have helped me in the past, and that gives me confidence for the future.

LENS self-treatment has been wonderful in many ways. An example: Until recently I have always experienced an awkwardness in the motor mechanics of reading. The simple task of visually moving from the end of one line of text down and left to the next was always imprecise and caused rereading, inefficiency, and frustration. Many decades ago I accepted this as inevitable and never searched for any remedy other than spending extra time and effort when reading. In the past few months, this problem has been lifted from me, and without any willful effort of my own. It "spontaneously" came to me that I could retrace backward on the same line I read and then drop down one line and continue reading left to right. This was an improvement but required conscious effort. A few months later I started to automatically do the retrace as most do in one integrated sweep. At first this result was exciting, distracting, and surprising. Subjectively, it seems as if I can also "see" the space around the lines of type. Weeks later, it came to me that my handwritten notes have a far more uniform left-adjusted margin than before treatment. This too was surprising, and it is typical of how people sense improvements as "just happening." The healing process is typically hidden.

When I am with a patient, I often say, "Are you ready for Len's work?" The double meaning always makes me happy. Clearly Dr. Ochs has discovered an energy health method of great utility. I am grateful to Dr. Ochs and Dr. Larsen; my patients often pass along their own gratitude to me.

FIVE

THE ADOPTED CHILD

ATTACHMENT DISORDER AND THE COMPROMISED BRAIN

With Sebern Fisher, M.A., M.S.W., L.M.H., BCIA

> *The truth is that the least studied phase of human development remains a phase during which the child is acquiring all that makes him most distinctively human. Here is still a continent to conquer.*
>
> JOHN BOWLBY

O ur last chapter began with the story of how attachments to other human beings can forge careers in healing. Nick Dogris knows he is a more skilled and wiser therapist because of AJ. He went on to invent his own healing system, called NeuroField, that is now helping many, many others. Mike Beasley knows he has walked through hell to help Julie. The trajectory of his life as a corporate CEO before his daughter was shot did not prefigure the extraordinary healer he has become. And my colleague Richard Smith has found a new lease on his professional life as a psychologist, and the beneficiaries are his North Country patients in New York State.

In this chapter, we explore more about how human beings come to love and care for each other under equally difficult circumstances—

because adoption implies that unknown continent that Bowlby speaks about above. This intense bonding of a parent with a yet-to-be-known child from another world (already a difficult place, or the child wouldn't have been given up) can lead to great hopes and dashed expectations, and a challenge to win through in the end with love and understanding. I believe this chapter is another installment on the theme of "a path with heart" known to the families—and to therapists—who have ventured on these difficult but rewarding journeys.

As we prepare to enter the difficult territory that follows, let's reassure and fortify ourselves a little by walking first into the territory of pre-, peri-, and postnatal child care with a positive model. A little boy or girl is conceived in an act of love and carried by a mother who is basically happy, supported by a significant other—or a family or community—and who feels safe, joyful, and optimistic. The baby has a relatively comfortable ride down the birth canal and is made to feel welcome and cherished by its parents. It has lots of cuddling and skin-on-skin time with Mama, along with nursing. Cradling and rocking to soothe from distress play their timeless roles. Above all, the environment feels safe to a wide-open new nervous system—that is to say, as yet unmyelinated* and undedicated neural tissue, that is nonetheless responsive to every nuance in the environment— and particularly on the emotional level. There is stimulation for the baby; little soft-foam "mobiles" dangle over the crib, lots of fuzzy toys. Each day yields new encounters, most of them friendly and affirmative. There are safe places to explore, romps increasing in distance, and autonomy—out away from "the mothering one" or the caregiver (be he or she mother or father, nurse or nanny, or some other role). The child's developing capabilities are met with commensurate responses and encouragement, and there are gradually escalating challenges and demands posed that keep interest engaged. The dynamic environment is linked to the child's developmental stage, and he or she doesn't have to deal with (neurotic) caretakers who keep making baby talk or in other ways infantilize a growing child.

---

*Unmyelinated means that there is not yet the fatty insulating layer around the neurons, which develops through the first part of the first decade of life, gradually refining and speeding up the child's coordination. A myelinated state characterizes the mature nervous system.

Eric Erikson and Abraham Maslow, very much influenced by some of the pioneering theorists you will read about in this chapter, believed the outcome of such humane and intelligent child rearing would be the socially contributive and self-actualizing adults of tomorrow.

Our First Experience of Feedback

The reader knows this story by heart and may have participated in such interrelationships as parent, as child, or, best of all, both. The healthy parent and the wanted child do a dance in which each offers feedback to the other. The parent delights in the child's efforts at vocalizing and playing, then talking or toddling. The child delights in the ambience of being wanted, being nurtured, seen, and heard, and of interactive play. In fact, the healthy child-rearing scenario is an example of how *feedback itself drives and encourages the developmental processes of growth,* and we see miracles of cognitive development, socialization, and language for these new arrivals to the human race. The feedback need not all be positive; in fact, it must be a judicious mix of positive and negative to shape the child's genetic expression and ready the biochemical environment for further developmental enterprises.

Adoptive parents are very often ready to embrace this same warm dynamism, even though the child is not their own. In fact, it usually takes genuine resourcefulness and generosity to become an adoptive parent. Adopted children are typically from families who cannot raise the child in the above-mentioned ways, or may not be able to take care of their own societal obligations effectively, let alone care for a demanding child (and yes, all babies are demanding, some much more so than others). The child may then be abandoned, institutionalized, or placed in suboptimal foster care. Prospective parents are barraged by bureaucracy and climb through mountains of domestic or international red tape. All this time, biological clocks are ticking, developmental processes within the child are crying out for feedback, for reciprocity, and once that phase is past, its original promise and potential may be lost forever. All of the nurturing and generosity in the world seem unable to bring the "reactive, attachment-disordered child" into normalcy.

Before we move into the really miraculous ways in which neurofeed-back can help redeem this difficult and frustrating situation, we should look at the nature of what is called "attachment" and how it becomes "disordered." We begin with ethology, derived from the animal studies of Konrad Lorenz and Nicolaas Tinbergen, and move to the developmental psychoanalysis of Freud and his successors (these latter, such as Melanie Klein and Heinz Kohut, described how the original bond between mother and child is inflected into object relations and the ability to encounter the world with freedom and security), to the discovery of the attachment process itself, as seen through the eyes of thinkers and therapists you will meet below: from pioneers such as John Bowlby to contemporary thinkers such as Allan Schore.

The Reactive Attachment Disorder (RAD) Child

The predicament has been known throughout history. Think of the fairy tales you know that have as the hero or heroine an orphan, a found-ling, a neglected child. From Cinderella, carrying out the ashes from the fireplace under the cruel eye of a "wicked stepmother," to Harry Potter, orphaned and living in a closet under the stairs with a heartless "Muggle" family, the human spirit is aroused and moved by the predicament of a human child neglected or abused. The rest of the story is about how such a child is "rescued" or brought back to empowerment and full human-ity. Therapists who treat the RAD child wish it were as easy as the fairy tales make it seem. At the end of our own story in this chapter, we will find that while conventional (perhaps Muggle?) remedies such as medica-tion or talk therapy often fall flat, and while neurofeedback is far from a "magic wand," in the hands of a clinical wizard, this instrumentality can have effects that border on the miraculous.

What if a child is born to a mother whose only income is from her body, used by men she doesn't really know (prostitution)? Or one who, at sixteen years old, gets into a compromising situation, and gets date-raped, but her fundamentalist parents say she has to have the child? She is now emotionally disowned by her family for sinful behavior—so there is guilt deep in her soul as she nurses, holds, or ignores the child. Without many resources, and scorned by society, she may be too anxious to nurse, and so crams a bottle full of condensed milk into the infant's mouth, while she herself eats junk food, smokes, and watches TV for escape, while the child spends most of its time screaming in wet diapers in a cold and barren room.

It was between two world wars that pioneering psychologists did the work showing how indispensible is maternal nurture and attachment to the growing infant and toddler. Lorenz and Tinbergen had already established the principle of "sensitive periods" in the development of animal species, from birds to primates. Innate releasing mechanisms, as they were called, appeared during certain windows in development and initiated intense bonding of an infant to a mother, or to another being that was perceived as a mother (we all remember the Psych 101 photo of Konrad Lorenz walking along in his farmyard boots, followed by a loving line of goslings).

This principle ran oblique to the hegemony of behavioral psychology in the twentieth century, which implied that a thorough knowledge of conditioning principles could explain, or allow psychologists to shape, any human behavior. It was a kind of ontological conceit, as if all learning lay in the hands of the mighty experimental psychologist who manipulated the reinforcements, extinctions (the cessation of behavior when reinforcement or reward is withdrawn), and punishments around an experimental animal—or a young human. (Some people were really thinking of raising their children in the human equivalent of Skinner boxes, so pervasive was this naive and inflated behavioral paradigm.)

Psychologists were taught not to infer inner or emotional states in their subjects but only to master a new vocabulary of operant conditioning, with its schedules of reinforcements, extinctions, and discriminative stimuli. But the experiments of Harry Harlow and his associates a few decades later on mother surrogates in barren environments showed that monkeys raised in uncomforting Skinner-box environments, apart from monkey mothers, had abundant pathologies. Those reared in total isolation— even if biological necessities were taken care of—were even worse off, with behaviors such as self-mutilation, rocking, and thumb-sucking.

John Bowlby (1907–1980) himself suffered from parental separation when he was sent to an English boarding school in 1914 at age seven. These institutions are not known for their empathic nurturance, and Bowlby, contemplating his feelings—that probably ignited his later career—said, "I wouldn't send a dog away to a boarding school at seven!" (Bowlby 1969, 1982). He felt there was something intrinsically wrong with how children were treated in his culture (and many others at the time).

Originally trained as a psychologist, Bowlby went on to earn a medical degree, became a psychiatrist, and then went on to postdoctoral training as a psychoanalyst. (In the late 1920s and '30s, Freud's theories were still controversial but of growing interest to specialists in human development throughout Europe and America, with the exception of Nazi Germany, which banned Freud's work because he was Jewish.) During World War II, Bowlby became interested in the plight of *Kindertransport* children who had been rescued from Germany or Nazi-occupied countries, perhaps lost their parents in the Holocaust, and now were essentially growing up in orphanages, usually without any close relatives for nurturance and support.

While accepting the importance of Freud's theories, Bowlby felt they lacked an empirical basis and came to disagree with Anna Freud and Melanie Klein, influential developmental psychoanalysts, that the children's main problems were sexual in origin and that they were afflicted by unconscious fantasies and inner conflicts (consistent with psychoanalytic theory). He thought the pathological effects were less abstruse and more immediate—the direct outcome of lack of nurture. Bowlby identified more closely with the work of another (renegade) psychoanalyst, Rene Arpad Spitz (1887–1974), a Hungarian physician who was himself psychoanalyzed by Freud but had also come to feel the purely psychoanalytic account was insufficient.

It was from Spitz's studies of institutionalized children, beginning in the 1930s, that the terms *hospitalism, maternal deprivation,* and *failure to thrive* entered the common vocabulary. The institutionalized ("unattached") child, Spitz showed, is usually smaller and weaker than normally raised peers, even with adequate nutrition. He or she is probably less coordinated and less exploratory, may seem vacant or unresponsive, and may play repetitive autoerotic or self-stimulating games. He or she may scream inconsolably, then rock or head-bang for hours, then be silent and unavailable. Often the child may be misdiagnosed as retarded or autistic.

Probably more than anything, the films that Spitz and his associates made of these fragile, extremely maladapted children and their comparison to normal children began to change the mind and heart of the world. You may still see these films on YouTube on the Internet if you wish to explore their emotional impact.

In the late 1940s, just after the war, Bowlby was commissioned by the World Health Organization to write its official report on the psychological state of orphaned and institutionalized children. The report led to the publication of his book *Maternal Care and Mental Health,* published in 1951. Bowlby's work would in turn influence developmental psychologists Erik Erikson, Mary Ainsworth, and Mary Mains on patterns of attachment and inspire the further work of innovative American psychologists such as Harry Harlow and Jerome Kagan, who explored tactile stimulation and facial recognition respectively. *Attachment* began to become an acceptable word in psychology (but not yet the forbidden-by-behaviorists "L" word—*love*). Bowlby and the attachment theorists would help change patterns of child rearing in which parents had been told, or had persuaded themselves, not to show too much affection to their children for fear of "spoiling" them. His work would alter the patterns of visitation in hospitals, schools, and boarding schools and even make sure that, when possible, institutionalized children would have caregivers to whom they could become attached.

Spitz and Bowlby had repeatedly said that the effects of severe maternal deprivation, neglect, or abuse were irreversible—*that is to say, even the best and most nurturing adoptive families were playing against a psychologically stacked deck.* The abilities and behaviors that most of us take for granted in healthy children and adults rest on a painstakingly acquired neurological scaffolding of attachment patterns, security, and familiar routines. This was the importance of reciprocity and feedback between innate mechanisms in the child and parenting skills in the adults.

But it was not until the end of the twentieth century and the thoroughly researched and documented work of Allen Schore, sometimes called "the American Bowlby," that the modern world began to understand the *neurobiology* of attachment disorders. His three seminal volumes—*Affect*

Regulation and the Origins of the Self, Affect Dysregulation and Disorders of the Self, and *Affect Regulation and Repair of the Self*—are regarded as the defining works on the subject of attachment and its effect on the nervous system of the child. And so just what is the "irreversible" part of all of this?

Children do not just grow "like cabbages." The exquisite intricacies on which later developmental achievements rest are fashioned in exchanges with caregivers. But what is affected are not just nice or nasty little personalities. It is the brain's very circuitry, important control and processing regions such as the orbital prefrontal cortex and its relationship to deeper, older limbic organs, such as the hippocampus and the amygdala, that is at stake, and, by extension, the intricate neurochemistry of the entire brain. We are talking here of how early experiences of human feedback between caregiver and child actually fashion the neural networks that enable us to become socialized humans. Common-sense attitudes and behaviors that we take for granted in the normal child are simply unavailable to the inconsistently attached child.

Schore called this "the dyadic regulation of emotion" and said in the clearest terms: "The development of synchronized interactions is fundamental to the healthy affective development of the infant" (Schore 2000). The intellectual habit of the time was to regard the child and its caregiver as two essentially separate entities after birth, ignoring what we now know as systems theory—that is to say, the rhythmic attunement and alignment, or lack thereof, between caregiver and child—and the fact that the two organisms occupy a common attentional and emotional space crisscrossed by lines of feedback and attachment.

I will first simplify for the reader an enormous corpus of work on the neurobiological consequences of neglect so that he or she will have a context for grasping both how difficult it actually is to treat these disorders and how miraculous it then becomes that neurofeedback can do anything at all.

As the infant scans the world around him or her just to see what kind of world he or she has landed in, the senses of vision, touch, and hearing are brand new and a little blurry. But the child's attention is charged with rudimentary kinds of questions: "Is it safe, is it comfortable, *does anybody know I'm here? Am I loved?*" These are not cognitive but affective queries,

What Is "Attachment Theory"?

1. Children between six and about thirty months are very likely to form emotional attachments to familiar caregivers, especially if the adults are sensitive and responsive to child communications.

2. The emotional attachments of young children are shown behaviorally in their preferences for particular familiar people; their tendency to seek proximity to those people, especially in times of distress; and their ability to use the familiar adults as a secure base from which to explore the environment.

3. The formation of emotional attachments contributes to the foundation of later emotional and personality development, and the type of behavior toward familiar adults shown by toddlers has some continuity with the social behaviors they will show later in life.

4. Events that interfere with attachment, such as abrupt separation of the toddler from familiar people or the significant inability of caregivers to be sensitive, responsive, or consistent in their interactions, have short-term and possible long-term negative impacts on the child's emotional and cognitive life (Schaffer 2007).

and not "conscious," as my words might make them seem, but a kind of emotional scanning of the postbirth world. The important part of attachment theory is to understand that the scanning is, in fact, instinctual, emotional, and subliminal in its agency; eager in acceptance but furious in rejection; and all the time reaching, as it were, for the caregiver, as the gosling follows the mother goose in Lorenz's studies during the "sensitive period." This emotional scanning will constitute the child's first experience of synchronized reciprocity.

No matter which hemisphere of the brain eventually becomes dominant (the left for about 90 percent of people, who also become right-handed), for the first 18–24 months of life, *the right hemisphere is dominant in all infants.* Before spoken language ever forms, there is another, affective language present: that of facial expression, expressive body language, emotional prosody of voice, all coordinated in the right, emotional, hemisphere. "The orbito-frontal" right cortex, says Schore, is "the senior executive of the emotional brain" (Schore 2000, 29). The amygdala, the fight-or-flight organ, develops intra-utero at five months.

The critical period for myelination, in which the neurons of the brain become insulated for rapid, foolproof conduction—and, as it were, dedicated, through being used repeatedly—is seven to fifteen months. As a result, said neuroscientists Kinney, Brody, Kloman, and Gilles in 1988 (Schore 2000, 29), the maturing limbic areas (often referred to as "the old mammalian brain") are "wired" to the orbital prefrontal cortex in ways that will endure. "Due to its location at the ventral and medial hemispheric surfaces, it acts as a convergence zone where cortex and subcortex meet. It is thus situated at the apogee of the 'rostral limbic system,' a hierarchical sequence of interconnected limbic areas in orbitofrontal cortex, insular cortex, anterior cingulate, and the amygdala" (Schore 1997, 30).

The limbic system also includes the hippocampus and regulates emotionally stored memories, which will in turn be brought up, unconsciously and almost instantaneously, to evaluate the significance of any new experience on the basis of past (emotional) experience. This system represents a circuit equal in importance to the often-cited hypothalamic-pituitary-adrenal axis (HPAA) of stress-related fame, and is, in fact, intimately connected to it, participating in every aspect of the "stress response." These fiber bundles, being myelinated in the first year or two of life, also have interconnections to the reticular activating system (or RAS), which is in charge of arousal states. It also reaches down into the autonomic nervous system (ANS). "Thus," Schore says, quoting Dolan, "in later life, the orbitofrontal cortex is necessary for acquiring very specific forms of knowledge for regulating interpersonal behavior" (Dolan 1999).

We know that there are also neurohormones working intimately with these systems to promote bonding (oxytocin) and to give pleasure and relief from pain (beta-endorphins). The activating and well-being neurotransmitters dopamine and serotonin play their part, along with the inhibitory neurotransmitter GABA (gamma amino-butyric acid). Acetylcholine is used in movement and exploration, and the adrenal-related norepinephrine and cortisol are involved in "fight or flight" or freezing in fear. These systems are all intimately geared to the orbitofrontal-limbic connection, and yet they have far-reaching influence through the rest of the brain.

We now know that the right hemisphere processes information so quickly that it verifies the old James-Lange theory of the emotions. When a sudden experience happens (you meet the classic bear in the woods), your emotional state is not just a cognitive one ("I think I see a large, dangerous animal and should vacate the scene"). Along with the cognitive perception, you are aware of the somatic events of gasping, pulse pounding, stomach churning, and possibly piloerection (hair standing up on end), and starting to turn and run, all mediated without a thought. (The fact that these reactions are so immediate they are truly *unconscious* is what has attracted so many psychoanalysts to attachment theory and its neurobiology.)

Ideally, in a healthy brain and nervous system, the right hemisphere is specialized in inhibitory control, so that your reaction to that suddenly appearing bear might not devolve into instantaneous shrieking and running away (a bad idea with any predator), but rather you begin speaking in a measured, solemn voice to the creature while holding your hands up (to look large) and slowly backing away (instead of running away like a prey animal).

This same neurobiological system, the orbitofrontal-limbic axis, is the key to the infant's rage (the amygdala is an organ that resembles the old daisy-pulling ritual: "She loves me, she loves me not . . ."). The amygdala has a simplistic dichotomous system, says the distinguished neurobiologist Karl Pribram, "that makes us very primitive creatures"— "I love you," or "Get away from me." Out of this zone comes the anxiety-ridden black-and-white thinking of the fundamentalist (about which I have written in *The Fundamentalist Mind*). Politically, this kind of thinking gives rise to "You're either with us or against us!" (Where have we heard that?) Most humans and most animals seem to be prone to such bipolar shifting back and forth, especially when the amygdala is aroused. The sadistic rage of the RAD child, and the tendency to torture animals or hurt younger children, is unfortunately also found in this domain. Along with that dichotomous complex comes seeing oneself, seemingly compulsively, do lots of bad things. Self-concept and its ongoing role in the affective life of a child—or adult—is thus established through this same circuitry, and forms a kind of background against which subsequent events may unfold.

There comes a time when people of such unfortunate backgrounds of trauma and abuse meet my eyes in the therapeutic context—this is often after we have worked together for a while. I then say to them, "Now we have seen where some of your problems come from, and that, with therapy, you can gain much more control over (your rage, depression, seizures, whatever)." People are often astonished to hear confirmation for how out-of-control they have felt. Cultural influences that stress guilt and shame may have exacerbated their feelings of unworthiness. Religious perspectives that stress the omnipotence and omniscience of God, along with concepts like "original sin," seal the wound. People may feel like miserable sinners who can't even control their own lives, or that God has failed them or rejected them.

But on a truly humanistic level, we should not be held accountable for our genetic predispositions, our poor nurturing, or our tormented childhood (nor should God). These things must be taken into account in the overall equation. Once you've been able to recognize the hand you've been dealt by fate, the next therapeutic stage requires what Buddhists call *upaya,* or "skillful means," to play it well.

Adoptive families sometimes feel they are struggling against impossible odds. Try as they might, their nurturing and supporting role is anachronistic. The sensitive period during which this child really needed nurturance has disappeared in the mists of antiquity (when the parents who conceived the child abrogated their—admittedly daunting—role). It is sometimes easy for the adoptive parent (not to mention the self-aware but still damaged child) to feel bitter. One of the criteria we use on our CNS questionnaire and subjective symptom checklist is, "Failure to learn from experience." I always wear a funny smile when I ask my clients to quantify how well they, or their children, are "learning from experience." I know when their numbers improve in this category alone that the overall prognosis is more hopeful.

As Freud correctly discerned over a century ago, when your conscious best intentions and resolves are thwarted, time and again your unconscious mind is working as a counterplayer. His method was psychoanalysis—but from my perspective, analysis is costly, long-winded, and more effective in the long term rather than the short term. Neurofeedback is much faster and doesn't go into the laborious details of how ambivalent you feel about your parents. And more than psychoanalysis, I feel it puts the power and the authority into the hands of the patient. Ultimately, both processes do what Freud called "speeding up the processes of maturation." Individually they're both effective. (The subject of how neurofeedback and psychotherapy can be integrated effectively must be the subject of an entire new book.)

I happily refer the interested reader to Schore's encyclopedic corpus of work. In fact, I feel the study of attachment could benefit all child psychiatrists, pediatric social workers, and mental health therapists. It goes without saying that a study of the neurobiology of attachment is indispensible for neurofeedback therapists who work with children.

Let's look then at some promising indicators of what neurofeedback can accomplish for RAD children and their adoptive families.

Neurofeedback for RAD—
Sebern Fisher, M.A., M.S.W., L.M.H., BCIA

The possibility that neurofeedback could help reactive attachment disorder was first opened for me by Sebern Fisher, a skilled neurofeedback practitioner from Northhampton, Massachusetts. I first heard her speak at one of Rob Kall's Winter Brain conferences in Palm Springs, California, in the late nineties. Sebern struck me immediately as someone who "walked her talk," as she began with an astute summary of the work of Bowlby and Schore before moving on to present her own clinical attachment disorder cases.

Sebern outlined what happens when affect regulation is impaired in the RAD child—or adult, for that matter: tantrums, lying, impulsivity, violence, cruelty; the list goes on. Children with impaired attachments become adult sociopaths, and if they are capable of childbearing, will probably treat their own children as they themselves were treated. (An image that is indelibly engraved on my mind since the '60s is one of Harlow's female monkeys that was raised with a surrogate mother—whether made of wire or cloth, I do not remember. Just like a human RAD woman, her urge to procreate was unimpaired; it was her ability to mother that left quite a bit to be desired. She didn't know what to do with her furry, hyperactive little infant, so she walked around listlessly, dragging the rumpled child by one foot. She lacked the instinct to nurse, cuddle, or groom it, but she knew she was supposed to keep the unfortunate little thing with her.)

Sebern's protocol was constructed to correspond with Schore's neurobiology of RADs. The focus was on the underdeveloped orbitofrontal cortex, and to institute brain wave training at both the orbital prefrontal cortex (a site called FP02, up inside the socket of the right eye) and T4—the temporal site above the right ear, and the closest commonly used site to the amygdala. Both sites could be treated independently, or the active and reference electrodes might be placed on both, for "dual site training." The goal is to use EEG biofeedback to establish a connection between uncontrollable emotionality (the amygdala) and the regulatory but underdeveloped and perhaps even physiologically atrophied right prefrontal cortex. Fisher said she was well aware of pharmaceutical and psychotherapeutic remedies but knew nothing more effective than neurofeedback to mend the connection. Eventually, one can see the difference in the trained sites on a qEEG.

Psychotherapy never hurts in such a situation, but it is probably the neurofeedback that drives the boat. Perhaps the healing agent is neural plasticity (chapter 2), in which old abandoned pathways are stimulated and resuscitated. Our science is not yet detailed enough to give us the answer. But the clinical stories below hint at the promise of good outcomes for many who previously would not have had a chance.

Gandalf the Dog

In 2002, my wife, Robin, and I had already begun our work with the LENS (neurofeedback technique) with animals. At around the same time as Hurricane Katrina, we lost our old Australian shepherd, Moondog, one of our first patients. Experiencing "empty basket syndrome," we hoped to adopt a homeless dog from Louisiana or Alabama. Instead we learned of a dog named Gandalf who had been adopted by a family that didn't really know thing one about sheepdogs (such as their active intelligence and intimate involvement with people).

So we learned that Gandalf had been locked in a crate for the first year of his life. He was given enough food and water to survive, but no interactive play, no romps or outings. A neighbor heard the forlorn barking and noticed his absence in the yard. When he was liberated and taken into care by Aussie Rescue, he was lying in his own excrement, with withered legs and a displaced hip—and a look of terrible fear in his doggy eyes.

When we first got him, we realized we had a tall order on our hands. This was the animal equivalent of an attachment-disordered child. He exhibited fear barking and biting, incontinence, and counter-surfing (stealing food from tables and counters). He had a fear of bearded men with hats—which I did not know when I first picked him up wearing both beard and hat.

It wasn't easy to get the electrodes onto Gandalf, as he repeatedly bit and snapped at the wires, or tried to leave the room in a hurry, unimpressed by all cajolery. When the map was printed, I was astounded by

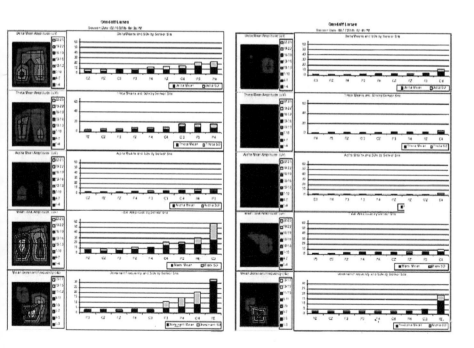

Fig. 5.1. Two LENS maps of Gandalf; the first when we got him, the second after fourteen treatments. Note the disappearance of the "hot spots" in the second map.

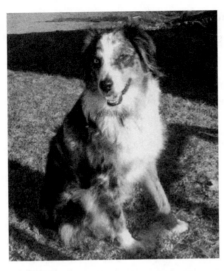

Fig. 5.2. Gandalf, our beloved shepherd

how it resembled the maps of children we had treated from orpanages around the world. As we will discuss in chapter 14, the left hot spot has to do with the image of oneself in the world and the right, the world itself: "Who am I?" and "What kind of a world is this?" (Or, "Why am I locked in this barren orphanage, or this crate? Could I be that unlovable?")

This case shows the undeniable continuity between animal and human—not just that their brain waves are similar, but that they react similarly to similar treatment—or maltreatment!

With six months of TLC and about fourteen LENS treatments, Gandalf was a changed animal. Robin took him to a series of dog-training classes, where his social behaviors—especially with other dogs—changed dramatically. Now, a couple of years later, people consistently comment on what a well-behaved little animal he seems to be, and he has completed most of his training to become a "therapy" dog. He loves to visit hospitals, care centers, and retirement homes.

The Wolf Boy Syndrome

> *His mind is with the wolves. He will howl at the moon for the rest of his life.*
> PROFESSOR DR. KARIZBAYEV ON "DJUMA"

The case we begin with reminds me of the famous feral-child case study by Dr. Jean-Marc Gaspard-Itard: *The Wolf Boy of Aveyron*. Captured in a wild and hilly region in the south of France, the scars on the ten-year-old's naked body showed the boy had had numerous scraps with wild animals. He was immune to the cold, which he proved by rolling naked in the winter snow. He had neither language nor socialization; he uttered guttural sounds, ate like an animal, and tried to climb the draperies like a squirrel or a monkey. He bit people when frustrated. Agile and determined to escape, he got away from his captors, only to return voluntarily a couple of years later.

Soon after his capture, he was examined by doctors and educators but was deemed to be ineducable. Only Dr. Itard had the will to take on the boy he called Victor. After a while Victor seemed to gain some comprehension of spoken language, but he was never able to speak. He died at the age of forty, and the careful study by Itard has been included in many psychology and sociology textbooks—as an example that clearly shows how indispensable socialization is in making a human being.

Djuma, the "wolf boy of Southern Russia," a much more recent discovery, was found in 1991 and had really been raised by wolves. He crawled on all fours, ate raw meat, and also bit people when frustrated. He could say only a few words: "Mother dead, Father dead." (His mother had probably died protecting him—from human murderers—before the orphan was adopted by the wolves.) Djuma, found at age seven, died at thirty-seven, socialized only to the extent of using the toilet and brushing his teeth—and speaking those very few sad and tragic words.

Professor Rufat Kazirbayev, who examined the boy, said, "Doctors had battled to re-educate him to act like a normal human being—but failed. They are now giving up the fight. His mind is with the wolves. He will howl at the moon for the rest of his life."*

Overall, the above cases were seized upon by the empiricists in psychology and social anthropology to show just how decisive nurture is over mere nature. What they left out until recently is that the real problem was that it was nature, maturing on its own timetable, that had gone awry

---

*For more on this, please visit this website: http://dreamhawk.com/inner-life/animal-children.

when the outer environment failed to nurture, and "draw forth" the child (which is what *e-ducare* means) during maturationally sensitive periods.

These stories are mentioned here to underline just how remarkable was the neurofeedback intervention below. The "Wolf-boy of Aveyron" was probably nine to ten years old when first captured, and Djuma seven to eight years. Fortunately "Ben" was four to five years old when serious socialization began. Ultimately, the combination of our patient's youth, the TLC of a couple of young, resourceful parents who adopted him, and neurofeedback, would win the day.

Ben had been born to a mother who was something of a local phenomenon. The mother and father were both very young adults, and *had both themselves been abandoned, and finally adopted, as children.* Both probably suffered from RAD. (We see how inadequate parenting perpetuates itself. "Right to Lifers" take note; there's more to making a socially contributive human being than preventing abortion!) There was a good chance of fetal alcohol syndrome, drug use, and extreme erratic behavior, both before and after her baby was born. Ben's mom was a welfare mother, living alone, and her baby was often screaming loud enough to wake the neighbors; Mom was elsewhere, like a bar or a Burger King, or some other unknown destination. When she was home, she was in a stupor. The baby was hospitalized for "failure to thrive." (An example where "hospitalism" was better than personal but inadequate care of a "natural" mom. The institutionalization may have actually helped the baby in this case.) But then Ben was once again returned to his mother.

Even after this, Child Protective Services did nothing, until an event that definitely got local attention. The three-going-on-four-year-old had survived neglect long enough to fall out of a third-story window all the way down to the street—around thirty-five feet—and lived!

Now the little family definitely got on on social services' (Child Protective Services) radar. Mom was soon deemed "unfit," and Ben was taken away. But what to do with such a child? A health-care professional who evaluated him at the time said, "He was definitely a 'feral child.' He didn't understand anything that was said to him, and had no language himself. When introduced to the bottle, he didn't know how to suck on it. He was not toilet trained and could not talk except to say 'no,' and to swear."

Ordinary foster care was inadequate to say the least! In fact, at one of the places Ben landed (temporary indeed), he somehow got ahold of matches and tried to set the house on fire. The foster father, in a rage, burned Ben, rather badly, to let the boy know, it seemed, the seriousness of what he had done. Now Ben was in the newspaper, and the whole community was aroused by the case. But what could be done?

Finally a young couple, recently married and with no children of their own, stepped up to the plate and volunteered to take the baby into foster care. By a strange twist of fate, the couple happened to be renting a cabin from Sebern and John Fisher.

"We could hear the baby screaming from the other end of the property," Sebern said. "The blood-curdling screaming began as soon as it was dark. It continued right up till midnight, whereupon Ben passed out. But he was awake in an hour or two, screaming some more, crawling around crying and saying 'No! No! No!' ceaselessly. He might suddenly dart from the house in the middle of the night and have to be retrieved. No one could affect him. In one of the foster settings he had tried to kill a sibling, a younger boy. He would bite, kick, scream. He would crawl around under the table, and eat his food like an animal."

It was very hard to get the neurofeedback sensors on him the first time. He had to be held tight by his foster father, who was, fortunately, physically very strong. The initial neurofeedback session, Sebern remembered, was barely ten minutes. But strangely, after that Ben slept for twelve hours, uninterruptedly. There could be no doubt something had happened.

Sebern offered low-cost or no-cost sessions for this oh-so-at-risk family. After a while, the bulk of the treatment was turned over to a practitioner named Catherine Rule, whom Sebern supervised. Progress took place against incredible deficits. It was slow, with setbacks, and yet oh-so-encouraging when it actually happened. Eventually the father got trained in neurofeedback by the Othmers and EEG Spectrum, and the family bought their own home-training unit. While the neurofeedback went on, there seemed to be progress. When the treatments decreased, improvement slowed; it was as simple as that. Eventually the time would come that this courageous couple would adopt Ben, even knowing his big-time problems, as their own child.

If I had known the full extent of Ben's history, I would have been doubly astonished by the handsome, well-spoken fifteen-year-old I met in the summer of 2009. The family had read *The Healing Power of Neurofeedback* and wanted to try the LENS form of neurotherapy. Ben still suffered from some developmental delays, executive function problems, anxiety, and distractibility. In taking the case history, I elicited the story of the thirty-five-foot fall and confirmed the part that TBI played in Ben's problems. As his parents and I talked, I realized I was in the presence of extraordinary people. Ben looked at the sandplay environment and all the little figures in my office. His eyes lit up: "I think I died and went to heaven," he said, and we all laughed. (I keep the toys and sandbox available not only for sandplay therapy but so kids don't have to sit in a chair feeling like a specimen while I talk about them with the parents.) Ben played in the sand with the glee of an eight-year-old; and this became quite important in his therapy.

I was given permission by the parents to talk with his previous therapists, and a few weeks later ran into Sebern at a conference. I asked her about her former patient, and since I was on the track of head injury along with RAD, I asked about the early thirty-five-foot fall.

"What a terrible sign of neglect," I said, "to let a toddler fall like that."

Sebern looked me in the eye. "Fall?" she said archly. "I think he was thrown!"

I was absolutely speechless. I realized that Ben's parents had not wanted to bring up this ultimate rejection by his birth mother in front of Ben. He had enough on his plate already. But the story did give new meaning to the word "rejection." (I believe the mother was subsequently incarcerated.)

Not knowing what to say, I asked Sebern in astonishment: "How long did it take to get him from 'feral child' to a viable young man with a few residual problems?"

"Well, it might have been a few hundred sessions, spread over a number of years," she said. "We saw important signs within six months."

I wasn't sure whether I marveled more at Sebern's kindness, or her uncanny skill as a therapist. The full sweep of what she, her colleague Catherine, and the family had accomplished was breathtaking; and the witness was the remarkable young man I had met. "I think it was the 'village it takes to raise a child' that did it," she said. (After learning the full story, I developed even more respect for these parents, taking on the burden of someone else's RAD child. Now they were bringing him on a 300-mile round trip to see me—to smooth out some of the rough places.)

I think we were able to help Ben a little with his cognitive problems and improve his energy in eight LENS sessions spread over about three months. Ben also took readily to the HRV training (HeartMath) that we did, and he said he was using it all the time.

For my own case, I matured a little more as a therapist, and marveled at the potential of the method we all practice, in its various inflections. Here was living proof of what Sebern had taught me in that first inspiring seminar!

Smaller Is Better

Joaquim was fifteen years old, short, but physically fit, and intense—he had a wicked little smile that emerged if he thought you were "putting him on" or trying to control him. His mother, who worked in the local public school system, said her professional specialty for years had been the "attachment-disordered child," and she had no lack of candidates in the local school district. About twelve years previously she had decided to "walk her talk" and adopt a child from Colombia.

She had helped other adoptive parents get children from the same drug war–torn streets of Bogota, and (sort of) knew what she was in for. But it didn't bode well that when she went to pick up Joaquim from the orphanage in Bogota, he was tied up like an animal. The workers said they had had to tie him to his bed because he was hard to control and sometimes violent to the other children.

Knowing a lot about the disorder did not necessarily make it easier to live with Joaquim from day to day. He learned his new language slowly. He was irritable, oppositional, defiant, and, as he grew older, insolent toward his parents and school authorities. He didn't seem to know the difference between lying and truth. He exhibited mood swings, irritability, and a kind of constant anxiety. Restless thoughts, he said, made it hard to sleep, and he would awaken exhausted and miss the schoolbus.

Schoolwork seemed very difficult to him, and he hovered right on the border of passing and failing all the time.

Within the first five treatments, the LENS neurofeedback and HeartMath, the family was noticing changes. "Thank you," his mom said heartfully. "He's not in a paroxysmal anger all the time. He actually thanked me for something the other day. Other people always told me he was polite, but this is the first time I saw it at home."

Joaquim began sleeping better, and it was a little easier to get him to the schoolbus on time. His energy improved, and he no longer lay around the house all weekend. But still he seemed depressed and surly. After a girlfriend jilted him, his depression became black. One session, I had an insight about his depression, based on experiences of my own. I looked at him and asked him how tall he was. Five-foot-two, he acknowledged, with his head down.

I said, having spent time in South America, "It's probably your Indian blood. That's something to be proud of! Those guys were little, but boy, were they strong and tireless. They climbed all over the Andes, and they built Macchu Picchu. They were probably twice as fit as the white men who enslaved them with germs, guns, and steel."

I acknowledged for Joaquim that at five-foot-six, I had always felt small for my age while growing up and had compensated for it by becoming an athlete: wrestling, gymnastics, and the martial arts—all of them good to build self-confidence in little guys.

In junior high school, I told him, I had begun to study jujitsu. Once while crossing the schoolyard, I had been accosted by the school bully, who was about six feet tall and outweighed me by at least sixty pounds. He brashly demanded I give him something of value that I was carrying. I was a rather shy and introverted kid, but I just got so outraged by his demand that I flatly refused and tried to go on my way, whereupon the bully grabbed me. I was as astonished as he was when what I had been practicing at home took over, and I suddenly had him on his back in a crushing wrist-lock. I hissed into his gaping face: "Don't you ever do that to me again!" (And he never did.)

Joaquim liked the story and the idea of the little guy reversing the odds. We continued our neurofeedback work, and he began really to relate to the HeartMath training. As the weeks went on, he was getting almost perfect scores on the games. He told me he was using the breathing and the HRV training almost every day. He did it while waiting for the bus, for classes to start, and then commencing his summer job—lifeguarding—all day long. He said the state he got into by regulating his breathing made him feel calm, clear, and focused.

Also gradually, on Joaquim's EEG the ragged edges and the ugly spindling smoothed out and came down. He passed all his courses. Joaquim's father, initially quite hostile to the treatment, acknowledged something was happening.

A therapeutic breakthrough came with a wrestling match. The coach pitted him against an opponent a couple of weight classes higher, and he was placed in a vulnerable position at the opening of a wrestling tournament. There he was, against a highly favored opponent, and with the whole school watching. At the beginning of the match, his opponent slapped Joaquim dismissively on the head.

Joaquim said, "I just continued doing the breathing, like you taught me. Inside, I went kind of cold and watchful. He was way overconfident. When he made his first move, I just kind of instinctively took him down, totally relaxed—but very, very fast. I pinned him in less than a minute."

From that time on, we had a kind of alliance. Therapy became a place for an empowering magic that would allow Joaquim to find his true potential. He no longer agonized about being the smallest kid in the class. He continued to improve. His parents said that he was like the child they had always wanted to have—but until now, never did.

Joaquim's mother was so impressed that she sent us the case described below.

The Kid from Krasnoyarsk

Krasnoyarsk, Siberia, is a very, very, cold place—except in the dog days of summer, when it is over 90 degrees Fahrenheit for a month and a half. Krasnoyarsk has permafrost that the summer heat doesn't touch, but various kinds of mining ventures have left large scars in the frozen earth. The main industry in Krasnoyarsk is fishing from the Lena river, which winds its way north to the Arctic Circle through the tundra. On the muskegs (bogs) that surround the city are the carcasses of great iron machines of industry and of war.

The old culture of the region is shamanic, and there is still a respectable museum of anthropology there, where the artifacts of the Yakut, the Chukchi, the Goldi, and the Tungus (indigenous tribes) are displayed: elaborate costumes with the bones of animals, hundreds of jingling bronze bells, and paintings of the spirit creatures of the shamanic pantheon. Now that the extreme restrictiveness of the communist regime has ended, the old ways are enjoying a comeback.

Not much is known of Kristina's mother, Natalya, except that in this unforgiving environment, she was barely making it. Vodka was the only solace readily available, and she did have a drinking problem; she also probably drank while she was pregnant with Kristina. And so it was that Kristina was born in a Krasnoyarsk orphanage—not a desirable international destination by most standards. At least the children were fed, clothed, and warm. They lay in adjoining cribs with a sheet, no blanket, twelve to a room. There were no toys in that room—there was an adjoining one that had them—a sort of playroom. Each child wore a kind of mu-mu, no diapers, and was whisked onto a metal basin when they had to "go potty." Beyond that, there were few amenities. Life consisted of daily routines, meals, and bedtime.

Rumor had it that when children "graduated" from the orphanage, around high school age, they were basically kicked out on the streets to survive one way or another. But it's one thing to be on the streets of Mumbai, or Guatemala City, and another to be on the streets of Krasnoyarsk.

To adopt their child, the American family had to complete reams of paperwork, then fly into Krasnoyarsk and pick her up from the orphanage. Kristina was adopted when she was just over a year old. She was "curious" and eager to play with objects, but she showed no emotion whatsoever.

Kristina, when we met her at the age of thirteen, had overcome any residual "failure to thrive" and seemed healthy and very athletic, emerging as the star of the school soccer team. But she was failing every subject, her bedroom was a mess, and her locker was worse. She was described by her family as irritable, oppositional, and extremely moody.

Around Kristina, inevitably it seemed that some kind of Russian soap opera was unfolding, and she refused reasonable, age-appropriate demands that were put on her. She lied frequently, and when confronted, she denied everything flatly; she caused mayhem and refused to acknowledge any part in creating it, her desperate mother said. She would often be cruel to her younger, much smaller brother, also adopted from Siberia, but "not as much trouble." Remorse seemed alien to her; she never apologized for anything.

Her parents brought her to us, not because they knew anything about neurofeedback, but because they were desperate and didn't know what else to do. When they met Joaquim's mom, she gave us a good recommendation.

Treatment started a little slowly with Kristina, and for a couple of months, it seemed, not much was happening. She was still flunking, she was still a royal pain . . . Then one day, on a kind of inspiration, I switched to one of Nick Dogris's "ramping protocols": the 1–8 Hz "Rocking the Brain," as it is called. These protocols only read the dominant frequency in the LENS from the targeted area, in this case delta (1–4) and theta (4–8) combined. They are only for the "hardy," that is, people with a strong underlying constitution and lots of energy. Kristina proved to be that way. Joel Lubar's protocol says that attention deficit (and Kristina certainly had ADHD) is determined by the theta/beta ratio. I chose this protocol because I wanted to use the LENS to "break up" theta, so that higher frequencies could emerge.

The next week her mom looked at me with absolute astonishment. "She's cooperative," she blurted, "even polite. What did you do?" Kristina was grinning like a Lappish elf. She didn't know what had happened either, only that she felt less like making trouble.

The progress continued over the next month. Lying was down from a 10 to a 2. Oppositionality also dropped, from a 9 to a 4. At one point Kristina astonished the family by showing remorse for something hurtful that she had done to her younger brother. But when one day the school suspended her from the soccer team for "academic probabation," the old Kristina came back: depressed, angry, defiant of the authorities and the school system that had kept her from her favorite activity.

A little psychotherapy was used here, because I know that Kristina and I have a bond. Sometimes I tease her like one of her peers, but mostly I respect and encourage her. I told her she was just going through the first of many frustrations in life. There would be more. But success, using a soccer metaphor, came from learning to be a "team player," and she had a strong team in her family and her counselors. You don't always get the best passes, but when you have the ball, it's your responsibility to play it. I reminded her that she had been through traumas that most ordinary American children never face in their lifetimes. Being suspended from soccer for a few weeks was nothing compared to what she had already gone through to get here. She looked at me wide-eyed, but she seemed to be taking it in.

By the following week, she seemed to have put the disappointment behind her—and in a little while was back on the team again, playing as well as ever.

At this point she plateaued in treatment for a while again, and again I tried a new protocol, the Dogris "Rocking the Brain" 9–12 Hz. The following week I again had the astonished mom: "What did you do? She is wonderful, more attentive and loving than I've ever seen her!" The treatment seemed to ameliorate a different level of her ADHD.

The great thing about Kristina is her underlying hardiness and resilience. When I see these qualities beneath—constitutionally, as it were— I know we are on a roll toward improvement.

A few weeks ago I had a conference with the school administration, principal, and guidance counselors. When I had finished giving them a brief introduction to Bowlby and Schore, they were all ears. One of the teachers said, "Everyone was saying 'lazy kid,' but I knew there was so much more to it. Thank you for the education—it could make *me* a better educator." The meeting concluded with the school board agreeing to paying for a qEEG—better to understand Kristina's problems. When the qEEG was done, it told us a great deal about Kristina's brain and its problems and paved the way to Z-score and ILF trainings (see chapter 13) that are continuing to make a difference for her.

Every time I meet the parents of an RAD kid, I tell them that they are my unsung heroes, every one of them, for attempting to do something that is against all the odds. Help a kid who otherwise had no chance at all—to at least glimpse the possibility of a normal life. In this sometimes cold and uncaring world, and knowing that the odds are against them, these parents still want to do something good. Of course their successes are hard-won and fragile, but they—and I—believe it is worth the effort!

We still don't know the exact mechanism of neurofeedback's efficacy with these children, but it may have to do with the neural-plasticity principle and the delicate art of coaxing a nervous system to find pathways it had forgotten it even had. What we do know is that it is a wonderful thing to succeed, even partially, in giving kids with a bad start a better opportunity to finish with grace and style.

SIX

AUTISM AND ASPERGER'S SYNDROME

With Mary Lee Esty, Ph.D., L.C.S.W., and Donald Magder, M.A.

Autistic Spectrum Disorder

The first important comprehensive theories were summarized by Austrian child psychiatrist Leo Kanner (1894–1981) during the 1940s. Kanner was the first physician identified as a *child psychiatrist* in America, and he published his influential textbook *Child Psychiatry* in 1935. It is generally acknowledged that with the contribution of Hans Asperger, another Austrian psychiatrist, who lent his name to the high-functioning children within the spectrum of the disorder ("Asperger's children"), these two pioneers defined the *autistic spectrum* and (more or less) clearly differentiated it from *childhood schizophrenia, dissociative identity disorder* (DID), and *affective disorders.*

Because the climate of the time was still very much psychodynamically influenced, particularly by Freud's psychoanalysis, there was a determined attempt to trace the disorder to disturbances or conflicts in the family environment or lack of affective contact in parenting—or, if the parents seemed unlike the stereotype that was being imposed upon them, even a "cold womb." The details of attachment disorder discussed in the previous chapter were still being worked out by mental health theorists, and while clearly affect regulation is a problem for autistics, very often their parents seemed committed to the well-being of their children, determined to provide a healthy environment and help them find a successful life adaptation.

Unfortunately, because of this prejudice and diagnostic stereotyping or "indissociation" between the diagnostic categories, many parents of autistics were cross-examined and made to feel culpable and guilty by well-meaning but insufficiently educated mental health professionals. In effect, we could say that these parents were victims of psychiatric or psychological fundamentalism, in an era that had few scientific or controlled studies on the subject and relied mostly on clinical or ideographic data: *Autistic (or attachment-disordered) children come from emotionally deprived conditions. Your child is autistic, therefore you must be a bad, inattentive, or unresponsive parent.* We can only lament and send belated sympathy back to such parents, who were often simply the victims of a social and behavioral science still in its own infancy.

It has been tempting, therefore, to look for causes in other domains, such as genetic defects, and the usual ways of identifying the same disorder in parents, grandparents, siblings, or other relatives has been inconclusive. So the search has gone elsewhere. Diet has been seen as a possible culprit, including factors that did not exist before what has seemed to some to be a modern "plague" of autism had been identified: excessive sugar and carbohydrate (empty calorie) consumption, food dyes and additives, avitaminosis from lack of essential or organic nutrients in food. A modern dietary approach proposed by Feingold has alerted the modern world to the dietary dimension of children's problems (since they likely don't eat any better than their parents, who may be addicted to SAD, or the standard American diet). Strong evidence has been brought forward that excessive amounts of trans-fats and the lack of omega 3-6-9 in the proper proportions is at least one of the offenders in the plague of autism and attentional problems, since the health of the phospholipid cell-membranes is clearly crucial to CNS functioning.

An additional environmental factor that has been proposed is the neurotoxins in pesticides, such as Dioxin, or "defoliants" such as Agent Orange, used liberally in Vietnam of which even small amounts in the body are highly disorganizing in certain animal and insect models. (See www.ejnet.org/dioxin and www.vba.va/gov/bln/21/benefits/herbicide.)

Others have brought up the onset of electromagnetic pollution in the form of electrical fields of various kinds on immature nervous systems or on those rendered highly sensitive by other factors. Generations of children (the reader very likely among them) received a kind of "double whammy" from watching TV: distracting, repetitive, and mindless stimulation masquerading as entertainment, along with bombardment by radiation from the electronic image-painting "guns" in the old-style TV sets. This has certainly alerted some parents to the potential dangers of children spending time glued to the "boob tube," a passive form of entertainment, in lieu of more interactive approaches afforded by normal play and peer interaction, or storytelling, reading, or games with adults (www .health4youonline.com/article_electro_magnetic_pollution.htm).

Whole groups of parents have become certain that their autistic children's problems began with vaccinations. While there is much debate about this among the professional medical community—and large-scale studies that seem to disprove the theory—many distraught parents point to a critical vaccination as the onset of their child's problems. The more dramatic cases tell stories in which the child is born healthy, has good Apgar scores (tests at birth of sensory and motor coordination), seems fine on the developmental path, and has a vaccination—and then suddenly the child's development is either arrested or, less frequently, begins a serious regression, losing gains already accomplished and sliding down the developmental ladder again into preverbal, asocial, emotionally dysregulated states.

A commonly cited culprit is the organic mercury-based preservative thimerosal that was used to keep vaccines fresh and ensure that pathogens (the microorganisms inevitably present in vaccines) were dead. The neurotoxic potential of mercury was ignored until evidence began to mount. Even then, according to good sources, pharmaceutical companies, driven by a motive in which profit was preferable to untold consequences for people's children, continued to market the vaccines.

After the American FDA worked to remove or reduce the amount of thimerosal in vaccines, the companies continued to sell vaccines to third-world countries, whose people very naturally wanted to vaccinate their children against really dangerous infectious diseases. Worthy epidemiological goals, such as helping eliminate diphtheria, mumps, or rubella (German measles), obscured the possibility that the vaccines might cause neurological deficits a way down the developmental path. Many physicians still feel the risk is not significant enough to be considered a problem, when the main motive was getting the vaccines out there to prevent epidemics (www.fda.gov/BiologicsBloodVaccines).

Treating Autistics at Stone Mountain

The people who bring their children to us have typically exhausted all other resources. They have consulted pediatricians, pediatric neurologists, psychiatrists, or psychologists. They have tried medications, psychotherapy, behavior therapy, cognitive behavior therapy, and maybe have themselves assayed the Feingold Diet or a course of chelation to remove toxins from the body.

Our first task is to understand the case as completely as we can, including family history, early experiences, the possibility of head injury, exposure to infectious diseases, pediatric autoimmune neuropsychiatric disorders associated with streptococcal infections (PANDAS), Lyme disease, diet and nutrition, and what has already been done, including regimens of medication, and what the child's reaction to each intervention has been. We may refer the family for a further workup, or a neuropsychological evaluation if it seems appropriate. We then do our own diagnostic evaluation including a LENS map, a qEEG, or, ideally, both—because each yields different kinds of information.

The qEEG, as we have discussed, is superior as an evaluational instrument because the reading is taken from nineteen sites simultaneously; in addition to the amplitude and frequency at any particular area (which the LENS map shows), it includes measures of coherence and connectivity as well as phase-lag. In addition, the qEEG is database driven, which means that each child is compared, in the evaluation, against a population or cohort of peers, age and gender-related. One can say that this child is "normal" in a statistical sense, in this or that area of EEG-related functioning.

Once all information that is possibly relevant has been gathered, we meet with our medical director for possible medical or physiological factors that might have been overlooked—a deleterious combination of medical side effects, or the possibility that there is a familial sensitivity to an allergen, or a clear nutritional or infectious problem.

A course of treatment is then planned based on the child's unique makeup and sensitivities. The early treatments usually involve an approach in which a fairly conservative treatment intervention is tried and the results carefully evaluated. In all this the parent or caretaker is enlisted as a collaborator or partner in the treatment process. With older children we do ask the child how she or he felt after the last treatment, but it is usually the parent who notices an increase or decrease of certain salient behavioral features: more or less annoying, anxious, avoidant, perseverative, better or worse sleep, temperament, ability to tolerate frustration, and so forth.

We are less concerned about having a correct diagnosis than we are about evolving a treatment plan that is partnered to the child's unique sensitivities and resources. Because neurofeedback treatment for the most part is not diagnosis based, we are less concerned about naming the disorder than about identifying the problem as acute or chronic, the precipitating factors, and the child's sensitivity to ordinary stimuli such as light, sound, touch, or responses to medication. These allow us to get a toe in the water, so to speak, and try an intervention.

The trajectory of responses to treatment is then carefully monitored. For example, does the child get better right away and hold that improvement for a little while, or suddenly get much worse, and then slowly—or quickly—get better? In general, if our first modality is the LENS, we expect responses to treatment within the first five sessions. If there are none, we suspect a hidden variable, a toxicity or an infection we have overlooked. If there are overreactions, we will cut back until the direction of the improvement turns positive.

Depending upon the age of the child, certain other variables will be monitored and explored: the addition of nutraceuticals, or changes in eating habits, discontinuation of a medication or taking a new one, or any environmental change. Parents often ask us: "What if my child is on medications? Does that interfere with the treatment or its results?" We usually respond that at least half our patients, including children, begin treatment on regimes of medication of some kind.

We also say, "If the medication seems helpful in some respects (and maybe not so good in others), continue on until your doctor directs you otherwise." We will not infrequently ask permission to speak with the prescribing physician, because beginning neurofeedback treatment, the child may suddenly get much more sensitive to the medications, and the side effects also multiply or worsen. Hopefully the physician or other prescriber will be sensitive enough to modulate the child's regime of medication accordingly (less is needed for a more sensitive and responsive nervous system).

A quick initial response to the treatment, the "honeymoon phase," is a wonderful thing, but with Len Ochs we often say, "Don't worry, it will pass." Then we settle down for the long, hard work of treating and watching the responses, treating and watching. There will always be ups and downs because of variables over which we have no control. But the goal is to hold on to the gains as long as possible, with the parent a cotherapist in the child's healing process, and using other modalities such as behavior therapy or cognitive therapy for learning disabilities, socialization training, and so on. Our philosophy is that since the child's autism is probably not a single-cause disorder, there is probably not a single cure. Rather, through mobilizing the child's central nervous system as an ally rather than an antagonist, all the other activities and learning opportunities in the child's life (made available through involved parents, school settings, and the like) will support the changes being made.

The following is an example of just how this approach might work with a living, severely compromised child in an extremely loving family. I am warmly appreciative and grateful to the S. family for allowing me to describe the case of their daughter, Emily (her real name), in as much detail as we have. It may offer some encouragement and hope for families with children who seem in equally impossible, no-win situations.

No Words but "No!"

At four years of age, little Emily is impossibly cute. She is petite, quite a bit smaller than her (fraternal) twin brother, Chris, blonde, and wears tiny wire-rimmed glasses that only she herself may touch. She is still in diapers, not toilet trained, while her brother was trained years ago. When she sees that my office is full of sandplay toys, she is visibly excited. But she grabs one after the other, in a haphazard fashion, puts it in the box, or throws it on the floor, and then grabs another. In one corner of the room, behind the couch, I have beautiful antique Czechoslovakian handmade puppets that are only for older children to play with carefully, but she makes a beeline for these again and again, despite (and likely because of) being told no. There are, in fact, lots of other toys available. When she is pulled back repeatedly from the only forbidden ones by her parents, she throws a fit, kicking and screaming and rolling on the floor.

"Ah," I say wisely to the parents, "another practitioner of tantrum yoga," and the laughter dispels the tension a little.

The first neurofeedback session is quite an ordeal because she is also quick and clever to rip the electrodes off her head as quick as they are put on. Her screams of "No! No! No!" fill the therapy center. Rich and Lola, her devoted parents, are very concerned, but they are determined that she will indeed get a treatment, because they don't know what else to do; they are at their wits' end.

Just after birth, she and her twin, Christopher, were both healthy and had normal Apgars. Emily was the second one out and quite a bit smaller. As the months of the first year passed, she crept and crawled, and soon stood and toddled, as he did. She began to talk, as he did. Then by the end of that year she had inexplicably begun to slide backward developmentally. He went on to toilet train; she did not. He did interactive play with other children; she did not—with her brother or any other children.

When we first meet Emily, her mood is quite unstable. She is restless, easily frustrated, highly willful. Her parents have explored up and down the East Coast, visiting every highly regarded pediatric psychiatrist and neurologist that was recommended. Finally an entire team of therapists at a Connecticut Center confirms the terrifying word they have been hearing at almost every place they have been: *autism*!

At that initial session, the parents and I come up with a strategy that will have to be employed for every session that she comes to for the first few months. We call it the "breakfast burrito." Emily is cocooned in a soft blanket that I have in my office, so that her arms and legs are trapped, and then she sits in her father's lap as I attempt to apply the electrodes. But she is resourceful and whips her head around uncontrollably to knock them off. Finally Lola has to hold the head of the uncontrollable little girl. Her screams reach the furthest part of the building, and my staff is worried that people sitting in the waiting room might think we are engaged in child abuse. Finally a couple of seconds of stimulation with the LENS is accomplished, and she is free to play in the sandbox again as we wind up the session.

It will take us months of treatment to make an initial map, as I am using the "stim" map because I suspect seizure activity to be present. She will, of course, not close her eyes for the treatment; she insists on keeping her glasses on (she wants to wear them all the time). The first EEG recordings are so full of artifact from movement and eye blink that they have to be repeated and then integrated to obtain what seems like a final map. The amplitudes and standard deviations are off the charts (see Emily' problem list on the next page). Still, after the paroxysmal rage, she calms down a bit after the first treatment and goes back to grabbing toys off the shelves.

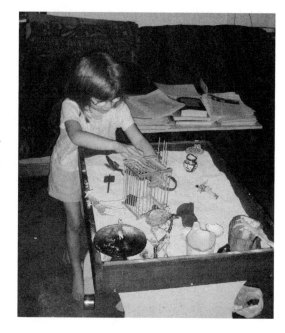

Fig. 6.1. Emily at chaotic play

Emily's Problems at the Time of First Treatment
(Highest Values on CNS Questionnaire)

Speech delay	10
Distractibility	10
Mood instability	10
Willfulness	10
Lacks toilet training	10
Eye strabismus	9

On the subjective symptom rating scale, Emily has 10s in the categories we will be tracking during treatment: mood instability, no language, no cooperative play, no toilet training, willfulness (followed by a tantrum when restrained or denied in any way). She does not make eye contact with adults and ignores questions or instructions that are offered to her. There is also a visual category, given by her opthalmologist: strabismus, in which the eyes often wander independently of each other and will not track or focus together. Though the parents face a 200-mile round trip from where they live in Connecticut to our center in New York, for the first few months, Rich and Lola are faithful about coming every week.

Other therapeutic modalities that are undertaken with Emily include sandplay, pediatric opthalmology, craniosacral manipulation, energy healing, occupational and speech therapy, special education, physical therapy, the HANDLE approach (the Holistic Approach to Neurodevelopmental Disorders and Learning Efficiency developed by Judith Bluestone), and nutritional therapy.

As the weeks pass, Emily's parents are equally faithful about reporting observations and detailing the amazing changes that begin to happen to their daughter. (Please also refer to plates 8 and 9 of the color insert to follow Emily's progress.) Reports begin coming back from the school and play sessions to which she is taken from people who have no idea what neurofeedback is. She is making more eye contact, saying more words than No! In classroom settings she joins activities rather than sitting apart.

She still requires the "breakfast burrito" to get her neurofeedback treatments, but her parents and I both notice it is a little bit easier to

SUBJECTIVE SYMPTOM RATING SCALE

Prominent Symptoms	Begin Date	2	3	4	5	6	7	8	9	10	11
Session Dates:	7/28/2006	8/4/2006	8/11/2006	8/18/2006	8/25/2006	9/1/2006	9/8/2006	9/15/2006	9/22/2006	9/29/2006	10/10/2006
1 Speech Delay	10.00	9.75	9.75	9.75	9.75	9.75	9.75	9.50	9.25	9.25	9.25
2 Attn/Distraction	10.00	10.0	9.75	9.75	9.50	9.50	9.00	8.50	8.00	8.00	7.50
3 MoodInstability	10.00	9.50	9.50	9.5	9.50	9.00	8.50	8.50	8.00	8.00	7.50
4 Willfulness	10.00	10.00	10.00	10.0	10.00	10.00	9.50	9.50	9.50	9.50	8.50
5 InteractivePlay	10.00	9.50	9.50	9.5	9.50	9.50	9.50	9.00	9.00	9.00	9.00
6 ToiletTraining	10.00	10.00	10.00	10.0	10.00	10.00	10.00	10.00	9.00	9.00	8.00
7 EyeStrabismus	9.00	9.00	9.00	9.0	9.00	9.00	9.00	9.00	9.00	9.00	9.00

	12	13	14	15	16	17	18	19	20	21	22	23	24	25
	10/13/2006	10/20/2006	10/27/2006	11/3/2006	11/10/2006	11/22/2006	12/1/2006	12/15/2006	12/29/2006	1/12/2007	1/26/2007	2/9/2007	2/23/2007	3/9/2007
1 Speech Delay	9.50	9.50	9.50	7.00	8.50	8.50	8.50	6.75	6.75	8.50	8.50	8.50	8.00	8.00
2 Attn/Distraction	7.50	7.50	7.50	7.50	6.75	6.75	6.75	6.75	6.75	6.75	6.75	6.75	6.75	6.00
3 MoodInstability	7.50	7.50	7.50	7.50	7.50	7.50	7.50	8.00	8.00	8.00	7.10	6.50	6.00	5.50
4 Willfulness	8.50	9.00	9.00	9.00	9.00	9.00	9.00	9.00	9.00	9.00	8.00	7.75	7.50	7.00
5 InteractivePlay	9.00	9.00	9.00	8.50	8.00	8.00	8.00	8.00	8.00	8.00	7.50	7.50	7.00	7.00
6 ToiletTraining	7.00	6.50	6.50	7.00	7.00	7.00	7.00	7.00	7.00	7.00	7.00	7.00	7.00	7.00
7 EyeStrabismus	9.00	9.00	9.00	9.00	9.00	9.00	9.00	9.00	9.00	9.00	9.00	9.00	9.00	9.00

	26	27	28	29	30	31	32	33	34	35	36	37	38	39	40	41
	3/23/2007	4/6/2007	4/27/2007	5/11/2007	5/25/2007	6/8/2007	7/6/2007	7/20/2007	8/3/2007	8/17/2007	8/31/2007	9/14/2007	9/20/2007	10/26/2007	11/23/2007	12/21/2007
1 Speech Delay	7.50	7.25	7.25	7.25	7.00	6.75	6.50	6.50	6.50	6.25	6.25	6.00	6.00	6.00	6.00	5.50
2 Attn/Distraction	5.75	5.50	5.00	4.75	3.50	3.50	3.50	3.50	3.50	3.25	6.25	6.25	6.00	5.75	5.50	5.00
3 MoodInstability	5.25	5.00	5.00	4.50	4.25	4.25	4.25	4.25	4.25	4.00	4.00	4.00	4.00	4.00	4.00	3.50
4 Willfulness	7.00	6.90	6.50	6.00	6.00	5.75	5.50	5.50	5.50	5.50	5.50	5.25	5.00	4.75	4.50	4.50
5 InteractivePlay	6.75	6.50	6.00	5.50	5.25	5.00	5.00	5.00	5.00	4.50	4.25	4.25	4.25	4.00	4.00	3.50
6 ToiletTraining	7.00	6.50	6.50	6.50	6.00	5.50	5.00	5.00	5.00	4.50	5.00	5.00	5.00	4.75	4.50	4.50
7 EyeStrabismus	9.00	9.00	7.00	7.00	7.00	7.00	7.00	7.00	3.50	3.50	3.50	3.50	3.50	3.50	3.50	3.50

	42	43	44	45	46	47	48	49	50	51	52	53	54	55	56
	1/18/2008	2/29/2008	4/4/2008	5/16/2008	6/27/2008	8/8/2008	9/12/2008	10/24/2008	11/21/2008	1/16/2009	2/29/2009	4/10/2009	5/15/2009	6/19/2009	7/24/2009
1 Speech Delay	5.50	5.00	5.00	4.90	4.90	4.50	4.00	3.90	3.50	3.00	3.00	3.00	2.90	2.00	2.00
2 Attn/Distraction	5.00	4.90	4.75	4.50	4.50	4.00	3.90	3.90	3.50	3.00	3.00	3.50	3.00	3.00	3.00
3 MoodInstability	3.50	3.50	3.50	3.00	3.00	3.90	4.00	4.00	4.00	3.50	3.50	3.50	3.50	3.00	3.00
4 Willfulness	4.50	4.50	4.50	4.50	4.50	4.50	4.25	4.00	4.00	4.00	4.00	4.00	3.50	3.00	3.00
5 InteractivePlay	3.50	3.25	3.25	3.00	2.90	2.90	2.50	2.50	2.00	1.90	1.90	1.90	1.50	1.00	1.00
6 ToiletTraining	4.50	4.50	4.00	4.00	4.50	3.90	3.50	3.50	2.00	2.00	2.00	1.00	1.00	0.00	3.00
7 EyeStrabismus	3.50	3.00	3.00	3.00	3.00	3.00	3.00	3.00	3.00	3.00	3.00	3.00	3.00	3.00	3.00

Fig. 6.2. The results of Emily's fifty-six LENS sessions spread over three years

get her in the chair, and her tantrums are a little shorter, and seem more manageable. She now begins to select sandplay objects more carefully and seems to be developing themes: one week it will be "houses," another week "animals." Sometimes she will get a boy and a girl. She sets up a little table and chairs and pours sand into cups as if it were tea. On Halloween she surprises us all by taking out a haunted house from my shelves, and a ghost, which she flies out the window of the house. She excitedly says the word "ghost" and giggles as he flies around the little house.

Soon parents and teachers are hearing more verbalizations, and there is occasional eye contact. She begins to express preferences for what articles of clothing she will wear that day—and her mother is fairly indulgent of her preferences as long as they are fairly close to what the weather or the occasion warrants. Soon she is asking for things she wants by name or pointing at objects and saying their names.

Below is a chronological sequence of responses to treatment, reported by Emily's parents (or school authorities via her parents). These first responses are detailed because they convey to the reader a more exact and nuanced way that an autistic child might respond to neurofeedback treatments.

How We Measure Clinical Change

- As in the "100-Person Study," Larsen and Harrington, *Journal of Neurotherapy,* 2007, clinical (subjectively reported) changes are compared to changes in the LENS map (objective measure).
- Improvements are confirmed by independent professionals in schools and clinical environments.
- We assemble a running narrative report, as below, which details parents' responses to the treatment. It is important to note they aren't always good.

8/4/06   Night of treatment not so good. Up till ten o'clock, temper tantrums up, but also more smiling and some verbalizing. Showed more emotion generally.

8/11   Mood unstable. During one meltdown Lola noticed something amazing, real tears present; before she would cry dry.

8/18 Refused to put diaper on, wanted to sit on potty.

8/25 Irritable, lots of meltdowns.

9/1 Got right into car seat, better for a while. First day back to school; covering ears again.

9/8 Using one-syllable words; says "Mom." Easier getting dressed . . .

9/15 Continues to show progress. Therapists noticing improved coordination. At school no fuss, hangs up coat, walks to seat.

9/22 Easy Friday night after treatment; Sunday cranky and emotional. People at school notice good things; independently sorting objects by color and shape.

10/6 A very good week. Sat on potty for an hour, reading a book! More cuddly, physically affectionate, gives Mom kisses.

10/13 Appetite increased, noncommunicative; rewinds toy over and over.

10/20 Right after session calm, relaxed, good-natured, continued over weekend. Toilet training continuing. Wanted to be naked all day.

10/27–11/10 Up and down, Not wanting to get into car seat. Wants to stay at therapy center (loves sandplay toys). Says "cat" and "camel" (appropriately) to pictures. Playing interactively with Christopher (brother). Runs around naked all the time (Lady Godiva phase). Was a tiger for Halloween. Wanted to keep on costume.

11/22–28 "Nature girl" still active, hard to keep clothes on her. Physical therapists say great progress, but osteopath thinks she has regressed, wants more allergy testing. Showing more emotion, squealing with laughter, curious.

12/1 Not a good week. Hard to get into car seat—high screeching. Tried sounds of alphabet.

A Summarization of Emily's Narrative Report

Concurrently with the narrative report above, you can see that each time, we ask for a numerical score on the (usually five, but in this case seven) clinical categories. We are also asking for copies of reports from schools, or from other therapists doing simultaneous interventions. We are remapping periodically. This progress can be seen in the accompanying graphs and charts (for our part, it is always useful to compare the clinical subjective symptom checklist, and other clinical notes, along with the EEG data). As you can see from the maps at the beginning and three years later, profound changes have taken place in Emily's brain.

In the interest of brevity, and, hopefully, clarity, we are going to summarize the middle and later phases of the narrative reports (below).

After seven months of treatment, in February 2007, the developmental psychiatrist ameliorated her diagnosis: *"mild* autistic spectrum disorder." Among the milestones of this period was that, for the first time ever, Emily saw herself in a mirror and started *acting*. That is to say, she "got it" that it was her in the mirror, and she suddenly had the ability to improvise on her self-image—not a small thing at all! There were more and more seconds of eye contact; she wanted to be tickled and to laugh together with Mommy (sounding less like autism). A few months later she was watching videos and seemed to track the stories and characters. Her parents took her to see a rather famous local healer who, although not a mental health professional, said Emily was not autistic. He had worked with autistics and knew what their "energy" was like. (This was in direct contrast to the diagnosis of a developmental pediatrician who said the child was definitely on the autistic spectrum.) Emily had always seemed kinesthetically and physically weak and uncoordinated. Now she became bolder—doing acts of derring-do involving walking on garden walls with good balance.

Within a month or two in the spring of 2007, Emily responded positively to her name and turned to look when someone greeted her. By eight months she was dressing herself and using qualifiers like "more." Her parents noted that she was able focus longer. The teacher noted that she sat nicely in assembly. At home she was more responsive to touch and stroking. By April of 2007, Emily was vocalizing frequently.

Her mother reported she was playing interactively with Chris, her twin. At an informal event she sat right in front of the musician, "mesmerized," and interacted with him during the intermission. By late April, the opthalmalogist reported that her astigmatism seemed to have normalized. Her vision now, corrected, was 20/20.

A teacher reported "paying attention better." She was playing inter-actively with other kids. Her toilet training was coming along well, both at home and in school. A very important event reported by the school psychologist: Emily had a friend!

By July of 2007, almost a year after she began treatment, Emily had entered preschool. She and Chris each had their own rooms. She played interactively, she got into chairs for meals or schoolwork on her own, and she sat waiting for the activity to start. When she was brought to Judith Bluestone (the founder of the HANDLE Institute), the autism special-ist noticed changes. She thought Emily had more attentional focus and made a greater variety of sounds. "Putting things away" in their place was noted. She was noticing when she was wet and didn't like it, making her more motivated to do toilet training.

Emily progressed in her ability to tolerate stronger neurofeedback (LENS) protocols. She responded very well to a Rocking the Brain (Dogris) protocol. By September 2007 she was in school five days a week in special learning programs. She was playing more interactively, and by October she was observed imitating others (playmates).

By November 2007, Emily was observed visibly reacting emotionally to significant events in stories that were being read to her (an atypical autistic response). Judith Bluestone was very "impressed by her progress." During this time her parents were also accessing craniosacral manipula-tions for Emily.

By January 2008, a year and a half after commencing treatments, Emily was responding better and better to treatments. She was babbling more and working harder on toilet training. She was able to concentrate on a board game. She liked it and knew her pieces and what their moves were. Reports said, "Very affectionate, lots of kisses and hugs" (this is defi-nitely not autistic behavior). She dressed voluntarily and chose her clothes. She sat next to a friend on the schoolbus. She was invited to a birthday party, and during the party she sat next to a friend and paid attention to the unfolding events in an appropriate way.

Because of the length of the trip to our center, by summer 2008, almost two years after starting, sessions settled down to a timetable of about once a month. Emily was now taking relatively high doses of treatment (ramping protocols: Rocking the Brain, Rocking the Spectrum) and was handling them pretty well. There might have been small ripples or aftershocks to the treatment, but they were short-lived: "Sharper and shorter," as Len Ochs says. It was now obvious there was a dimension to her behavior we had not been tracking: object constancy—with an OCD complexion. After breaking her favorite barrette, she was inconsolable (just as she couldn't ever be separated from her glasses and would even try to wear them while sleeping). The loss of the barrette was intolerable, but then over.

Plate 9 of the color insert reflects Emily's final improvements, mentioned in the symptom checklist below. There was a nice steady improvement (lower on scale) between sessions 46 and 54. We were now using stronger protocols such as Dogris's Rocking the Brain and Rocking the Spectrum (multiple stims in different frequencies and measured from different ranges—delta, theta, alpha, beta).

Emily's Problems as of August 28, 2009

Speech Delay	2
Distractibility	3
Mood instability	3
Willfulness	3
Lacks interactive play	3
Lacks toilet training	1
Eye strabismus	0

In a few months, Emily was reading whole sentences: "I see a Mommy!" The speech therapist noted that she was able to speak of what she read and saw in a book. Toilet training was languishing, and there was a "smearing" incident. Still, there was a feeling of progress. Her original obstinacy and oppositionality had now refined into an absolutely definite idea of her choosing her own clothing for the day. She socialized well with her fellow kindergartners. There was continuous steady progress. Her parents noted that it was "a steady improvement in all dimensions." She read simple children's stories. She colored and named the colors she used. She was able to register and name emotions occurring in other children (not an autistic feature). She was trying to string words together.

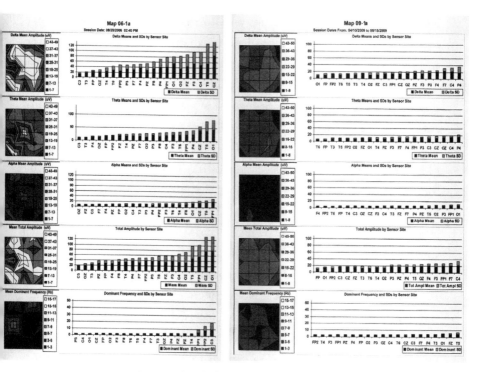

*Fig. 6.3. Emily's before and after topographic
brainmaps, three years apart*

By January 2009, Emily was putting together more words and sentences. She named people. She would hear the word "pink" and be able to spell it. She was able to say what she wanted. Toilet training seemed by now "almost complete." She could dress herself and write her name. In February 2009 she won the "student of the month" award. Her picture appeared in the school newspaper. She melted this therapist's heart by giving him a hug and a kiss and climbed into his lap to see her map on the computer.

At this point the improvement we have all been waiting for begins: toilet training. It is slow, but definitely, over months, moving in the right direction. Finally comes the day, between her fifth and sixth year, when she is completely toilet trained. Her parents, teachers, and I are ecstatic. Emily is coming of age.

What is remarkable about this chronicle is that the nuances of developmental progress—or lack of it—are noted in detail. In any genuine sequence of healing there are ups and downs of progress. But if the parents, and the clinician, are careful about what is happening, there is overall progress, which is all these committed parents can hope for. It is as if we were all working with exquisitely complex processes with their phasic shifts that seem like progress or regression—and both are part of the process. Ultimately, what happens is what we are witnessing now.

A more complete human being comes into my office these days. (This is being written in December 2010.) Emily is still cute as a button, still wears her wire-rimmed glasses that give her a slightly elvish look. She heads right for the sandtray and enacts a drama, great or small, that absorbs her, and at times her own play-acting of the characters makes her squeal with delight. (Study any developmental text and you will find role-taking as a rather advanced stage of cognitive development.)

Because I am very appreciative of the many other therapeutic modalities that these resourceful parents have accessed, I am guarded in ascribing all or even most of Emily's gains to the LENS treatments. Her parents, however, ascribe to the LENS a central role in their daughter's healing, and continue faithfully to make the long commute back and forth to our center. They warmly endorse the LENS as a "catalyst" that not only empowered her healing but made all the other modalities they accessed "work better."

We still do not know much about the complex of factors that brought about Emily's sudden regression, and there are no obvious candidates, since her parents deliberately resisted vaccinations because of warnings they had received from other families in their network. For my own part, as a mental health professional with over forty years working with children and families, I can vouch that there was no lack of nurture in this family, nor nutrition, as they eat healthfully, and there is an overflowing abundance of caring and love. My private suspicion, based on things I saw in the EEG, was that Emily suffered from some kind of atypical seizure disorder that masqueraded as autism. It is presented in this book to note that symptomatology can be deceiving when there is severe CNS dysregulation, and children's nervous systems are eminently fragile and yet eminently plastic.

Learning from Emily

- Even a firm diagnosis of autism is not immutable.
- Seizure disorder may masquerade as tantrums or perseveration. These would be called subclinical seizures.
- With the seizurelike instability of the cortex resolved, developmental milestones can be within reach and repaired, so other lost abilities can be developed.
- Lots of patience, love, and warmth are humus for the soul to grow or regrow itself.
- Families like the S. family are the true heroes of our story!

Tom: Asperger's Syndrome
MARY LEE ESTY, PH.D., L.C.S.W.

Tom was twelve years old in the spring of 2009 when he and his mother came to the Neurotherapy Center of Washington to explore the possibility of Flexyx Neurotherapy System (FNS/LENS) treatment for the symptoms of Asperger's syndrome. He was formally diagnosed in 2008 and had struggled with the social problems throughout elementary school. He had already benefited from and was continuing in counseling, socialization group, and tutoring. However, lack of eye contact, indifference to appearance, difficulty making transitions, and rigidity about food and activities remained problems, and he did not respond to being touched. Tom's mother learned about neurofeedback from two friends and their therapist referred Tom to Dr. Esty.

Tom's response to treatment was immediate. His mother writes about the first treatment: "When it was over and my son opened his eyes and looked directly at me and said, 'Wow mom that was cool,' and from that day on he now looks at me or anyone he talks to." At his socialization group the next day he talked more, participated actively, and made eye contact. After the second treatment he cracked a joke spontaneously (actually a funny one), then smiled at his mother, something he had never done before. Tom's mother wrote this about events after the second treatment: "The second was the one when I knew this was going to be a cure for my son. He had not, nor would he even try to ride a bike. After a treatment he said to me, 'Mom, I want to learn to ride a bike!' Two hours later he was riding a two-wheel bike all by himself." As treatment progressed he became aware of his mother's feelings and would comment on them in relation to his behavior and he began to hug his mother.

During one relatively brief period he developed temporary side effects. He began humming constantly, putting his hands to his mouth, reminiscent of previous tic behaviors, and he seemed to become more noise sensitive again during treatment. These side effects faded and gradually organization of his school binder greatly improved, as did his handwriting. Five months after starting treatment Tom visited his grandparents, who were astounded with the changes in him. "Like night and day," they declared. Conversation was easy with lots of give and take. In school he was volunteering. Most impressive was his statement to his mother, "I wish I wasn't as afraid to do things." He got his wish: fears began to have less hold on him. As these changes were sustained, we reduced the frequency of treatments to once every two, then every three, weeks.

Two major events reflect the magnitude of Tom's progress. First in Tom's mother's words: "I went to the school to pick my son up and ran into his school counselor. She stopped and told me that she and the other teachers are amazed at how well my son is socializing with his peers and that one of those peers approached her and told her that my son was just like them now." The surprising second event was the day Tom asked his mom if she was busy on Saturday night because he wanted to go to the school dance. He still doesn't want to cut his long hair however. Tom's mother now describes him as "a thriving teenager with friends of his own age group."

Very early on, Tom's mother had felt that something wasn't right with her son and she embarked on a long journey to find help for him.

It was his eyes. He always looked lost and he struggled with everyday tasks that came so easy to most kids. Once he started school it was apparent that he did not fit in with the other kids and was having difficulties with learning and making friends. When he was in the third grade a teacher diagnosed him as being ADD or ADHD and said he should be medicated. I took him to a psychologist and I was told he was fine. Well, that year passed and then the fourth grade, no better, and then the fifth grade (still struggling). Then one day my mother was watching a news show and came across a special on Asperger's and saw the similarities between the child on the show and my son. With initial denial I started researching Asperger's on the Internet and the more I read the more I realized that this is what my son had.

Thanks to Tom's mother's determination and the increasing availability of information about neurofeedback, Tom's life is now, and will always be, very different from what is traditionally expected. His mother glowingly describes the situation now, after thirty-four treatments, each half an hour in length, by saying: "Life couldn't be any better."

Indigo Children's Project 2010
DONALD MAGDER, M.A.

In May of 2010, a minister in Westland, Michigan, who is also an advocate for autism, called me to see if I would donate my neurofeedback services to his group of parents whose children were autistic. The name of his group is the Indigo Children's Network.

I offered to work with the parents from the network and those that responded to a *Detroit News* newspaper article, which had expressed my interest in helping this subset population. The result was that I ended up working with over twenty children, who ranged on the PDD spectrum from Asperger's to severe and nonverbal autism, as well as four individuals with ADD or ADHD. I treated these children for six months, from June through December of 2010.

Specifically, with fourteen of these children I used the LENS system, because these were the children that had the greatest difficulty sitting still; as well, they were rated as being the most severe on the spectrum.

I also made sure parents did not tell other third parties that their child was starting treatment with LENS, in order to get a more objective view of any changes that might occur. (Because there is a tendency for parents to look for changes, they are not always the best reporters.)

The biggest litmus test of the success of this program is that six parents (40 percent of the group) are still coming to see me, now as paying clients. Some say they "never want to stop the treatments," and some travel from as far as two hours away to get to my office. In one case, a parent stayed behind in Detroit for an extra three months after her husband had moved to Tennessee, solely in order to be able to continue with her child's LENS treatments.

Though I had worked with a few autistic children in the past and saw some profound changes using the LENS system, I was not prepared for the number of parents who were hugging me, almost crying, at the positive changes they were seeing. Within four weeks, often after changing the treatment protocol (known to LENS practitioners as the offset), the stories started coming in.

In fact, I came up with a new category for my notes, called "The Nevers." Parents were saying that their child had never done this or that, or never said things a certain way, or never acted a certain way before.

For example:

"My son did the chores without prompting. He never did that before."

"Never counted to twenty without being prompted."

"He is using 'I want' statements. Never did this before LENS."

"Saw him being silly for the first time."

"Said his first five-word sentence, 'Hi, Dad, how are you?'"

And so on.

Third-party comments sounded like this after one to two months of treatments:

Amazing, amazing, amazing! I cannot believe how calm and cooperative your child is. She understands about 90 percent of what we are doing now!

ABA THERAPIST, AFTER NOT SEEING THIS CHILD
FOR ONE MONTH OF LENS TREATMENTS

Jesse is not playing with "little people" anymore. Interested in group activities and has made really good progress.

TEACHER AT JESSE'S PARENT-TEACHER CONFERENCE

I am very pleased with his progress. He would not even look at me before.

TEACHER AT SPECIAL-ED SCHOOL

Out of the fourteen parents that worked with LENS, ten feel they received great benefit from doing LENS for their child. The greatest improvements were in the following areas:

Expressive Language

- Almost across the board, these children started using more language. Three parents heard their child use a five-word sentence for the first time.
- Names of siblings and dogs started popping out. I began telling parents that LENS is "a verb machine," as phrases like "I want" and "the girl is running" were reported by many parents, instead of the child just pointing or only using the word "girl" to communicate.
- Frequency of communication as evidenced by one parent's comment: "My child now says one sentence every ten minutes instead of every half hour."

A Sense of Understanding

- Parents reported that they could "see the wheels of thought turning" for the first time. A sense of understanding, or trying to understand what was happening, appeared, rather than just having a robot-like response to the world.
- A parent noted these changes: "We could see the child trying to process her thoughts. I thought it was just me seeing this, but the occupational therapist saw the same thing."
- Another parent said, "He is starting to enjoy identifying things now."

Impulse Control

Many of the parents reported that their children displayed better impulse control; their ability to sit still in a doctor's office or at home improved. Specific comments include:

- "Not agitated in restaurants any more. He is just a new kid! Best haircut he ever had. He sat still the whole time."
- "When he has a meltdown, it is much shorter in duration."

A Sense of Playfulness

A sense of play and playfulness started coming out with about six of the children; an impishness the parents had never seen before. Also symbolic play appeared for the first time; some children started singing with less inhibition. Specific comments include:

- "He started telling 'knock knock' jokes."
- "He exhibited teasing and playfulness. He pretended he had a mustache by putting his finger below his lip."

A Sense of Self and Self-Assessment

Some of the children defended themselves for the first time with siblings or by saying the word "no" more often. They had a better sense of what they wanted and how they wanted it. One parent said that LENS was filling in the developmental stages the child had missed when younger. Specific comments include:

- "Went into a store all by himself and picked out the CD he wanted. He started showing an amazing amount of initiative."
- "Started watching less TV and dancing more."
- "Picked out a Dumbo video all by himself!"

Self-Expression

Drawing, paintings, and singing were in evidence as treatments progressed. The children colored more within the lines of the drawing and drew better and clearer shapes. Often, prior to the LENS treatments, the children had only scribbled. Specific comments include:

- "He wrote the name 'Harry Potter' by himself on the dry erase board."
- "She is singing all the time."

These are the main changes I have seen these past six months. It has been a life-changing experience for me, and I am now convinced that LENS can play a vital role in helping the brains of these children connect the dots. One child in particular improved so much since the first treatment (as if a "cascade effect" of connections started happening) that his mother felt like she had a brand new child.

The Story of David B.

The following is a case history of the first six treatments of a sixteen-year-old Asperger's client (rated "moderate" on the Asperger's scale); I will call him David B. Though this example covers only six treatments, the comments and behavioral changes depicted herein are indicative of those experienced by the majority of clients that have come to see me. Typically in the course of treatment, developmental stages, long dormant and delayed, would start to surface and integrate into the child's personality in the months to come. It is important to note, as of this writing (one year later), that these changes have become permanent for David B.

As exciting as it has been for the parents (and me!) to see these changes, it must be noted that they may appear to be "small" changes to the average onlooker. But to a parent of a special needs child, they are profound changes indeed.

Upon assessment, David presented with a lack of social skills and self-awareness. His communication was brief and his words were stilted and short. He had to be told to do everything. He is involved with Special Olympics. Specific comments on his behavioral changes are noted below.

First Treatment: No Change
Second Treatment: No Change
Third Treatment: "A bit calmer"
Fourth Treatment: "Showed initiative in doing chores for the first

time! He wanted to find a song on the radio that he liked. Has *never* done this before!"

Fifth Treatment: "Really becoming independent! I can see him starting to think!" His grandmother said that David is talking all the time. "First time I have seen so much communication."

Sixth Treatment: "Showing amazing independence. I do not need to tell him to do anything anymore! I am absolutely thrilled at the results my child has been getting with LENS. What is so amazing is that the results have come so quickly. I am a registered nurse and this is by far the best intervention I have ever done for my child."

SEVEN

ATTENTION DEFICIT DISORDER AND ITS COUSINS

With J. Lawrence Thomas, Ph.D.

In the world of pediatric diagnosis, it is always an open question whether the child who has problems in coping and maturation is to be given a diagnosis of ADD, ADHD, PDD (pervasive developmental disorder), or perhaps a combination. Unlike the neglected or abused children with attachment problems we discussed in chapter 5, and like many of the autistic or Asperger's children from chapter 6, the home environment may be intact, even very comfortable. The biological parents may be devoted to the child and its well-being; there may be an absence of traumatic events, abandonment, or failure to nurture, so the mystery persists as to the cause of the child's problems. Additionally confusing is that symptoms may overlap, so that children who clearly merit the autistic diagnosis also seem very attentionally disturbed and have clear learning disabilities. Kids who are clearly ADHD also seem oblivious to ordinary social learning environments and seem autistic at times.

The box on page 144 might be helpful for understanding how pediatric psychiatrists and developmental psychologists parse out their diagnosis.

Diagnosing ADD

Pervasive Developmental Disorder (PDD): Usually the child has shown failure to meet developmental milestones from an early age and may have had compromised Apgar scores. Fails to initiate eye contact with adults or others, unable to creep (usually earlier) or crawl, unable to sit upright or stand upright. Lateness in walking and talking, seems more immature than nursery school peers. The PDD child may be late to toilet train, weak in appetite, and generally have poor energy.

Attention deficit comes in many shapes and forms, but is broadly divided into two categories: With hyperactivity or ADHD, the child shows restlessness, irritability, and curiosity, it seems without satisfaction, and is ceaselessly in motion. The inattentive type does not show the above hyperkinetic behaviors but is difficult to engage in tasks, is dreamy, disorganized, and compromised in memory or with learning disabilities (LD). Older children in this latter category have difficulty keeping track of things and have poor executive functions that involve planning, sequencing, and organizing. They don't seem to know how to persevere even at simple tasks like getting dressed, brushing teeth, or remembering to go to the bathroom.

Autistic spectrum children may exhibit the above features, but they are often observed to have more extreme variations: failure to respond when an adult comes into the room or tries to engage with them, rigid or wooden when held, failure to snuggle, repetitive or rocking behaviors, content to sit alone and rock, or perhaps more serious head-banging or self-mutilation. In addition, there may be disturbing features such as eating refuse or inorganic objects, self-stimulation that is difficult to stop, making the same noise, or asking the same simple question over and over without noticing the answer that is given, becoming disturbed when the environment is changed in any way, or seeming more oriented to objects than to people.

Attentional Deficits and Motivation in Children (and Adults)

While autism seems to include attentional pathology, ADD overlaps with, but does not include, much that is present in autistic spectrum disorders. The ADD child, hyperactive (ADHD) or not (inattentive ADD), shades all too easily into normalcy, leading us to wonder if the entirety of modern American culture itself is not attentionally compromised.

In the early twentieth century, William James pointed out that attention was the pivotal mechanism not only of consciousness but of learning, character development, and creative life fulfillment. James was familiar with the writings of Swedenborg, who said that our rational or attentive faculties only follow that which we "love." Put in more modern terms, attention follows motivation. That is why you never have to coerce or browbeat children (or adults) to pay attention to something in which they are intrinsically interested or that they love (cartoons, video games, spontaneous play).

One of the great mysteries, then, of the so-called ADD child is that he or she can *hyperfocus* in one area of interest and be totally distractible in another. While playing *Nintendo,* the child is so focused that you cannot distract him no matter what you do. But when he is asked to pay attention to an English or math lesson, he is hopelessly distractible.

Anyone who has worked with or seriously engaged an ADD or ADHD child knows what we are talking about. When engaged, the child is rapt, on line, intelligently pursuing a learning dialogue. When the motivational structure of the child is not engaged, he or she (more usually he) is definitely not very present. That is to say, to use a simple metaphor, when the fuel or "juice" of the child's "loves" or motivation is available, there is no limit to the absorption in the learning task. When the child has no "juice" for the activity, there is a drying-up, a paucity of attention and availability.

In chapter 14 we will peek in a little more depth into that mysterious grotto just behind the frontal lobes, where more primitive structures than the cerebral cortex are located—the anterior cingulate gyrus, or cortex (ACC), and the anterior insular cortex (AIC). Both of these lie exactly on that cusp between "in control" and "out of control," such as thinking repetitive thoughts that you might rather not think (OCD) or switches such as the AIC that operate on the basis of salience (literally, "what grabs you"). Beneath and nearby are the nuclei of the thalamus, such as the nucleus accumbens, which is one of those pleasure centers that can have rats pushing levers till they expire (a kind of rodent "shop till you drop" situation). It's obvious that pleasure leaks out of these nuclei, through tracts both myelinated and unmyelinated, to the ACC and AIC. So it is possible to find very serious addictions, say to *Nintendo* or pornography (may depend on your developmental stage), among people who are otherwise quite inattentive. Unfortunately the AIC is involved in sexual arousal, so there could be quite a torrid little "love nest" going on in that dark, moist cavern—and without any visible partner at all! One woman patient claimed she just couldn't get the attention of her porn-addicted husband—who was also badly ADD—even while sporting the latest revelations from Victoria's Secret. The inner preoccupation trumped the real thing.

Learning and motivational psychologists have explored these territories for decades. How do we get the children "on line" to enlist their motivation and thus "follow their bliss" right into schoolwork or homework? Unfortunately, if the motivation-gaining maneuver is too transparent or obvious, it may not work at all. (Young as they are, children understand about bribery!)

This dilemma brings up difficult questions about how similar or different are "motivated" and "unmotivated" learning. The maturational part is that, with normalcy, we expect a cerain amount of attentional "disposable income," so to speak, so that, in the long-term best interests of the children (or adults), they realize (consciously) that it is to their benefit to pay attention, even when a particular task is distasteful or boring, because the learning is embedded in a structure in which they realize that they have much to gain overall.

Let us contemplate the varieties of ways in which this works:

1. Totally spontaneous, *motivated* immersion, in which the child or adult is rapt with an experience. The passage of time recedes to the background, and pleasure suffuses the experience.

2. Culturally sponsored attention, in which rituals and lore, myths, and stories are imprinted on the child without much coercion or effort. As Joseph Campbell and Jerome Bruner point out (Campbell 1972; Bruner 1986), in "mythical" or narratizing consciousness, the culture knows how to encode information that naturally talks to the brain.

3. Culturally coerced and institutionally supported learning, in which the child is presented with a learning experience that, like it or not, they must participate in. There are moderate rewards (a letter grade or a diploma) and significant punishments (flunking or expulsion). (Until fairly recently there was also aversive conditioning in the form of the birch rod or ruler!)

Like it or not, category 3 is counted on as the backbone of our institutional pedagogy, and the threat of punishment, humiliation, or rejection is deemed motive enough, rather than the obvious charms of primary or secondary reinforcement—immediate and juicy rewards. While psychology knows positive reinforcement produces stronger operant behaviors than punishment or negative-reinforcement protocols, these are usually used only in the primary, early years of education, as we sing little songs, play, and tell stories to our children, all of which have intrinsically motivating and attention-engaging properties. With maturation, a more in-control or measured self-discipline, in the name of achieving culturally sanctioned goals, is the norm.

Think for a moment of the sad case of the suiciding schoolchildren in Japan. Anyone who has lived in Japan has seen extraordinary lavishing of love and unconditional positive regard on the younger child. As the child matures, however, and moves on to the Japanese equivalents of junior high or high school, increasingly demanding obligations are placed on him or her, and there is not much tolerance for failure. An extremely high-context society, which is based on a terror of failure to compete or really failure to fit in, begins to grind its terrible jaws. In a society in which social humiliation traditionally ended in ritual suicide, this is exactly what those children do.

Back in our own society, think of the plight of the English schoolchild who may, like John Bowlby, be sent at the age of seven to a regimented, impersonal context in hallowed (Gothic) halls, where social humiliation and, until recently, corporal punishment rule the day. In fraternities or the military it is *hazing* that (supposedly) converts child to adult. Indulgent and personal parenting may yield, in these "initiatory" developmental periods, to strict and impersonal rules and punishments. But like the punished monkeys in aversive conditioning experiments, children threatened with harsh punishment or ostracism may become neurotic or very depressed.

There is a fourth, more positive model of higher education, which I believe should characterize all evolving and flexible modern societies: the self-directed learning or self-actualization of Maslow, in which people gratuitously and sincerely put themselves through an initiation of learning, in which they practice an instrument or a language for many hours each day or work into the wee hours of the night on a new equation, a solution to a problem in chemistry or biology, or a novel, poem, or work of art.

The attention-deficit child is probably more likely to emerge in learning contexts such as number 3 above. Learning may become onerous or fearful for children. Operant conditioning may work against the child or learner, so that math or history (or gym with that fascist bully of a coach) has a permanent negative association. The whole subject (math is a common one), or the classroom, or the school itself, is associated with an avoidant pattern in the learner so that he or she procrastinates—or plays hooky. Learning freezes up and distractibility prevails.

Very often, the entire process takes place below the level of consciousness, so that the children—or, later, the adults—are not aware of just how avoidant, distractible, or disorganized they are. They just feel helpless or hopeless whenever that particular task or subject comes up. This can become phobic in intensity, so that paying attention becomes impossible (the term *paying attention* itself is telling, as if there is an economic or attentional *resource* to be yielded up, but the child may feel inwardly impoverished, or as if he or she has nothing to give). Various coercive techniques backfire. The punished child fears the punisher and the place of punishment. Then, in a psychological involution, the adolescent and subsequent adult introjects the standoff, so the hated and feared authority inside, which Freud called the *superego,* is resisted and sabotaged. And thus we have created the habitually self-sabotaging and locked-up person. The key word here is *habitual*. Any behavioral pattern, often repeated, gets ingrained.

Enter biofeedback. The task is morphed into one that is so easy or effortless that attention flows naturally to it. It should be innately pleasurable, so that the alienated or stuck (ADD) child just naturally enjoys it. Pac-Man and other computer games thus are used to snag the attentional mechanism at stage 1 or 2 above. This does not really take that much, and we think of the studies in which isolated monkeys found it pleasurable to watch another monkey merely "doing its own thing" in an adjoining room, or even a model railroad train going round and round on a track. So biofeedback or neurofeedback commences with simple tasks in which something changes—color, size, shape. A car runs on a track toward a distant landscape, a balloon flies higher, a little guy comes out and jumps up and down, and there is the sound of applause!

The LENS is different. I believe that because the learner does nothing voluntary or volitional whatever, the learning is thus subliminal, and happens by itself. The most a person may feel is a mild sense of well-being after a session. Sometimes a headache goes away, or a pain is lessened. At least the situation is painless and neutral or slightly positive, and the slow-yielding rewards must accrue over the next period of time. For discerning souls in need of help, this is often enough. Over the weeks and months of training, whichever kind of feedback is used, a kind of neurological internal logjam is gradually broken up and disassembled, and small successes may accumulate into visible behavioral gains.

As the attentional mechanism is freed up, there may be more economic currency or resources made available, and the whole topic to which the pattern of avoidance has developed now seems more approachable. In the best outcomes, there is a natural resumption of motivational reward, so that it comes to resemble those tasks that were effortless in the first place (and thus easily became the goals of hyperfocusing). People keep coming back because their lives are getting easier; they exert less effort, in effect "paying less" while still paying attention. Learning is less of an ordeal. They are in less discomfort than they used to be—and they know it. They will thus seek the context or the curious, playful learning that makes them feel better.

We should now return to brain wave theory. Speed of functioning seems related both to skill and reward of mental activity. The pharmaceutical approach prides itself that a brain on Ritalin or Dexedrine functions better. Stimulate the brain and nervous system, in a global way, and it finds the world interesting again. A level of mental functioning that previously seemed impossible to the ADD child is now accessible. Once the energy has been made available, at least as the theory goes, new habits develop, and the intrinsic reward mechanism spelled out above takes over. Unfortunately for the pharmacological model, there is something also called state-dependent learning, so that when the medicine is withdrawn, the learning also regresses to its previous state. With neurofeedback, it seems, this is less likely to happen because there is no global inundation of medicine and no withdrawal.

The Theta/Beta Ratio

For several decades now, neurofeedback has helped neuroscience in general understand which brain wave patterns foster optimal attention and learning. That is, there are some brain waves that foster sensory "capture-and-hold," in which the inner cognitive processes reach out to the external learning opportunity and import the new information into the nervous system. Since the work of Lubar (1999) and Monastra (2000), this understanding has been geared to the frequency of the brain activity, and substantial evidence has been acquired that it is the ratio of beta (12 Hz and higher), compared to theta (4–8 Hz) that tells the attentional story. Gibbs and Knott (Gibbs and Knott 1949), early EEG researchers, had shown during the 1940s that the EEG gradually speeds up in the course of development, so that by the time the child is encountering (and hopefully mastering) increasingly complex or abstract subjects, there is lots of beta accessible for that process of attention, and "sensory capture and hold."

Infants spend much more time in sleep than adults, and even in their waking brain waves, the slower frequencies predominate. Delta (5–4 Hz), those the huge, slow, lazy ocean waves, prevail when the "control center" (the brain-dominated CNS) is quiet, and vegetative processes, digestion, and physiological repair are carried on. When delta is missing in the EEG, this can be a sign of disturbance of sleep architecture and inability to sleep deeply and recuperatively.

Theta (4–8 Hz) comes gradually to predominate in the waking EEG as the young child grows and represents immersion in what Freud called "primary process thinking." This type of affectively driven cognitition contains elements of wish-fulfillment and narcissism and is also called "magical thinking," because it substitutes fantasy for outer reality. An excess of theta implies an inner world in which surges of pleasurably toned endogenous activity predominate over any information or learning requests from the outside. Because it is self-contained, it is considered autistic in nature. Theta arises effortlessly, especially when compared to the (effortful) higher frequencies involved in active learning (beta, 12 Hz+).

Simplified, the theory implies that paying attention requires a more activated, sped-up brain. Physiologically, resources are utilized, the simplest earmarks of which may be blood flow and glucose metabolism—the very processes that are studied in many brain-imaging techniques. And we have all heard it said that the activated brain is an energy hog, utilizing up to a quarter or a third of all the available blood sugar or oxygen in the body, to keep its level of functioning high.

Hence the paradoxical use of stimulant medications to help ADD and ADHD. At first glance it seems counterintuitive that you would give more "speed" to an already revved-up, hyperactive kid. But here's the rub: while the child speeds around restlessly *in search of stimulation,* his brain waves are dominated by slowed theta. The medical approach goes right for the gusto, using a pharmaceutical agent to change the theta/beta ratio—that is, to support the attention-focusing mechanism. And we have all seen it work, at least in the short term. Speed up the child's brain so that the processing itself is less effortful, and tasks that before seemed impossible, or simply distasteful, may now seem pleasurable. For children who can tolerate them, stimulant medications produce the most dramatically visible effects. But those effects, experience also shows us, wear off, and with them, the positive mood aspects as well; the medicated children (or adults) slip into a refractory period in which they become easily angered and frustrated, and even ordinary life, let alone paying attention, becomes compromised. So the pharmaceutical companies developed sustained-release versions of Ritalin and Dexedrine to prolong those high-functioning states. And indeed they do, but at what cost? The cumulative effect of stimulant medication seems to be that the brain does not work so nicely or smoothly when the pharmaceutical is withdrawn. In effect, the stimulant robs Peter to pay Paul. The speeding up has come at a price, and certain resources (brain nutrients) are exhausted.

Neurofeedback for ADD

Coming back then to neurofeedback, which uses natural means to get the brain to speed up on its own: yes, resources are also consumed in this process, but the neurobiochemical environment has not been tampered with. Even better, if the neurofeedback is done with an already nutritionally supported brain, there are nutritional "deep pockets" to draw upon, neurotransmitter precursors from which the brain fashions its own agents for speeding or slowing. Notable among these precursors are the long-chain fatty acids such as omega 6 and 9—to balance the omega 3s, especially docosahexanoic acid (DHA), which specifically crosses the blood-brain barrier; the whole family of B vitamins; vitamin D (and with it K); and substances such as phosphatidyl serine, which support the phospholipids ecology of the brain. More on these nutrients can be learned in the following source: Brown, Gerbarg, and Muskin 2009.

Several different protocols that affect the theta/beta ratio are "reward beta," say 15–18 Hz, or "reward beta, inhibit theta." When I first studied with Siegfried and Sue Othmer, they often used this protocol, with the caveat that too much beta can leave the person (child or adult) with a kind of hard-edged mental focus that almost resembles children's reactions to stimulants. Another problem is that theta has indispensable functions in our mental lives. It is the brain wave that seems to help the hippocampus consolidate certain memories, putting an emotional stamp on them: "important" or "unimportant." Theta is also involved in creativity, imagination, and understanding the emotional inflection of a speech or drama, or even a facial expression.

The Othmers found that if beta training "winds the brain up too much"—and indeed it can, from my own personal and clinical experience—

the use of the Lubar-pioneered SMR training (also called low beta, 12–15 Hz) at Cz or C4 (the contralateral point to C3 where mental-focus training was often done) "calms it down." We remember SMR or sensorimotor rhythm was first observed above the sensorimotor cortex of motionless cats waiting expectantly for a mouse, so they can pounce in an instant. Sterman found training the cats to this rhythm made them less likely to have seizures even when dosed with a seizure-inducing chemical called monomethylhydrazine, which was causing convulsions in NASA technicians and astronauts working around, or aboard, space rockets. Lubar had reasoned that if SMR worked to reduce convulsive activity and promote immobility, it might work for ADHD children.

It did, and it became one of the most commonly used neurofeedback protocols. It is also one of the best ways to reduce seizurelike activity in the brain.

There are some types of ADD that do not respond well to the protocols mentioned above. Some, with irritability and restlessness, *are actually associated with an excess of beta,* especially high beta (22–28 Hz). The presence of these waveforms can indicate that the brain is irritated or inflamed, and the behavioral sequelae of high beta are insomnia, irritability, hypervigilance, and, when found temporally, anger. Sometimes there is a well-recognized "earmuff" pattern of the high beta localized in the temples (T3–T4). This is sometimes, but not always, associated with trauma or abuse. We have seen it more than once in adults who told us their fathers used to "box their ears" for misbehavior. Here alpha training (8–12 Hz) to soothe the high beta might be indicated.

But there are also subtypes of ADD in which the alpha is much too high in amplitude, ragged in appearance, or badly placed in the head. Alpha, as we have established, is neutral on the gearshift, midway between high and low, and the default rhythm, in which the brain is idling or doing nothing. The alpha of meditators is often a beautiful, smooth undulating sine wave of about 10 Hz. But when there is very high alpha posteriorly (say 30+ microvolts) with a ragged appearance, it can betoken a type of inattentive ADD, or anxiety, or both (anxious inattention). High alpha found frontally is usually not regarded as good for cognition and may represent extreme rumination. Slowed alpha anywhere on the head, especially around 8 Hz, may signal compromised cognition.

One very encouraging fact is that whenever large-scale ADD interventions have been conducted, there are substantially good results across the board. One might look at the work of Vince Monastra and the wonderful Yonkers School Project with Linda Vergara (the principal, whose own child had ADD), Mary Jo Sabo, and Joel Lubar. The logistics of this program were so formidable that despite the early encouraging results, funding ran out, and the school administration changed; so there was no completion, and no publication came out of it.

Dr. J. Lawrence Thomas Uses HEG: Blood Flow to the Brain with a Case of ADD

One form of biofeedback that seems to provide a direct allocation of resources to the brain is hemoencephalography (HEG); more on this later, but in this promising approach for ADD, blood flow—with its accompanying oxygen and glucose—is simply redirected to the frontal area of the brain. Inundated with nutrients and oxygen, the frontal cortex begins to perform much better (and the EEG is likely to speed up). The pioneer of the method, Hershel Toomim, when I interviewed him at the age of ninety-plus, had a mind that showed few if any signs of aging: "I just put two and two together. Most higher functioning, including executive functioning of the brain, takes place in the frontal area. If I could teach people to increase blood flow to that area, more cognitive resources would be available, and they would 'feel smarter.'" (The complete interview with Dr. Toomim, which I conducted at the Denver 2010 meeting of the International Society for Neurofeedback and Research [ISNR], along with Dr. Jeffrey Carmen, a clinical psychologist from upstate New York, probably the most highly regarded clinician who uses this method, is found in chapter 13.)

I was recently able to observe the clinical use of HEG in action in the office of one of my colleagues, Dr. Larry Thomas. The ten-year-old boy in the chair was the son of a United Nations staff member who said that because of ADD she had almost had to withdraw the child from an elite private school in Geneva. Now he was at a comparable one in New York, which had boded equally poorly, until the child had started with

Dr. Thomas. On a break from seeing patients myself, I was curious to see what the neuropsychologist, who also does complete neuropsych exams on both children and adults, would do.

The first part of the training I observed was HeartMath, in which the child sat for about ten minutes, regulating his breathing. First the little boy brought life and color to a garden scene, then flew a balloon over obstacles, all by regulating his breath—and underneath it, affected indirectly, was his heart-rate variability, or HRV, on a screen. The goal is to have a smooth, undulating sine wave, with amplitudes as high as possible. Children will often have a 10–30 bpm, or beats per minute, variability with each breath. (Even as a stand-alone, this method is so effective with schoolchildren that in 2005 HeartMath Institute won a million-dollar grant from a conservative congress during the Bush administration, because the institute presented studies showing its efficacy for ADD and reducing behavior problems.) By the end of just this part of the session, the boy appeared very calm and still.

HeartMath is one of the oldest heart-rate variability training methods in the field, but it also adds something others do not: a mental focus on the heart itself, along with focusing on positive thoughts and appreciation. The ideal "coherent" breath rate (the one that produces the highest HRV, while reducing cardiovascular stress) varies with the age of the child, but the general range in child or adult is from 5–7 breaths per minute. The simple but effective biofeedback programs are just to help the child or adult get it right. With enough practice, the learning extends to natural breathing, increasing its efficiency, with accompanying physical and mental benefits.

But the HRV training was only Dr. Thomas's entreé to the HEG training. An age-appropriate movie with talking animals and slapstick events was put on. The child's only task was to keep watching the movie (and the movie came on strong and clear when the child increased blood flow to the frontal lobes).

As we watched the movie strengthen and fade, I conversed quietly with the mother. She told me that Dr. Thomas's training regimen had been dramatically effective. Her son was no longer in danger of being kicked out of school and had improved his grades from near-flunking to

Bs and an occasional A. More positively for the home environment, it was no longer a battle to get him to sit down and do his homework; in fact, sometimes it was so easy that the mother would gear up for the traditional fight, only to find the homework already neatly and quickly done.

The combined method of breath training first and HEG second assures that the child is already calm (without tranquilizers!) and that there is sufficient blood-borne oxygen available for the brain to speed up its processing. And of course, best of all, there is no refractory period, because the stimulant medication is now gone and the brain is no longer exhausted and frazzled. This child's mother left me in no doubt that she considered Dr. Thomas's intervention effective for both her child's academic performance and his personality in general (no more tantrums when the medication wears off). "It helps the person consciously to calm down and focus, first," he said. "Then when they start the HEG training—it's a little more subtle, they have to change their blood flow to their brain—they're calm and ready to go. The combination is great." I had to agree after I heard the glowing report from the mother that it was working.

A comparable process is happening with neurofeedback or EEG biofeedback, perhaps a little more slowly, because the brain has to deliver its own resources without being shown exactly how. In the beginning, longer training times can exhaust the child or adult brain in order to meet the training goals. Likewise with the LENS, and we have found that when the stimulation—or the training time—is too strong or disruptive that behavior deteriorates, and there is a setback in clinical improvement as well.

Angelo Bolea, a skilled practitioner near Washington, D.C., uses very short training times—three minutes or five minutes—especially in the early phases of training, and gets good results.

In general, we have found that the younger the child, the easier the biofeedback or neurofeedback "fix." That is to say, the younger ADD child has not yet developed the compensation mechanisms, avoidant patterns, and subterfuges of the older child or the ADD adult. But children and adults of whatever age can learn to speed up their brain metabolism naturally through biofeedback and thus overcome both motivational and attentional deficits in the way we have described above. In other words, without the use of artificial means (the stimulant medications) the brain has been fooled into adapting its own functioning to the learning environment. Motivation has been coaxed through the affectively neutral or mildly pleasurable learning reflected in the biofeedback task, and this in turn will transfer to the other learning tasks that await, rather than each new learning challenge precipitating a struggle or no-win conflict.

Neurofeedback Saves a Family

> Sam scored off the charts for memorization, pulling
> information back, with a few prompts, set after set.
> The neuropsychologist could not believe it. But I believe
> it was because the neurofeedback really primed his
> organizational abilities and memory.
>
> J.S., MOTHER OF SAM

We conclude this chapter with a clinical case from our own experience, which also has dramatic features. The referral came from Dr. Julian Isaacs, a veteran neurofeedback practitioner in California. He had qEEG mapped two boys, he said, aged eight and ten years, who were both ADHD and badly out of control. The mother who had gone to him for mapping was a business executive and single mom (she had her hands full). Dr. Isaacs said he was just gaining some respect for the LENS and knew that was our major modality—but these boys, from clinical observation and the qEEG, were both definitely ADHD.

The first time the family came to see us at our upstate center, J.S., the well-spoken mom, sat down with me while the boys ran around outside screaming, already going where they weren't supposed to and getting into mischief. As she talked about what her life was like, she broke into tears.

It took the all wiles of my charming associate, Alexandra Linardakis, and me to get the two boys, one after the other, into the treatment chair and mapped. While we were focused on one, the other was wreaking inevitable mischief in the background (we had just a tidbit of Mom's daily dilemma).

Since the family lived in New York City, Alexandra (Lexsea), one of my senior clinicians, who was there every week, did most of the treatments, while I saw the boys about once a month. Lexsea was wonderful in the difficult task of managing the boys in an office suite in which there were many other therapists doing quiet and serious work with their clients. The two boys, with their nanny, less often their mom, would arrive like a veritable storm, and she had to invent ever-more-skillful ruses with art projects and play to keep them from ruffling the urban therapy center. We had regular phone sessions with the mom. The boys had the usual ups and downs, periodic reports of dramatic improvement and others of sliding back. There were also unsolicited reports of improvements and breakthroughs by school officials, child-care workers, and family members.

Mom said, "I'm impressed enough so I'm going to do this regularly for myself based on what I've seen with the boys." We conferred a little and did a map, which, not unsurprisingly, was not so dissimilar to the boys' maps. Mom confessed that despite her high level of professional functioning, she suffered from some attentional problems herself. We were off and running to a whole-family intervention.

Interview with J.S.

STEPHEN: Thank you so much for taking time away from you busy life to talk to me. I'll nudge you every now and then with questions, but I really want to hear you tell your story.

J.S.: I'm the mother of two boys. When I brought them in a couple of years ago, they both had prediagnosed learning issues. My older son, Sam, then ten, had auditory and visual processing issues, ADHD, and dyslexia. Mark, the younger one, then eight, had ADHD, dyslexia, and OCD. Together, it was a lot!

I was really on my own on this. The doctors wanted to recommend cocktails of prescription medications, and I didn't want to do that. The boys' dad didn't seem interested; he just wanted to have a good time when they visited. I had researched the alternatives, and that's how I found biofeedback.

When I saw it working with the boys, I decided to try the neurofeedback myself to see what it was like.

What a great payoff! I had no idea how much it would help me, and thus would help them. As caretakers, sometimes we forget to help ourselves!

STEPHEN: I encourage people to do that if they can. Then they can relate to what their children are experiencing.

J.S.: I know there were lots of ups and down, roller coasters, not straight-forward progress or instantaneous miracles. The first month or two, it was just "keeping the faith, baby!" and being very methodical, doing appointments. Then I noticed they were a little more organized, there was a little less conflict between them. Those outbursts that were so difficult for a single mom to manage calmed down.

STEPHEN: How long did that take?

J.S.: I would say about a month. Then we settled down to being able to see what was happening with each child. My older one was har-dier. The younger one was totally different, very sensitive, so we reduced treatment.

STEPHEN: I have to say you were very good about keeping track—phone or e-mail.

J.S.: We would monitor the treatment that day or the next evening. That's when the response to treatment was exhibited. We would know if one or the other was having a meltdown and not being able to hold himself together. Often we would we reduce the treatment, and that worked a lot better. After six months I would know the moment we left the session if it was right; they would be more organized and calm on the way home.

STEPHEN: An observant parent helps us tweak things just right.

J.S.: Yes, absolutely. Over time it kept compounding. They became able to manage their own reactions to things, which is hard for an ADHD kid. Then when we had been doing it a little over a year, I had to have them tested for a new school system, and we were sent to a neuro-psychologist. Sam scored off they charts for memorization, pulling information back, with a few prompts, set after set. The neuropsychologist could not believe it. But I believe it was because the neurofeedback really primed his organizational abilities and memory.

We came every week pretty faithfully. I think it supported them. They are both on the lowest dose of one kind of medication, and they are very high performing in a mainstream setting now. I think the neurofeedback helped us do the minimum we had to do.

STEPHEN: I'm so happy for your little—er, now bigger—guys. Could you describe what you experienced doing it yourself?

J.S.: The surprise for me was that it was enhancing my own capacities, not only mentally but emotionally, so that over time I was able to hold it together, not only for myself but in being a parent, riding the roller coasters of emotion that kids naturally experience. I was much more steady and capable, not only at home but at work. There was a time when my obligations almost doubled, with hiring and all that, and I started coming twice a week because it strengthened my capacity to hold it all.

STEPHEN: Would you share a little about what you do?

J.S.: I do all the strategy and all the human resources elements for a Fortune 200. By that I mean "succession planning." I oversee all the recruiting. If we're hiring the CEO, or the president of a division, I do that search and am responsible for hiring that person. I also do learning and development, you could say, the performance management, across all our business units. And then I run all of the diversity components, or programs, including goal-setting for our company.

A pretty high-profile job; my performance is either obviously successful—or obviously not.

STEPHEN: Wow! I thought I knew how to juggle. All that and the kids, basically by yourself?

J.S.: I became more discerning with the kids and less affected by it emotionally. I used to feel exhausted, exasperated, and a bump with them would throw me for a loop. I think the neurofeedback strengthened my core self. I could see it:

"They're having a fight right now! That's what's happening."

I was able to let it kind of roll off my back; I was more detached emotionally. I often found that the exact same problem that would have caused a meltdown before, even the same intensity, wouldn't affect me the same way.

STEPHEN: Did you notice reactions, yourself or the kids, getting sharper and shorter?

J.S.: Yes, but I also had more of a purview. When I started my neuro-feedback, I didn't have all those pieces, and so that's when I started coming twice a week. It helped me grow my capacity. When I look at executives, it's about their capacity to hold all the information and to be efficient with their time. It's about being able to make the decisions you have to make today and to plan your work and not to be swept away emotionally. That kind of discernment really fell into place with the neurofeedback.

STEPHEN: I think we're talking about multiprocessing. Kids–work, work–kids; each one stretches you in a different way.

J.S.: I don't know if I'd be able to do the kind of work I do today without it, as dramatic as that sounds, because of the capacity issue. I could feel myself growing. I was starting to feel anxious about whether I could do it all. I did it until I felt I achieved a certain level of capacity, then I backed off.

I don't know if I told you what I do after I come here. I do fifteen minutes of meditation to pull what happens in my head down into my heart. It's about broadening my awareness.

STEPHEN: That's so cool. Do you feel something happen when you do that?

J.S.: I do the breathing, the HeartMath. From an executive standpoint, I notice that when I've increased my capacity and my ability to process things, I get to see what is the top end of someone else's capacity.

I look across the team and where they are, and I see where they're bumping up against the top, and where they're not.

I've added the heart meditation to keep from having too hard an edge and being too much in my brain. I have a little more compassion, not such a hard edge. I see all the chess pieces, and I'm moving them with more softness.

STEPHEN: Is there an intelligence of the heart?

J.S.: If I move people with the heart intelligence, they get inspired to be the best they can be, and you can move them into a place of just believing in themselves and giving their best; so I find myself surrounded by loyal people who want to give me their best.

STEPHEN: I'm learning from you with every word. That's superb! Do you have any last words for parents who might think about neurofeedback for their kids?

J.S.: I highly recommend doing it. If I were talking to another parent who was considering neurofeedback, I would encourage them to do it together.

I think I received something more on that other level than that mental or executive place. You know, it was a deepening of my motherhood; a leap of faith to try an alternative method. I had a lot of naysayers, including the psychiatrists who were treating the boys with medicines, and the schools, which were special-education schools, and whose teachers looked at me like I was crazy. But, you know, we all did this together, and we all three came out on the other end feeling stronger about ourselves. And I felt really good about my motherhood.

EIGHT

THE WONDERFUL WORLD OF ANXIETY

With Paul Botticelli, L.C.S.W.

Things in my mind, or brain, are now rounder. Before they were much more jagged, like spikey; and now they are rounder, softer, and that's a good thing!

LOIS, AN ANXIETY PATIENT

According to the NIMH [National Institute of Mental Health], 40 million people, about 18 percent of the population, suffers from anxiety disorder, whereas only about a third of that number, 6.7 percent, suffer from major depression.

THE ARCHIVES OF GENERAL PSYCHIATRY, 2005

Anxiety and Stress

I would like to start this chapter by saying just *a few nice things about anxiety* (before the other shoe drops). Anxiety seems built into us to get our attention, and it works beautifully up to a certain point. Bad or inattentive children can be made to pay attention by threatening punishment or social humiliation. A test or deadline looming up can mobilize anxiety. So can important occasions such as weddings or other ceremonies, particularly those where a person is singled out or may have to stand in front of lots of people. Public speaking, is, of course, one of the most common instances in which anxiety appears (in this instance, it can either mobilize intense focus or be really disabling).

I once was sitting with the famous mythologist Joseph Campbell before he was due to speak to a small rural audience. A trained psychotherapist, I thought I sensed he was anxious. "Joe," I said, "you speak to larger, far more prestigious audiences than this one. Surely you're not anxious?"

"Of course I am," he whispered. "I always am before a lecture. If I'm not anxious, then I get really anxious! Wait'll you see what I do with it!"

When he started talking, there were feats of historical and mythological memory, awesome scholarship, verbal and poetic pyrotechnics *de toute sorte;* he wowed the audience. We went out to dinner afterward. He had refused any alcohol with lunch, before his talk, but now he was sitting in front of a large fireplace in a four-star restaurant with friends. As he sat there with his Glenlivet (his favorite Scotch), he twinkled at me. "See?"

"Oh, yeah, I do, I do!" I said, full of admiration.

"I do some inner alchemy," he said. "It's just excitement rising—anxiety can be energy in disguise!" I got it. Prone to anxiety myself, I have been using Campbell's approach ever since. Whether in public presentations—or even while doing extreme sports that contain inherent anxiety, like trapeze, karate, rock climbing—I think of my friend and smile inwardly, saying: "If I'm not anxious, then I should be really anxious!"

On another occasion Campbell talked about a yogi he had met in India who was one hundred years old. He owned nothing, went naked most of the time, and depended upon gifts of alms for his daily food. "Anxiety doesn't eat me!" the old man would say waggishly. "Oh, no; I eat anxiety!"

Anxiety: The Great Awakener

I once knew a professional man, Arthur, who seemed incapable of anxiety. He was very well informed; he would read the newspaper for a long time each morning. He ran a consulting firm, and he would chat amiably with the staff, sometimes for hours. (They liked him, but there evolved a kind of lackadaisical atmosphere in the office, which meant that not much got done.)

In the afternoon he would take a long lunch, with a few drinks, and in the evening get caught up in going to a bar to watch sports on television. His wife, who carried all the anxiety in the family, wondered if he was alcoholic, but it seemed to be more the atmosphere and the nice big screen for watching the games (he had a small old TV at home) that he craved. Income tax returns were never done on time, but there seemed to be no great concern about any of that. He came in for a brain-mapping only under duress, prodded by family members, and with the urgency that the business was sliding slowly but inexorably downhill and his firm might get evicted from their premises.

Arthur's brain map, even though he was an intelligent man, showed an abundance of slow-wave activity, lots of theta and some frontal delta. Alpha itself, and the higher-frequency brain waves, were almost nonexistent. It was a kind of "Walter Mitty" syndrome. He was leading a fantasy life, not a real one. I suggested that he might want to get a good physical to see if there were a thyroid problem, or see a psychiatrist to be put on stimulants, because the situation was deteriorating. I suggested frequent neurofeedback and lots of brain nutrients, as well as a program of moderate physical exercise. But Arthur went about his usual existence without a change and didn't follow through with appointments.

When he lost his business for nonpayment of rent, he got an extra mortgage and thought he would work at home. I though this was a bad idea and told him so: "Your main problem is, ultimately, *a lack of anxiety,* and probably some metabolic insufficiency." He did a few more infrequent and desultory neurofeedback sessions, but we never could get him up to 10 Hz alpha as a prevalent frequency, or much beta, especially frontally.

Ultimately, Arthur's daydream existence caught up with him, and his house was about to be foreclosed. He finally called me up with some excitement in his voice: "I think I have some anxiety—it woke me up last night."

"Great," I said. "But this treatment works kind of slowly. I don't think even if you came in three times a week it would save your house. You'd better think about stimulant medication—here's a prescribing psychiatrist's number." (I knew he still wasn't anxious enough about his predicament to come regularly. He didn't, and he is now living in an apartment on Social Security—*all for lack of anxiety!*) His wife still works, and she loyally stays with Arthur—after all he is a very gentle, pleasant man.

Anxiety wakes us up, figuratively and literally. It says, "This is important, and until it is resolved, you can't think about anything else at all." In an important article entitled "Who Says Stress Is Bad for You?" *Newsweek* kind of blows the whistle on the medical fundamentalism that says, "Stress is the number one killer!" *Anxiety can also be good for you*—and here is where biofeedback and neurofeedback come in—*if it is managed successfully.* The very *idea of stress* sometimes stresses us out!

The Human Stress Response

The stress response was discovered by a clumsy biologist. On his way to do endocrine experiments on rats, the now famous Canadian biologist Hans Selye would inevitably drop some of the animals and then chase them around frantically with a broom until he got them back into the correct cage. Then he injected the rats with substances both experimental (various drugs) and placebo (saline solution) with equally clumsy zeal. The rats all developed "general adaptation syndrome," even the ones who received the neutral saline solution, starting with multiple ulcers, enlarged adrenals, and immune dysfunction. If the stress continued, these symptoms were followed by complete exhaustion and then rodent death.

The term *general adaptation syndrome,* coined by Selye, means that the stress response is adaptive. His rats' bloodstreams surged with adrenaline, then with cortisol. For a little while the rats had amazing physical energy—the basis of survival—plus heightened senses and memory. But when the stress persisted, the neurons began to shrivel and the synapses degenerate, particularly in the hippocampus and prefrontal cortex. "Acutely stress helps us remember some things better," says Bruce McEwan of Rockefeller University. "Chronically it makes us worse at remembering other things, and it impairs our mental flexibility" (Carmichael 2009).

And different strokes for different folks. Psychologist Salvatore

Maddi's studies of 430 employees at Illinois Bell during a major crisis showed that two-thirds of the group suffered terribly—strokes, heart attacks, depression, obesity, divorce. But one third remained healthy, found new jobs, and adapted somehow. What distinguished these guys? Had they grown up in peaceful, psychologically healthy circumstances? Not necessarily; large numbers of the healthy survivors had had tough childhoods. But their parents convinced them they were the hope of the family, and so they had to survive! "That led to their being very hardy people," Maddi said in the *Newsweek* article. "They had grown from the stress."

I also became very interested in Robert Sapolsky's baboons. Among the dominant males he studied were some of what were called "totally insane son of a bitch"–type baboons, whose anger, effectively, was their power. Next to them in the hierarchy, however, was a group of alpha baboons who didn't seem to need to be angry all the time, nor did they fight often. When they did pick a fight, it was one they could win. They enjoyed all the privileges of being high in the pecking order, had all the same competition for females and power struggles, but the stress didn't seem to faze them. Sapolsky would joke they were the "Zen baboons." These baboons were healthier than their angry counterparts.

Sometimes I work with the chronically angry, who suffer from irritability and explosiveness. Not infrequently, their brain waves are in the high-beta range, particularly in the anterior and posterior temporal lobes (known for their connection with emotion, among other things). Also not infrequently, such people were physically or emotionally abused in childhood. The high beta seems to betoken a state of hypervigilance, waiting for that other shoe to drop or another bomb to go off (if they had a military career). This EEG work confirms the gist of the general adaptation syndrome: these people are often in a state of hyperarousal that has become chronic; they can't turn it off even if they want to. In our office, where we see a lot of New Yorkers, we joke about the "high-beta queens" who are nervous urban, often professional, women who can't stop talking—even though the content of what is being communicated is repetitive, going around and around. Asking them to calm down or slow down does nothing, but we have seen again and again that after, say, ten or more visits, and without quite knowing how, *they do slow down.* Their family members subsequently report not feeling so sucked into the cloud of anxiety.

Not to neglect the male side of things, we have also seen really angry human "insane SOBs" gradually become more like Sapolsky's Zen baboons. When they calm down, their physiological problems, such as high blood pressure or acid stomach, calm down as well—and they mostly get their needs met!

In the *DSM IV,* anxiety is found in many disorders with other names, such as depression (as in "anxious depression"), OCD, PTSD, and so forth. It also comes in many other forms, from "generalized anxiety disorder," in which the anxiety seems to attend every aspect of life, to highly specific forms in which the anxiety is due to certain situations: about anything from public speaking, to sports, to performing musically. When the anxiety is intense and focused on these symbolic situations, and is irrational compared to the threat of the situation, we call them "phobias." Think of the many Greek names for the things people fear: *claustrophobia* (fear of being closed in, or trapped), *agoraphobia* (fear of the "marketplace," or going out in public). There is the famous movie *Arachnophobia* (fear of spiders), which, of course, the movie exploits to a high degree with giant spiders; then there is fear of things so seemingly silly only Monty Python could make a movie about it: *alektorophobia* (fear of chickens)—or those who could be said to be "chicken of the chickens"—Colonel Sanders, beware!

Sometimes anxiety becomes so intense it shades into panic disorder. Here the ordinary physiological symptoms that accompany anxiety (butterflies in the stomach, heart pounding, shortness of breath, dry mouth, and clammy skin) become so severe, the person may feel he or she is about to die. Panic attacks are known to account for a fairly large number of visits to the emergency room. Physicians routinely screen for it among genuine physiological emergencies, and Valium becomes one of their most frequently employed emergency room drugs.

Anxiety Central

So anxiety has its purposes and fits into the ecology of human survival. It alerts us to what is important and necessary to our well-being. But we have all at some point felt how crippling and uncomfortable it can seem. The musician fumbles his notes or forgets passages. The public speaker becomes inaudible, stumbles over words, loses her place in the speech. There is one point in the old "Peanuts" cartoon in which Lucy is offering five-cent psychotherapy. When she elicits what Charlie is afraid of, she finally says brilliantly: "Pantophobia! Charlie Brown, you are afraid of everything!" That is to say, anxiety can move into the core of our being and occupy center stage. There may be a mixture of generalized anxiety and phobia—or one of its variants.

The earliest popular "tranquilizers" were for anxiety: Librium, Valium, Xanax (in the benzodiazepine family). These drugs did indeed decrease anxiety for many people, at least while they were in the system, but they also proved to be quite addictive, and people claimed they felt "stupider," were forgetful, and made lots of mistakes. The SSRIs, such as Prozac and Zoloft, nominally antidepressants, were also found to inhibit anxiety and panic as well as depression. This goes along with the concept of anxiety-driven depression, which we consider in a subsequent section.

The following case is of Yveline, a teacher whose anxiety became so bad that it threatened to ruin her career. All her friends insisted she go on medication. She was desperate, but having had an early bad reaction to medications, she was determined not go down that road again. This case is chosen because it communicates how anxiety feels and where it comes from.

Relieving Yveline's Anxiety

Yveline had lines from worry on her face when she first came to us. As a public high school teacher, she often faced classrooms of thirty-five distractible wise guys. At her best, she had an irresistible sense of humor and great warmth, and she won her students over. At her worst, she could barely keep it together as the little hooligans went after her or simply got more and more unruly. A major problem was that she often felt hyper-vigilant, like jumping out of her skin, and she had insomnia with anxious rumination. The combination had her exhausted and at her wits' end.

I recommended a combination of HeartMath, the LENS, and psychotherapy, because I knew there were interpersonal issues at home having to do with the extreme anxiety. (Her spouse was actually very supportive and tolerant, but he was himself exhausted at the toll anxiety was extracting from Yveline.) When anxiety is severe, central, and chronic, it affects all those around us and can easily and readily ruin relationships—even whole families, depending upon how badly it is managed.

Within a few weeks the HeartMath breathing and exercises were actually helping a great deal. She was a quick learner, although she reported trouble in the beginning because her diaphragm was frozen up and wouldn't let her take a deep breath. This had to be worked with substantially, but since she had had acting lessons some years ago, she knew what she had to do to get sufficient oxygen (the term *angst* in German means "constriction"). She would practice breathing on the forty-five-minute commute to school each morning. Eventually she was able to breathe coherently during class and even when, or precisely when, the teenagers were at their most unruly.

I predicted that if we could get her sleeping well again, it would really help things along. A combination of melatonin and silimarin (milk thistle) was suggested and used nightly during the early weeks of treatment, while the neurofeedback did its work. It took about three weeks before it really swung the balance, but, astonished, she reported longer and longer periods of uninterrupted sleep. Now she had more stamina and didn't feel on the edge of a nervous breakdown any more, but still the anxiety persisted.

Yveline had not reported any dreams for years, but now they came. Many were turgid, uncomfortable, almost nightmarish, pointing to an area for further exploration: early-life traumas, and something usually quite inaccessible to talk therapy: perinatal anxiety on the part of her mother. She had tried earlier to get to this through talk therapy, but it had gotten nowhere. But neurofeedback seemed to be "stirring the pot" so that we could see the contents of the anxiety stew come bubbling to the surface.

The place from which the anxiety welled, in a ceaseless flow, it seemed, had no words to describe it. It was silent. But we both knew it when we had gotten there. Quite simply, World War II had separated her Russian parents. Pregnant and alone, her mother ended up in a displaced-persons camp in Poland. It wasn't quite a concentration camp, but it was filled with terrified displaced persons from many cultures disrupted by the war. It was into this bleak landscape that Yveline had been born and in which she spent the next couple of years growing up until the war's end in 1945.

Talk therapy does not reach down into this zone, because language skills were acquired only later, along the way. And we both believe that what she was experiencing was not her own early-life events, but her mother's emotions while she both carried and nursed the young infant. Some people do not believe in such transmission of primal emotions, but many do (and convincing clinical cases have been collected in Dr. Thomas Verny's *The Secret Life of the Unborn Child*). Mainstream psychiatry and psychology are now becoming fully aware that *the emotional condition of the mother while she is carrying her child communicates to the child.* Her mother was, in fact, inundated with anxiety from shortly after the time Yveline was conceived until well after her birth. There were events in the world far too large for her, or anyone, to do anything about. Before becoming a practitioner of clinical neurofeedback, I had encountered such cases, and I always felt helpless as a psychotherapist. Guided imagery and hypnosis could sometimes help, but the anxiety would bubble up again.

I believe the LENS form of neurotherapy is effective precisely because it cuts to the primal level, even well below rewards and punishment and operant conditioning. I believe it even can help with classically conditioned phobias and fears.

"Okay," I said to Yveline. "This stuff is so deep and so old, we need a miracle; neurofeedback, do your stuff."

Of course, nothing happened—at least right away. We kept on. Psychotherapy allowed Yveline to explore her conflict-ridden relationship with her mother, who had passed on some years before. "Mother was dominated by anxiety," she said. "It affected everything she ever did. I swore I'd never be like her, but I think I am—and our two anxieties are like a witches' brew. We were never able to enjoy each other at all!"

In psychotherapy we also found ourselves doing relationship counseling to help save her current partnership from the fate of the two previous ones.

But months went by and Yveline's anxiety began to come down, notch by notch, on the subjective symptom scale. She was sleeping better and remembering her dreams, and their complexion gradually began to change from no-exit scenarios to more ordinary ones. The coherent breathing exercises had become part of her life. In the beginning, the HRV would go crazy when I asked her to do a prominent part of the HeartMath regimen—which was to *think of something positive* (I have seen this again and again with traumatized people, and often will leave it out of the instructions until much later down the pike).

We remapped several times, and the most recent mapping showed some really substantial changes in the high beta that dominated certain central areas of her brain.

The shift came when I caught Yveline memorizing a script in the waiting room. "Humph," I said. "Memory a little better?" "Oh, yes," she said, smiling sweetly. "I told you I've been getting parts in plays and going back into acting. In a couple of months I'll be doing a one-woman show based on a script I wrote!"

"You're cured!" I said and stalked out of the waiting room—only to peek my head in a moment later. We laughed and hugged. "I was going to ask you if I could come a little less often," she said.

"Tapering off is a pretty good way to do it, so we don't go cold turkey, which sometimes backfires," I said. "I think we'll both know when it's time to stop."

A little cloud of worry seemed to sweep across her face. "As long as I can come back in if I get really anxious!"

"It's a deal," I said, and we both laughed again. (And after we finished up two years ago, she hasn't been back!)

Anxiety-Driven Depression

Although, as I described at the beginning of this chapter, anxiety disorders in our culture seem to enjoy a greater prevalence than major depression, what was left out of this figure is a factor called "comorbidity," or the occurrence of both together. According to some estimates, this may be as high as 50 to 60 percent, and statistical analyses show that this overlap group is at much higher risk for suicidality. However, there is disagreement on which comes first—the chicken or the egg, anxiety or depression.

What is known is that when anxiety shows up earlier in life, followed by later depression, this is probably a much higher-risk patient than either disorder alone (Aina and Susman 2006).

The topic is well explored in the psychiatric literature, and I bring it up here because I think neurofeedback has a unique contribution to make to the conversation. For years, conventional wisdom has placed depression with underarousal and anxiety with overarousal, and the rule of thumb still holds in some cases. Prescribing physicians often want to speed up the depressed brain with stimulants or SSRIs like Prozac or dual-action antidepressants like Wellbutrin, which work on both the serotonin and epinephrine reuptake systems—keeping more active in the bloodstream so as to lift the patient's mood.

But in some depressed people, we would find over and over again much higher frequencies actively present in the brain. Frontal alpha or even SMR (low beta) or high beta that was quite high and almost never came down was often associated with a state of anxious arousal that led to exhaustion. It was the exhaustion that was experienced as depression. In this disorder, "there is no rest for the weary." The rumination and worry go on and on, thought tends to run circularly, and the same issues are rehearsed over and over, but with no resolution in sight. So irritability, explosiveness, insomnia, and fatigue are found all together (a little like the patient described above, who also felt she was depressed because she had so many catastrophic and dark thoughts—but they were, in fact, transformations of primordial anxiety).

There is, in fact, a right frontal activation that is said to be a particularly dangerous and volatile configuration that leads to hopelessness and suicide. At the same time the traditionally optimistic left frontal hemisphere is underaroused, and the homologous site (F3, F7, or Fp1) is unable to compensate for the well of anger and despair that boils out of F4, F8, or Fp2. This is Richard Davidson's theory, which is fairly well regarded in neurofeedback circles. The same configuration that is found in reactive attachment disorder (chapter 5), in which the right frontal cortex is unable to manage emotions, is also found in these agitated-depression patients.

So protocols in which the brain is encouraged to speed up or reward alpha would be decidedly counterproductive. Len Ochs says he has not found positive results from concentrating the treatments on either the left or right frontal areas; instead he follows the maps (including sometimes suppression maps to balance and calm the entire brain system—with the frontal areas coming along naturally). Traditional feedback protocols do inhibit alpha and higher—or any high-amplitude—activity, no matter what the frequency, in the right frontal, orbitofrontal, or prefrontal areas and uptrain the more optimistic left prefrontals that also promote clear thinking and better executive functions.

Lynda and Michael Thompson report a case that matches what we are describing in their comprehensive *The Neurofeedback Book*. The patient, called "John," was a twenty-five-year-old university student who, whenever he sat down to study, was inundated by ruminations. He complained of a low-grade depression (dysphoria) with anxiety. His main distinguishing feature was right frontal high beta in the 23–24 Hz range, averaging about 8.4 in ηv (the symbol for "microvolts") in amplitude. The left hemisphere at the homologous location was less than half the amplitude of the right 3.1, while the theta (rated at 6–10 Hz in their study) was the inverse in amplitude, 4.2 on the left and 2.4 on the right.

The Thompsons comment: "The client's mental activity relating to worrying and ruminating seems to correspond to a high amplitude, high beta activity. This may be a subtype of ADD in that the client is internally distracted by these thoughts and not attending to external stimulation. When the client becomes calm and focused, this excess high beta activity [in the right frontal region] decreases" (Thompson and Thompson 2003, 170). The successful intervention was accomplished by righting the imbalance and also uptraining SMR (sensorimotor rhythm), the range right above alpha (8–12Hz). Their range was 11–15 Hz. "Higher alpha" and SMR are associated with "relaxed alertness." They also taught John a metacognitive strategy, training up the 17 Hz that emerged when the patient was actively engaged in problem solving.

Once again, the general rule that applies to neurofeedback training protocols is not only to balance out the frequencies that aim at the middle (in theory, right around 10Hz) but, perhaps more importantly, to open the gateway to mental flexibility that allows one to settle into the appropriate state for the activity that is underway. The LENS specializes in this flexibility, but I believe that other traditional neurofeedback protocols do so as well—by asking the brain to try something else or bump out of its parking place.

Sometimes anxiety-driven depression and fatigue are not to be solved on the level of the brain. We have seen both as the consequence of infectious diseases, such as neurological post-Lyme symptoms. My own reaction to a flu or virus coming on is often racing thoughts and physical restlessness (leading to anxiety, insomnia, and fatigue). In these cases, there is no substitute for a thorough physical examination and a quest into the physiological causes that might be responsible—with appropriate medical treatment.

One head-injured patient, after a couple of years of LENS training, calmed down emotionally, recovered her cognitive and executive functions and her memory, but her high anxiety persisted. The EEG showed an extremely high alpha that would not budge. However, her HRV score showed that she had a lot of tachycardia (rapid heartbeat) and premature ventricular contractions. When people have this kind of deep visceral anxiety, it often shows up in extreme irregularities in the HRV—which in a healthy person is a nice sinusoidal wave, with ten beats per minute or more between the low frequency and the high (say sixty-five beats per minute at the low end and seventy-five or more at the high end). If the wave looks jagged or irregular, this is often a sign of anxiety. At this point I might either interrupt a session or ask the person to make a mental note of what they were thinking at the point that the disturbance entered the HRV. Almost invariably, they were breathing along, doing the exercise, when a rumination about an anxiety-producing issue came surging along on the stream of consciousness.

I then say, "Good! Now we're doing biofeedback! Lets see how long it takes you to come back to a nice sinusoidal or coherent wave. And then let's do it again, and again, 'proprioceptively' (internally) attending to the results." With the aforementioned patient, though, the HeartMath training proved almost intolerable for her, making her more rather than less anxious. (I think this had to do with an extreme hyperarousal of the sympathetic nervous system, the fight-or-flight branch of the autonomic nervous system or ANS.) Finally, with NeuroField, Z-score treatments, and finally with ILF or infra-low frequency neurofeedback, this patient began to feel more stable and less anxious.

These days I often tell people that anxiety is their ally (just like Tom Brown, Jr., who, in his books, makes the cold North Wind his ally, so that he could endure winter in the wilderness without warm clothing). I do the same with anger. Think of either, or both, as a kind of raw uprising of energy that we can learn to use or channel. Anxiety is often trying to get our attention about something, and anger is often an attempt to release or transcend a frustrating situation. Act the feeling and the energy out physically, so that it doesn't stagnate: pound a pillow, vocalize, feel the energy in your body and in your energy field. Above all, don't let it become chronic, unexpressed, and hence stagnant, because of the undeniable results of studies on prolonged stress—which destroys neurons and carries a raft of health problems with it. If talk therapy or life strategies and counseling fail to help your anxiety enough, consider biofeedback— or, best of all, a combination of both. It really works directly on some of the core issues in the dynamic life of the nervous system.

Does Anxiety Have a Shape?

As I have been working on this chapter, the LENS professional user group has been abuzz with conversation about anxiety. Some clinicians submitted that the LENS made their anxiety patients worse, and Ochs himself in some cases was advocating stopping treatment, at least for a while, before "stirring the pot" too frequently.

I had noticed the phenomenon myself. If you pop people out of their parking places and give them a lot more energy, they could become quite anxious. One woman with a histrionic tendency threw a fit and alienated a section of her family. I shamefacedly consulted with the psychiatrist who had referred her. "Oh, she's the Princess and the Pea," he said, referring to the fairy tale, where the delicate creature feels the pea under twenty mattresses; every single medication, or even life stresses, threw her into a hyper mode. "Don't worry about it!" I still did, and she stopped soon after—but later referred her children to us, so we knew that she believed in the power of the method.

We know that anxiety and sleep disturbance are intimately connected. It is possible that people's sleep can be disrupted by anxious rumination following treatment. We then back down, try another treatment modality, or recommend coherent breathing with yoga or t'ai chi for a while, then try neurofeedback again. During the user-group dialogue, the following case surfaced, declaring that the LENS could be used very effectively on anxiety, even in the early sessions. I include it because of its simplicity and clarity.

Calming Obsessive Thoughts: The Story of Lois
PAUL BOTTICELLI, L.C.S.W.

Lois is a woman in her mid-fifties who is married to a clinical psychologist and is the mother of their two adult children, She has worked as an office manager in her husband's private practice for the past eighteen years. Lois initiated treatment with LENS because of the following complaints: anxiety; obsessive, ruminative thought processes; disturbed sleep; low energy; mental distraction; negative mood—that is, she reported that she always felt down and that she was allowing way too many things to occupy her mind that were "silly," in that they were not really important, but she found herself obsessing about them anyway. Lois also reported that she felt her functioning was not up to par.

Because of her responses to the sensitivity questionnaire, and because of Lois's constitution, as a relatively thin woman who eats very little throughout her day and reports being sleep deprived daily, I chose to perform her first mapping with a least stim (LS) map (a "weak" mapping procedure used with sensitive patients).

Her first mapping session consisted of only three sites, to see how she would respond going forward. Lois reported no discomfort during the mapping sequence but did report that she felt a "bit more focused" throughout the week.

Her next mapping took place seven days later and included six sites, also with no reported discomfort during the mapping itself. However, Lois did report that she woke up at 2:00 a.m. with a migraine headache. She took Fioricet for symptomatic relief and went back to sleep; she reported that the headache was not as "debilitating" as other migraines she has experienced throughout her life.

The next day, she reported being "hyper" at the office and was told that she was definitely more irritable. This hyper state maintained itself throughout Saturday night, and she woke up at 4:00 a.m. Sunday morning feeling "very wide awake" and stayed alert, with no headache and no anxiety, throughout the rest of Sunday.

It is not clear to Lois that the LENS mapping of the six sites was the cause of her headache, as she also had spinach and feta cheese during an evening meal, and these foods had been a known migriane trigger for her in the past. Regardless of the ambiguity surrounding this headache experience, I decided to limit Lois's next mapping to four sites.

It should be noted that Lois has reported no similar negative experiences throughout the rest of her mappings and treatments. We have just completed her third map and are halfway through her third course of treatment.

In summary, Lois has reported that since the completion of her first round of mapping (four sessions) and treatments (five sessions), she continues to feel "much less anxious" and "much more functional." She reports that she no longer obsesses over little things and can sleep much better, and she has reduced her use of Xanax from four half-doses throughout the day to one half a dose taken proactively on what she describes as "high demand" days (her typical dose is one half of a 0.5 mg pill).

Conclusions

Paul Botticelli did very well estimating the sensitivity of this case and how something as innocuous as a least stim map could be used, not just for mapping, but for treatment (the two must always be considered together). There would be no question that if he had used "stim" or even "high efficiency" (HE) protocols, the results would probably not have been so good. That is to say, if people are precariously poised and partially exhausted, it doesn't pay to push them too hard. This would be one reason why the LENS or any other biofeedback procedure might backfire.

~~~~~~

NINE

NEUROFEEDBACK TREATMENT OF OBSESSIVE-COMPULSIVE DISORDER

D. Corydon Hammond, Ph.D., ECNS, QEEG, BCIA-EEG

The OCD demons have haunted me all my life. . . . This distorted self is the only one I have ever known. . . . And now, who am I to become? I am both eager and afraid to meet her.

ANNIE, AN OCD SUFFERER, IN A "LETTER TO MYSELF"

The Nature and Symptoms of OCD

Symptoms of obsessive-compulsive disorder (OCD) may be roughly grouped into obsessions and compulsions. Obsessions are repetitive and anxiety-provoking thoughts, images, or impulses. Common compulsions are about contamination and illness, fears of harming others or oneself, doubts about whether something occurred, religious obsessions, sexual obsessions, obsessions about one's body, and obsessions about the need for symmetry or exactness. Compulsive behaviors often include cleaning or washing rituals, checking compulsions (e.g., checking that the door is locked, that the stove has been turned off, or that a mistake hasn't been made), counting, ordering or arranging things, or hoarding.

Individuals with OCD typically feel unable to control their thinking and compulsive behaviors. Sometimes they will insightfully realize that their fears and behaviors are unrealistic, and other times they will believe that they are quite justified. If they are prevented from engaging in one of their rituals, they will become highly distressed and anxious. Many times persons with OCD have a large number of things that they avoid, such as touching certain things or people or going certain places, and they may have great difficulty making simple, everyday decisions. Occasionally an individual with OCD will be preoccupied with physical defects or imperfections, which is called body-dysmorphic disorder. OCD symptoms will most commonly begin in early adolescence or early adulthood; about 2.5 percent of adults are estimated to have OCD. In addition to anxiety, other clinical conditions (referred to as comorbidities) can be associated with OCD, such as depression, phobias, Tourette's syndrome, and bulimia.

Innumerable neuroimaging and quantitative EEG (qEEG) brain-mapping studies have been done establishing that OCD has a strong biological basis. In this chapter we will not describe the numerous technical details of the findings in these studies of the brain. We will simply summarize by indicating that there is a very robust body of research demonstrating both cortical and deep subcortical abnormalities in brain function in OCD. Of particular interest to the reader, however, is the fact that the brain research informs us that OCD is not a unitary problem. It appears that there are at least three subtypes of OCD. What are the implications of this for treatment? It means that treatment will be most likely to succeed when it is individualized to the unique patient.

In this chapter we will begin by briefly reviewing the symptoms associated with OCD and the common treatments that are available, and we will then discuss cases where neurofeedback and the Low Energy Neurofeedback System (LENS) have been used in treating OCD. Although we do not yet have carefully controlled scientific studies of neurofeedback with OCD, I believe that the reader will see, both from previously published case studies (Hammond 2003, 2004; Surmeli et al. 2011) and from the new material presented here for the first time, that the preliminary data is quite encouraging and that neurofeedback holds promise as a treatment modality for this very debilitating and difficult condition—especially in comparison to some of the other treatment alternatives that are being used.

Pharmaceutical Treatments for OCD

Medication Treatment

Medication is the most commonly used treatment for OCD. Although a wide variety of drugs are used, SSRI antidepressants are among the most common. In a review of psychiatric drug treatment of OCD, it was found that the most effective of the medications produced a 1.33 standard deviation (a statistical measure) improvement in a comprehensive measure of OCD symptoms (the Y-BOCS: Yale-Brown Obsessive Compulsive Scale). Some other medications produced only half this much improvement. By comparison, in results from three OCD cases that the author treated with neurofeedback (where previous medication treatment had proved only mildly helpful), the levels of improvement on the Y-BOCS were 3.7, 3.0, and 2.2 standard deviations, without any of the cases needing to remain on medications. The latest published research (Surmeli et al. 2011) on neurofeedback treatment of OCD found that 92 percent of thirty-six drug-resistant OCD patients showed improvement. More impressive is the fact that the improvements cited in this paper were twice as much as the improvements found for the most effective medication (Ackerman and Greenland 2002) used in the treatment of OCD in a series of twenty-five drug studies. However, on follow-up after an average of twenty-six months, only 53 percent maintained their improvements.

One of the drawbacks of the common practice of treating OCD with antidepressants is that they frequently have side effects (e.g., dry mouth, sedation effects, impotence, loss of sexual desire, dry mouth, blurred vision, dizziness) as well as a very problematic withdrawal syndrome (psychiatrists prefer to more tactfully call it a "discontinuation syndrome") when a patient tries to stop taking the medication. Additionally, research has shown that positive results from antidepressants are commonly overrated. Research (Kirsch 2010; Moncrieff 2009; Pigott et al. 2010) actually shows that antidepressants on average have only an 18 percent effect or less over and above placebo effects—something that has been referred to as the "dirty little secret" in the pharmaceutical industry and with the FDA. In fact, recent research suggests that overall the only significant effect over and above placebo effects is found in the most severely depressed patients (Kirsch et al. 2008). We should add that the 18 percent effect is often regarded as an overestimate of the efficacy of antidepressants because of sneaky research designs that drug companies often use to purposely bias the research outcomes in their favor (Hammond 2007a). Remember that drug companies are very financially motivated to design their studies in ways that minimize placebo response in the placebo control group and maximize the possibilities that their drug may be shown to have an effect.

Similar problems have been found in the effectiveness of anxiety drugs. A review of the research (Khan, Khan, and Brown 2002) on three anxiety medications found (even without taking into account the inherent methodological biases in research design) that less than half the time (48 percent) was medication treatment superior to placebo.

It is the author's belief that there is an overemphasis on medication treatment of mental health problems, including OCD, and that in general the public and even many professionals are very unaware of the limited effectiveness that psychiatric medications commonly have. The public is generally not aware that Food and Drug Administration (FDA) approval of a new drug requires the drug company to produce only two controlled studies showing a statistically significant difference between the medication and placebo, even though a statistical difference in a study with hundreds of subjects may not translate into clinically meaningful changes. Even more startling, however, is the fact that there is no limit to the number of studies that can be conducted before they come up with those two supportive studies. Thus even if there have been a dozen or more studies with negative results, those studies simply do not count. In addition, we must note that the safety of new medication treatments cannot be known with any degree of certainty until they have been on the market for several years, and more than two-thirds of new drugs are withdrawn from the market within three years of being released (Hollon 2005).

Despite the very modest effects of medication, there is evidence that quantitative EEGs have potential to assist in predicting medication response in treating OCD (Prichep et al. 1993). One study (Brody et al. 1998) also found that a certain brain pattern predicted positive treatment response to behavior therapy and a worse outcome from treatment with Prozac. Unfortunately, such research seems to be rarely applied in clinical practice by the majority of psychiatrists or physicians. Of course, a serious drawback of medication treatment is what occurs when the patient stops taking the medication. Although medication is sometimes helpful with an OCD patient, one study (Pato et al. 1988) found that 89 percent of patients treated with even the one medication shown to be the most effective in reducing OCD symptoms relapsed after they quit taking their medication.

Other Psychiatric Treatments

When psychiatrists become desperate because pharmacology approaches are not producing significant improvements, they many times recommend neurosurgery or electroconvulsive therapy (ECT). It seems to me that ECT is rather like taking a fine Swiss watch that is not working and then banging it roughly on the desk several times. Occasionally the watch (and the brain) will begin to function better. However, this is a very callous way of treating the brain. When neurosurgery is done, they will often perform cingulotomies, which involves boring a hole in the upper forehead and using a laser or gamma knife (radiation) to destroy a section of the brain. Using a somewhat liberal criterion of having produced at least a 35 percent improvement in symptoms, such psychosurgery has been found to benefit only between one-quarter to one-third of patients (Dougherty et al. 2002; Jenike et al. 1991), even though most of these patients have to remain on medications following the cingulotomy. One psychiatrist (Rauch 2000, 169) summarized these results well when he said, "For neurosurgical treatment of OCD, the overall rate of efficacy is quite modest, the costs are high, and the risks are considerable." More recently, psychiatry has been using intense magnetic stimulation of the brain (commonly for thirty-minute sessions, five days a week for four to six weeks), but this remains unproven with OCD. It is thus apparent that current psychiatric treatment of OCD through either medication or surgery has very strong limitations.

Greist's (1990) review estimated the degree of symptomatic improvement with serotonin drugs as being only 30 percent. Goodman et al. (1992) similarly found that symptom amelioration in OCD treatment with serotonin uptake inhibitors is about 35 percent on average and that only 50 percent of patients experience this partial symptomatic improvement.

Behavior Therapy Treatment

Behavior therapy commonly uses exposure and response prevention techniques to treat OCD. This treatment consists of exposing patients to very anxiety-provoking stimuli (such as things they believe would contaminate them) and then not allowing them to engage in the rituals that would usually follow such exposure, despite the distress that they experience.

Foa and Franklin (2001) reviewed research and believed that about 76 percent to 86 percent of patients *who complete treatment* make improvements, although an earlier review (Foa, Steketee, and Ozarow 1985) of behavior therapy treatment found that in more than 200 patients, 51 percent reduced their symptoms at least 70 percent. Thus a behavior therapy approach to OCD treatment shows clear superiority to medication or neurosurgical approaches. It is the author's experience, however, as well as that of other professionals, that exposure with response prevention treatment is very emotionally difficult for patients. Naturally, most patients dislike this very unpleasant, rigorous treatment, and it appears that about one-quarter of patients are unwilling do what is required or sabotage it through overt or covert avoidance. Nonetheless, if patients are willing to repeatedly undergo these very anxiety-provoking experiences, it appears that between three out of four or four out of five patients will obtain significant improvements. It must be pointed out, however, that behavior therapy has proven less successful with individuals with obsessional OCD where they do not have rituals. With these persons, behavior therapy has been estimated to result in improvements only 50 percent of the time.

It is informative that several neuroimaging research studies (Baxter et al. 1992; Schwartz et al. 1996) have documented that following successful exposure and response prevention treatment, there are positive changes in brain functioning compared with individuals who did not change as a result of this treatment. These results suggest that there is more than one path leading to Rome, so to speak. There appears to be a reciprocal interaction process wherein if we intervene with neurofeedback (which we are about to describe) and produce improvements in brain function, this will often translate into emotional and behavioral changes. On the other hand, when cognitive behavioral therapy forces the patient to engage in avoided behaviors while being unable afterward to engage in rituals, when it is successful, it also appears over time to produce biological changes in how the brain is functioning.

Because there are limitations and unpleasantness associated with psychiatric and behavior therapy, some clinicians have begun looking to neurofeedback as another treatment alternative for assisting patients with OCD.

Neurofeedback Treatment of OCD

Only three previous papers have been published on the use of neurofeedback with OCD (Hammond 2003, 2004; Surmeli et al. 2011). In Hammond's case reports, two cases of OCD and another case of obsessional OCD were very successfully treated with qEEG-guided neurofeedback. Follow-ups at six and four years following treatment on two of these cases (the other case moved away to another state and has been lost to longer term follow-up) have confirmed that they remain basically symptom free. These three consecutive cases were the first OCD patients treated by the author using neurofeedback. As noted earlier, Surmeli and colleagues (2011) found that 92 percent of thirty-six drug-resistant OCD patients treated with qEEG-guided neurofeedback showed improvement, although on two-year follow-up only 53 percent had maintained their improvements.

Figure 9.1 displays the changes on the Minnesota Multiphasic Personality Inventory in the twenty-three-year-old man with OCD (Hammond 2004). For readers not trained as psychologists, the scale on the left side of the graph shows the degrees of statistical deviation (T-scores) from norms. Only 2.5 percent of persons score above a T-score of 70. Thus the reader can see the very substantial changes that occurred following neurofeedback. The Pt scale (Psychasthenia scale) measures anxiety, obsessional worrying, self-criticalness, and perfectionism. It declined from 115 T-scores to 60 T-scores after sixty-two half-hour neurofeedback sessions that were guided by a qEEG. His score on the Y-BOCS improved from 16 to 3. Since completing treatment he has married, completed undergraduate college studies and an advanced degree, and is happy and normal in his adjustment.

It is common for psychiatric studies to consider medication treatment successful if it produces at least a 35 percent reduction in symptoms. However, in Hammond's three case reports, patient symptom reductions on the Y-BOCS were 84.6 percent, 72 percent, and 81.25 percent. In these cases the length of treatment was 60, 62, and 93 sessions (mean average 71.7 sessions), and the author suggested that successful treatment appeared to require 60 or more sessions. Since that time, however, the author has found that successful neurofeedback treatment

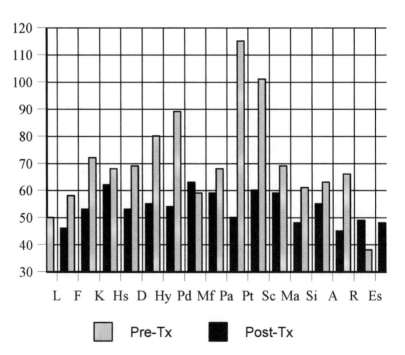

Fig. 9.1. Minnesota Multiphase Personality Inventory pre- and post-treatment changes of a twenty-three-year-old man with OCD

of OCD has often occurred significantly faster using the LENS.

LENS neurofeedback (Hammond 2007b; Larsen 2006; Ochs 2006) is a unique and passive form of neurofeedback that produces its effects through feedback involving a very tiny electromagnetic field. This feedback, which is only 1/400th the strength of the input one receives from holding a traditional cell phone to the ear, is delivered in one-second intervals at a time down electrode wires while the patient remains motionless, usually with eyes closed. However, unlike a cell phone signal, this feedback is adjusted sixteen times a second to remain a certain number of cycles per second faster than the dominant EEG frequency. Preliminary research and clinical experience have found that LENS rivals and in some cases may surpass more traditional forms of neurofeedback in the treatment of conditions such as traumatic brain injury (Hammond 2010a), fibromyalgia (Donaldson, Sella, and Mueller 1998; Mueller et al. 2001), ADD/ADHD, anxiety, depression, insomnia, and other conditions (Larsen 2006; Larsen, Harrington, and Hicks 2006). LENS has even been used to modify behavioral problems in animals (Larsen et al. 2006).

Several Cases of OCD Treated with LENS

Case 1: Daniel

The first OCD patient that I treated with the LENS was a twenty-one-year-old married man who had experienced OCD symptoms for eight years. He suffered with anxiety, and especially social anxiety, with a fear of touching or being touched by people. This greatly reduced his social interactions.

The patient's mother wrote a letter three months after he completed treatment in which she described his life prior to beginning LENS treatment. The patient and his mother have given me permission to reprint it, and his name has been changed to preserve confidentiality.

We noticed Daniel's OCD symptoms around the time of puberty, when he was about thirteen years old. He had always had a high sense of morality, of right and wrong, but it became intensified at this point. He became very conscious of doing the right thing religiously and never felt as though he was being "good enough."

He also became very hypersensitive to people and their comments to and about him. He could not endure teasing and would take offense easily. His friendships pretty much dried up during the next few years because he felt like others were always making fun of him. He would come to me repeatedly and ask if he had done something wrong or had acted inappropriately. One example of this was when he came to me and said he had seen a picture of Britney Spears in her underwear on the Internet. He was horrified because he couldn't get the image out of his mind and felt like this would keep him from pursuing a mission for his church because he was not worthy, after viewing the photo. I talked to him repeatedly and tried to assure him this was normal and that he had done nothing wrong. It would seem to be okay for a couple of days, but later I would find out he was still obsessing over it.

Another example is when he would hear swear words and then couldn't get them out of his head. He would be in agony and he always had a stressed look on his face. You could just see by looking at him that he was in constant turmoil. His relationship with his father became very difficult at this time. Daniel would let me hug him most of the time, but he would pull away if his dad ever tried to do so.

If he had a problem with one of his peers at school, he would obsess over it, going over it again and again. We would discuss things and I would think I had gotten through to him, only to find out later that he was still thinking about it. I was so weary of his feelings, of his constant need for reassurance, especially since it didn't ever seem to clear up the problems. He was fearful of homosexuality or any reference to it. He has an aunt who is a lesbian and he had adored her, but it became increasingly difficult for him to be around her. He had a young niece and nephew, and while he loved them dearly he found it difficult to hug or hold them, especially his niece. She was four at the time, and if he saw her in a swimsuit it would throw him into a tailspin. He couldn't be near them if I was changing a diaper or bathing them.

We took him to a counselor when he was eighteen and preparing for a mission with our church. This counselor saw Daniel a couple of times but never diagnosed him with OCD. He proceeded on his mission [at age nineteen he left home to voluntarily serve as a missionary for the Church of Jesus Christ of Latter-Day Saints], but the situation got out of control there, and he was diagnosed by a psychiatrist at that time with OCD, hypermorality, hyperreligiosity, and social anxiety. At this time he was put on the medication Prozac, which helped the problem slightly, but he could never really adjust in Mexico, and six months later he came home. We got him back in counseling, and he also saw a psychiatrist for medications. He tried several medications, including Xanax, Zoloft, Seroquel, Cymbalta, and Lexapro, with some positive results. However, they only made his life livable, but he had no real quality of life."

Daniel was asked to rate his symptoms each week on a 0–10 scale, where 0 represented the absence of a symptom and 10 would represent the most intense level of the symptom that he could imagine. At the completion of twelve LENS sessions during a six-week period, his average symptom rating had decreased from 4.5 to 1. After sixteen LENS sessions he cut back his dose of Lexapro (an antidepressant) by one-half. In the next session six days later, his average symptom rating had increased to 2.8, but by two days later his mean symptom rating had further declined to 1.3. After twenty-three sessions Daniel was off all medications, and after twenty-eight LENS sessions he was essentially asymptomatic. At that time his mean symptom rating was 0.17, after which it remained at this insignificant level or below. Six more sessions were done over the next seven weeks (a total of thirty-five sessions) in the interests of reinforcement. His total score on the Y-BOCS had decreased from 22 to 3 (an 86.4 percent improvement, and an improvement of 3.2 standard deviations). These changes have been maintained at nine-month and twenty-eight-month follow-ups that have been done independently with the patient and his mother.

Case 1, Daniel: Pre-Post-Follow-up OCD Outcome Measures

Test	Y-BOCS	Mean Symptom Rating
OCD mean and SD	24.7 (SD = 6)	
Pretreatment score	22	4.5
Posttreatment score	3	0.17
SDs Improved	3.2	
Percent Improved	86.4 percent	99.96 percent

Even more gratifying than the changes on the Y-BOCS and subjective symptom ratings was a letter from the patient's mother three months following termination of treatment. She wrote:

We heard of Dr. Hammond and neurobiofeedback, and Daniel and his dad and I went to see him. After talking to him, Daniel felt like he would like to try Dr. Hammond's treatment. He began treatment in June. Within the first three weeks we noticed a change in Daniel. At first we thought we were just imagining it because we didn't feel like we would see results so quickly. However, when I asked Daniel how he was feeling, he said he had already noticed a remarkable lessening of the constant anxiety. From that point on, it was a matter of positive and quick progression. Toward the end of September, Daniel felt like he felt good enough to start coming off of his medications. We were amazed by this because that had been the lifeline that let him maintain whatever sense of normalcy he had, but he felt like he could do without it. The results of coming off the medications were difficult, but more because of the physical side effects of these strong medications, and not so much because of the mental or emotional effects. He continued in treatment until the first part of December and then felt good enough to stop [neurofeedback].

It's difficult to put into words the difference we see in Daniel. To watch the anxiety and stress leave his face for the first time in eight years was amazing. His countenance changed entirely, and you could just watch the peace that he finally felt. He became a carefree person, joking and laughing with ease. He would play with his niece and nephew, wrestling around on the floor with them. I would watch in amazement as he played with them, marveling at the change in him. He no longer became so easily offended, and he didn't feel like everything that anyone did to him was a personal slight. I would say it was like someone had given me my son back, but this was a person I didn't really know. It was like we had been raising our son in black and white, and suddenly someone turned on the color button and we had this incredibly beautiful picture where we had only had darkness. I love to hear him laugh, because it has been so long since he had done so when he was suffering with OCD.

Daniel made a comment to me when he first started seeing Dr. Hammond. He said, "What will it be like to say I *had* OCD?" And now we know. This is a person who has been let out of the prison of his mind and been set free to enjoy a life that is carefree and he can meet head on without the suffering and the insanity of OCD. In our wildest dreams we never felt that we would get the results we did with the neurobiofeedback. It exceeded our greatest expectations, and now we look forward to watching our son continue to grow and live a life without the struggles he had previously experienced.

Case 2: Annie

Annie was a thirty-year-old single woman suffering with OCD. She had been on Paxil for ten years. She received thirty-two sessions of LENS neurofeedback, during which time her various symptom ratings declined from an average of 7 to zeros and ones, and she quit taking Paxil. Her symptomatic improvement has been maintained at eighteen-month follow-up with three reinforcement sessions occurring during the year and a half at stressful transition times such as starting a new job. She remains medication free. Annie's treatment is described in her own words, which she has given me permission to share:

I remember vividly the morning I woke up thinking *nothing*. I had been treated [with LENS neurofeedback] maybe ten times. Staring at the ceiling, I searched for a thought to obsess about. I couldn't find one. I burst out laughing. Sure, that seems like a strange reaction. But I'd never encountered such a morning—ever.

Even my earliest childhood memories are inextricably tied to my OCD. I didn't know it then. We didn't even have anything to call it; though I was painfully aware that I was different. I wasn't one of the classic OCD sufferers you might find counting stairs or checking to see if the stove was off for the millionth time. Perhaps if I had been more typically obsessive-compulsive, my struggles might have been detected earlier.

As a young child, my parents used to call me a hopeless perfectionist. I was the only child my mother ever saw who would destroy her own creations. She often tells me how many drawings and projects she rescued from the trash. My sisters used to call me vain. It took me a full forty-five minutes each morning to do just my bangs. And there was the unfortunate incident when I was in fifth grade. My attempts to create perfectly coiffed hair resulted in me actually literally burning my bangs off. All I knew was that unless I had things "just right," all hell would break loose. I remember with embarrassing clarity the screaming tantrum I threw as a ninth-grader because my mother sent me to school before the getting-ready "process" was completed.

Raging obsessions and compulsions about my appearance weren't my only difficulty, however. The same drive that made me spend hours in front of the mirror also compelled me to seek a standard of control in my relationships that was ridiculously outside the norm. While I was a naturally friendly and bright child, my obsession to have the perfect conversation or perfect friendship stunted me immeasurably. I could barely start a conversation . . . and when I did, I had no mental boundary on when I should stop. My peers found me intimidating because of my misdirected emotional intensity, and I did not make friends readily.

By the time I was in high school, what could have been written off as quirks about appearance or social awkwardness could no longer be ignored. At seventeen, I punched a guy for touching my hair. Not just punched, either. I pinned him down and beat him as hard as I could. It's a fortunate thing that I was neither coordinated nor strong. He laughed it off, but I knew something in me was unhinging. None of my friends would group date with me. I was so obsessed by the prospect of something going "wrong"—which it invariably did—that I never enjoyed a social function. Neither did anyone else around me. Such events ended with me at home on my bathroom floor, hysterical. I knew logically how I should act, but the reality was that I couldn't make my actions fit within any normal social boundary. No one else carried a comb and hairspray around *all the time*. No one else flew into a rage at a small misunderstanding. I knew it. But I couldn't stop myself. I lived with a constant battle raging in my mind. Actual reality and reality as I needed it to be fought bitterly for mental space. I fought bitterly with everyone I knew. Still, much of my behavior was chalked up to teenage hormones and general awkwardness.

My poorly constructed house of cards finally collapsed when I entered college. Circumstantially, everything I obsessed about and couldn't control was all neatly contained on one campus. The social phobia I had developed because of my inability to relate normally to people ran rampant. My roommates were mystified by my passionate mood swings, rages, and inability to attend class.

It was a miserably wet, snowy winter that year. I couldn't go out. I literally couldn't leave my dorm room to go to class because by the time I had walked to campus my hair would have been ruined. Logic told me I had to go to class, but logic seldom won in battles against the OCD. I simply couldn't last the day that way. The stress I endured because I looked and felt imperfect drove me to distraction. The only relief—compulsively going home to redo it. Once an honors student, my GPA plummeted to a 1.97.

When I realized that my problem was going to get me dismissed from the university, I was determined to find a secondary safe zone—one that would allow me to stay on campus through the duration of my classes. When the stress of the day started to overtake, I would simply duck into the restroom until I could cope again. The perfectly contained stall was the only place on campus

I could go to quickly order my world. Eventually, I knew the location of every bathroom on campus and which were the least likely to be occupied. But like Pavlov's dogs, I began to react physically to this mental exercise. Convinced I had the longest-lasting UTI ever, I finally consented to see a doctor. I can only imagine that it was the opening my parents had hoped for. Any prior conversations about seeking help for my mental state had met with almost violent resistance on my part.

That doctor's appointment would change everything. While I thought my difficulties were deeply and carefully hidden, my insightful physician must have seen me for what I was—a twenty-year-old girl on the verge of mental collapse. I was prescribed Paxil. Right or wrong, I never bothered to read the packaging and took the prescription I believed was for my UTI. I felt remarkably better. I couldn't understand why. I refilled the prescription. Curious, I finally read the information. Paxil: prescribed for OCD, social phobia, and depression. I was crushed and angry. I hadn't asked for medication for any of that! But I was also incredibly relieved. After a full month of medication, my moods had already stabilized considerably.

I continued taking the medication and began my intense, personal study of my own mental health. What was wrong with me finally had a name. My "perfectionism" was raging OCD. The pieces fell together at last. I felt I knew myself for the first time. And I could stop feeling such immeasurable guilt for my thoughts and feelings. Relative control settled in. My grades improved. I improved.

Fast forward through a decade of life, loss, triumph, struggle, clarity, and heartache. A family member began pursuing neurofeedback for her son. I watched carefully as he began to change. Small changes turned into huge strides. Whatever this was, it worked. Frankly, I was content with my managed self. But I was also at an age where I was thinking of marriage and children. Paxil is not a drug you can take during this process, but I also was acutely aware that life without it was nonnegotiable. The monstrous self that had once driven me would come back, full force. It wasn't a reality I was willing to accept. Something else would have to be done. With some skepticism and secret hope, I consulted with Dr. Hammond. The promise of a life without OCD and without medication seemed impossible. I set my expectations on simply cutting my dose in half. If that was all that came out of it, it would be enough.

I wrote a letter of sorts to myself the night before my qEEG. It reads, in part:

"The OCD demons have haunted me all my life . . . altered my ability to be in relationships, destroyed friendships, and cost me jobs under often humiliating conditions. I can't say I'm not grateful for the grace and strength these experiences have afforded me. But I will say that I have suffered sometimes almost unendurably under the weight of my own thoughts and actions. It's difficult to describe myself to people who do not suffer this way. I have yet, in all my searching, to find a way to put into words the 'needs' that drive me—my own will grated against logic and reason. I have conquered many of these foes with a match of will and strength. There is still a marked duality within me that I have only managed to merge for the purpose of daily life. Am I who I might have been without these struggles? Surely not. Would I trade it? I cannot say.

"And now, who am I to become? I am embarking on a process that may take my crutch and replace it with a wellness I have never known. I will no longer be a chemically altered version of myself, but instead a self I have never met. I am both eager and afraid to meet her. I will have no more excuses for my failures. They will be entirely my own . . . as will my success. I will have nothing to blame but myself for what I become. And the prospect of that terrifies me. This distorted self is the only one I have ever known."

We discovered quickly that I was extremely sensitive to the LENS feedback. Cumulatively, I have received only seconds of treatment. And still, I improved in ways that I didn't think possible. After only twenty-three treatments, I began the painful but necessary process of detoxing from my ten-year Paxil treatment. That was, by far, the most difficult part of the change. Mentally, I still felt better than I ever had; physically, it was extremely challenging. The first few weeks of tapering often had me questioning whether I should stop taking the medication at all. To say that I felt horrible is a kind understatement. But I wanted to challenge the neurofeedback process. I wanted prove that I could manage without the medication as well as I had managed on it. That seems almost laughable now.

I had no idea then that in a few short weeks I actually would be the person I had written about only weeks before—an unaltered, though much-changed self. Obsessions and compulsions that had been a part of my core for years fell away easily, almost imperceptibly. My confidence skyrocketed. I could, at long last, think and reason clearly. I reacted perfectly normally in social situations. All my hopes of being a "normal" person were realized. OCD and medication free, I am fundamentally myself for the first time in my life. In every sense of the word, I am a captive—liberated.

Case 3: Dewayne

The third case of OCD treated with LENS was a twenty-two-year-old college student. He began treatment with mean symptom ratings (on a 0–10 scale) on obsessions and anxiety that were both 8.5. These ratings had reduced to 4.5 after only five LENS sessions, to a rating of 3 after eight LENS sessions, were only rated a 1 after thirty-two sessions, then mildly increased to 1.5 during a two-week period associated with final examinations at the university, and then remained at a rating of 1 after thirty-seven sessions. A total of thirty-nine LENS sessions were completed, and on two-month follow-up the symptoms remained at this negligible level (a reduction of 88 percent), and on a year and a half follow-up he had maintained about 75 to 80 percent of his improvements.

Conclusions

The average length of treatment in the three cases the author has previously reported (Hammond 2003, 2004) that were successfully treated with qEEG-guided neurofeedback was 71.7 sessions, and in the case series by Surmeli et al. in 2011, the average treatment length was 100.4 sessions. In comparison, the mean length of successful LENS neurofeedback treatment in the three cases described was 34.3 sessions, which was only 48 percent of the length of the traditional neurofeedback treatment. Both the Surmeli group and this author have had cases of OCD where neurofeedback has not proven successful. We do not yet know what percentage of the time neurofeedback will be successful in the treatment of OCD. However, the available results in treating OCD with neurofeedback are clearly encouraging. The author believes that neurofeedback offers an important additional treatment alternative for this debilitating condition.

TEN

TRAUMATIC BRAIN INJURY

With Harris McCarter, Ph.D., Michelle Luster,
Mary Lee Esty, Ph.D., L.C.S.W.,
and D. Corydon Hammond, Ph.D., ECNS, QEEG, BCIA-EEG

Head Injuries from the Mild to the Severe

In this chapter we consider head injuries from the mild to the severe, but you will learn from the cases presented herein just how severe "mild" can feel to the sufferer. The human brain is not only the most complex entity in the known universe, it is also the most exquisitely intricate in organization. To develop this organization includes all of those maturational processes we discussed in chapter 5, where we looked at how easy it is for them to run awry without proper environmental response and nurturance. In chapter 6 on autism, we looked at how subtle disruptions, from sources unknown, whether genetic or chemotoxic, prevent the personality from maturing normally. How easily disrupted are those delicate mechanisms that are built, one on another, to allow us to enjoy the full complexity that is human—even when we have no obvious cause of the disruptive agency. Attentional mechanisms, perhaps milder in their impairments, still disrupt lives (chapter 7) and our ability to cope effectively.

In traumatic brain injury (TBI), we have a brain that is mostly "working okay" until the auto accident, the fall on the ice, the blast explosion, or, more insidiously, the toxic exposure. As we will see in some of the accounts that follow, life must always be reckoned again, from that point onward. In our first story, when the TBI happens in childhood, the damage may include those developmental aspects already mentioned. Our first narrative also shows how such problems may blight or alter an entire lifetime, until they are addressed. Because sports injuries have such currency these days, an entire separate chapter is devoted to these (chapter 11).

The sequelae of TBI, child or adult, may include difficulty with organization, time management, sleep, mood instabilities, energy, planning, pain, and headaches, shading into chronic fatigue and fibromyalgia. Also, things we don't normally think of as connected to head injury, such as digestion, immune functioning, endocrine regulation, and even sexuality, may be affected. People lead a compromised existence some describe as "a gray room" where all is "cloudy and confused," as one of our clients described the post-TBI state. People then may lead lives of quiet desperation until help arrives—or never arrives. Worst of all, they are accused by employers, or managed health care, or no-fault insurance, or even their doctors, of malingering or making it up. Yes, it is "all in your head," as the callous dismissal goes; it may indeed be "in your head," but it is not the outcome of a bad attitude. It is because an extremely delicate, intricate neurological environment has been disturbed, and it runs too fast or too slow, it fails to talk to its other parts, or all the neuronal voices babble at once.

It is not that health care providers are uncaring—it's just that they may not know what to do. As discussed in the chapter on TBI in *The Healing Power of Neurofeedback,* medicines that may work fine for uncomplicated depression or cognitive problems may backfire when the origin of the symptom is a TBI. Cognitive remediation and psychotherapy may be helpful, or contrarily may run up against problems that seem stubborn and unyielding because the brain is not repaired. And TBI is the chameleon of the *DSM IV;* people may think it is anxiety, depression, OCD, even psychosis.

Fortunately neurofeedback seems almost tailor-made to deal with these problems. In fact, the first published paper in a peer-reviewed journal demonstrating the efficacy of the LENS was based on a controlled study with TBI in the *Journal of Head Trauma Rehabilitation* (Schoenberger et al. 2001). Also, since my earlier publications and presentations were on the state of the art only up to 2005, a lot of important work has been done since that time, and some of that work is presented in this chapter, reflecting the deepening awareness in the neurofeedback community both of how pervasive head injury is and how neurofeedback can help in ways that, in my experience, nothing else can. In fact, neurofeedback works like a catalyst, helping all the other forms of remediation, be they cognitive, occupational, or self-help, work much better.

Like it or not, human beings are born not only with the largest brains in the animal kingdom but with developing bodies that seem uncoordinated or unprepared to protect that oversized head from injury. Our very first case demonstrates how head injuries acquired early in life can blight that life. Michelle Luster (who agreed to let us use her real name) has given us a beautiful but painful account of how this process works—and yet how neurofeedback in the hands of a caring and skilled provider, Dr. Harris McCarter, gave her a chance for rehabilitation for which she had spent decades searching. Mary Lee Esty's successful treatment of a youth with TBI who was misdiagnosed as psychotic is another example of the efficacy of neurofeedback for people seriously misdiagnosed. My colleague Dr. D. Corydon Hammond has provided some cases with extremely dramatic features—like being crushed by a runaway 30,000-pound chip-seal crusher. This (University of Utah) medical school professor has provided some cases for this book that are exemplary in being documented with before-and-after brainmaps and clinical and psychological testing.

Prologue
HARRIS MCCARTER, PH.D.

In March of 2010 I was contacted by a young woman from the community college across the street from my office. She was a psychology major, and her advisor, Richard Seymour, knew I had a special interest in learning disabilities. When I spoke with her on the phone, I learned that she was from an inner-city community where I had worked extensively earlier in my career, at the time when she would have been a child there.

I was familiar with the burdens that poverty and other social inequities placed on children struggling to survive and develop in that environment. I had watched many of her peers, as they were drawn down into a world of violence and despair. Within minutes of meeting her, I was struck by the unusual courage of this woman, now thirty-six, who was still determined to get an education and to provide for herself and her children, despite the poor hand life had dealt her.

Early in our work together, Michelle mentioned that in order to graduate, she would have to complete what her college called a "Capstone Project," and she came up with the idea of writing about what she was learning from our work. This led her to do her own research on the effects of traumatic brain injury, and what she learned deepened her ability to be a partner in the work we did together. As the treatment progressed, she became more and more able not only to do the research and writing the project required of her but also to cope more effectively with the circumstances of her life, all of which then fed back into the therapeutic process to make it more effective. What follows is an excerpt from the paper she wrote.

My Journey Through Brain Injury
MICHELLE LUSTER

When I was young I experienced a head trauma while playing outside catching bubbles with friends. I fell down my cement basement and fractured my skull. I was rushed to the hospital in a cab, and the doctors told my mother that I had cracked my skull, but I should be okay because they couldn't see any damage to the brain. I was hospitalized for three weeks after that for further evaluation, but they still could not see anything that would delay my learning process. The only scar was the one on my forehead from the surgery.

The first thing I am able to remember from the experience is doctors surrounding me while I lay in a hospital bed. The doctor asked me if I knew my family members' names. Then I was given a series of short tests that included some occupational therapy to determine if I had any damage to my brain. My mother said she remembers the therapist saying that I couldn't remember the entire alphabet, and I would slur my words. However, due to a trauma like the one I suffered, it was expected that, as time went on, I would be fine, and it was okay for me to return to school. In middle school, when I had assignments, the teacher would sit me in the back of the class-room and overlook my situation. It was very uncomfortable to participate in class because I felt stupid. She asked me if I felt that my writing class was too difficult, and she also asked me to read samples for her. I stumbled over words when I began to read out loud, and my classmates would call me names and laugh at me. I felt out of place and frustrated, discouraged, due to the fact I couldn't keep up with the other students.

As I went on to high school, my mother still never got me any help for my learning disabilities, so I was put into smaller classes, but that still didn't fix the problem. I noticed my reading skills were declining, and I wasn't able to comprehend things I read. My spelling in high school was not on grade level, and I was unable to remember little things that really counted to me. My poor performance in high school caused me to become very depressed and angry at myself. I started to gain a lot of weight because this was the only way I could find comfort. I started to pay less attention in school, and pay more attention to seeking acceptance from my peers.

I started to fail in all my subjects. In math I wasn't able to solve a math problem due to the fact that my reading was poor and I was not able to make connections. Reading was a major problem for me. I would sit in class and pretend to understand, but I was clueless. When reading I was stumbling over my words, so I got to a point in class that when it was my time to read part of a passage, I would read it real fast so it seemed like I knew the words. I hated spelling; it was a struggle for me because of my bad memory.

I noticed things about my writing, but I really didn't pay attention to the signs and symptoms of my problems, such as the fact that the words I was writing down were backward, and so when it was time to study, I couldn't understand what I had written. Even so, following high school, I made the decision to go to college. I wanted to better myself, and I believed I was capable of doing so, in spite of the trauma I suffered when I was younger.

I was determined to learn regardless of my learning disability. In the fall of 1994, I took one course at Urban College to get the feel for the col-lege experience. Unfortunately I did not continue to go to Urban College because of the distance and location, but I didn't stop trying to pursue my college education. In the spring of 1994, I entered Roxbury Community College. I completed three semesters, but I did not like my learning experience there, because I felt out of place and frustrated, discouraged, and uncomfortable due to not being able to keep up with my classmates. Also, the classes were too large, and the professors never gave students individual attention. My grades went from As and Bs to Cs and Ds. It made me feel as if I was back in high school all over again. At that point I decided I no longer wanted to continue my education.

Following RCC, I took a long break from school because I became intimidated by the atmosphere. During my three-year break from RCC, I realized that I was missing something in my life, and that was education. I had to finish what I had started. I wanted to be a positive role model for people like me who had some type of trauma and who felt that their education was over.

After doing my research, I went back to college in 2001, but this time I went back to Urban College, where I studied human services and got my associate degree as a human service major. Over the next five years, I wanted to build on this education. I wanted to go back to school, but unfortunately I could not continue at Urban College because I had completed my degree there. I was scared of going back to another college due to the experience I had at RCC, but instead of letting RCC hold me back, I went to a faculty person at Urban College for support in picking another college that would help me be successful in my life and my education. That's when I applied to Cambridge College to attain my bachelor's degree in psychology.

When applying to Cambridge College, I was scared that I would not get in. Luckily, I did. I remember the first class I took was in critical thinking. The professors had us pair up into groups and do assignments together, which was good because I really didn't have to do anything on my own. The hard part of that class was when I had to take notes. Just like high school, I was unable to take notes, so I could not do my homework, and I got a low grade in that class. Writing 101 was no better, because it was a great academic challenge, and I felt that I was not really ready for that. I dropped out of that class twice. At times, the classes were very difficult, and I would drift off into space. But many of my professors were very supportive, which made my learning easier. I have to say that one professor in particular really helped me by arranging a class climate to be one that I could do better in. This was Professor Seymour. He made me feel better about myself and my academic potential beyond high school because he guided me to the help I needed. Professor Seymour was the first to see that there was something wrong with the way I was doing my class assignments.

Now, here I am at age thirty-six, still struggling to read my five-year-old son a bedtime story. No one knows how hard it is to hear yourself read out loud while stumbling over simple words, or to hear your five-year-old child tell you that you can't read. One day I was sitting down at home, watching an episode of *Housewife,* when one of the kids on the program started to talk about a learning disability and how his grades were falling due to him not being able to keep up. What hit my heart was how his mother was very supportive by telling him that he could be any type of lawyer he wanted to be, and that she would support him. Those words made me cry because my mother never seemed to be supportive around my education.

During my second class with Professor Seymour, we were discussing how the brain works and its different functions. At the beginning of class, he told the class that when he was younger, he was diagnosed with dyslexia. At this point, I decided to step out of my comfort zone and have a talk with him about my situation and the difficult time I was having understanding the classwork. I told him that I felt as if I had a learning disability. I asked him if he knew where I could get tested, and he told me that he had a good friend that dealt with the brain and maybe he could help me or give me some information on how to get the service I was seeking.

Professor Seymour gave me Dr. Harris McCarter's telephone number, but I was scared to call him at first. I put the number down but forgot about it. When I finally reached the point when I felt I could not go any further, I remembered him. But I could not find his number, so I started to feel hopeless, until I saw that Professor Seymour was teaching the "capstone" class. I signed up for that class, and I was able to talk to him about his friend, so he gave me the number again. This time, I called him, and we set up an appointment for me to come in to see him. I went to Dr. McCarter's office, where we talked about my learning disability. He asked me what type of insurance I had, and I replied that I had Mass. Health. He told me that he did not accept Mass. Health. At that point, I thought any hope that I had was out the door, until he turned to me and said he would treat me anyway. That was in March 2010.

At that point, I felt as if God had heard my prayers. Dr. McCarter explained to me that he did not know if it would work, but he would give me ten treatments; if it worked, he would continue the treatment. He said he was going to make a map to get a better understanding of what was going on in my brain. He hooked me up to the computer with wires attached to my ears and head. Then he made a map of my brain. After he looked it over, we had a discussion about my diagnosis and what he had seen on the map. He said that part of my brain was sleeping due to the trauma I received from the fall I had when I was younger. He wanted to wake up that part of my brain that was affected by the trauma. He did that by using a treatment called LENS neurofeedback.

I have been seeing Dr. McCarter for about six months now and feel that the treatments have made a big difference in my life and education.

After the first treatment I didn't really notice much change, but after the second, I started to notice how I was able to remember what happened when I was younger, how my injury came about, and other things from my childhood that I told about in this paper. Also I started to be able to remember where I put things. For example, before the treatment I would put important things down and have no idea where they were, but after the treatment I would know exactly where they were. Or with mail, I would wonder: "Did I mail that?" But now I remember, "Oh, I have to mail that," and I go do it. Or with appointments, I usually had to write them down and have someone call me and remind me, and even then I would forget them. But now I remember them without even writing them down. I know what I have to do, and I get there.

Another example is being able to remember things that happened. There had been a misunderstanding between me and the people in charge of my Section 8 housing. They had made a mistake and were going to throw me out of my home because I couldn't remember my side of the story to explain it. Then the treatment started, and all of a sudden I could remember exactly what happened, what day it was, what time it occurred, who was involved in it, and what was the process I took. I was able to remember all that very well, told them everything, and they said, "You're right." They went back and saw everything I said was all there in the record, and that's what saved me from losing my housing.

My organization became better too. I was able to organize things properly. Whereas before I just put things wherever, now I could have a place for things, like I put my bills in one place and my schoolwork in another, or like I could organize things in alphabetical order, which I couldn't do before. Before I couldn't find things, and it would make me really angry. Now I can find them. In school, my writing is more organized too. This paper is a perfect example of that. If you read any of my old papers, you would say, "What in the world?" My motivation also changed. There were times I didn't want to get out and do nothing, but since the treatment I enjoy going to the gym and working out. I do things more. I have a social life.

The more treatment I was getting, the better I was getting, but when I have a break in treatment, things seem to go backward. An example of this is my headaches. Before treatment I used to have migraines every day. They would last two days to a week where I could hardly do anything because my head was really hurting. Sometimes before treatment I would take medication, but the pain was so bad it wouldn't touch it. I couldn't have any light, I couldn't have anyone say anything to me; I had to have complete silence and darkness. Any little noise would make my head pound. I had to isolate myself. My son couldn't be in the house with me, and I would be crying because it hurt so badly. Then, soon after the treatment started, the migraines started getting less. With more treatment I started not having any at all for many weeks and months. But then we had to interrupt some treatments, and that's when they started up again. Last week I had two of them.

Some other things haven't changed as much as I would like, like my procrastination or my ability to remember what I read. My understanding of reading is definitely better but not what I would like it to be. My ability to read to my son has improved only a little, but it is getting better;

just like my communication with others is not where I want it to be, but it's getting a little better—where people can at least understand the point I'm trying to make.

"Error marks the place where learning begins." Through my journey with traumatic brain injury, my feelings are that people with this type of disability may have the same capacity to handle information as those without it, if given the proper strategies to do so. Therefore it is especially important for teachers to be aware of each student's strengths and weaknesses in order to help them to become successful in their studies. I believe this is true. Due to dealing with my disability, I believe now that we have choices and we can change any situations that we are in by voicing our opinion and asking for changes to suit our well-being. I have made many mistakes in my education and in life generally, but now I'm very aware of how to make positive changes.

Notes on Michelle's Treatment Process
HARRIS McCARTER, PH.D.

I began Michelle's LENS treatment by making a map with no feedback involved (least stim map, using an Atlantis system). Using the amplitude sort from this map, I began treatment with very brief (brief map) feedback. I started out doing seven sites per session, but she reported that this made her feel wired, causing her to go on compulsive housecleaning binges when she got home. We cut back to three sites, which eliminated the binges but also reduced the benefits she experienced. For a long time, we settled on four sites per session. We experimented from time to time, and she has recently come to prefer five. Treatments have been once a week, but with frequent interruptions of a week or two, and one of the striking features of the treatment has been how much she has benefitted despite these interruptions.

Michelle and I continue to work together. We don't meet as regularly as either of us would like, and what we do is definitely a work in progress, unfinished and sometimes even disappointing. I don't want to overstate what we have been able to do. Michelle is still frustrated by the limitations of her memory and of her difficulties in making herself understood at times. The adversities of her environment still impact her life in ways she can't control. But in June she will receive her college diploma, having mastered challenges that seemed impossibly overwhelming only a year ago, and fulfilling a lifelong dream.

Furthermore, her life has been enriched in ways neither of us anticipated, although I have come to see them as typical of the type of life change that is promoted by the LENS. She has been able to remember more and more of the events of her past and to assemble these puzzle pieces into an increasingly coherent picture of the story of her life and who she is. During one session, as I affixed the electrodes to her head, she told me of attending a neighborhood reunion and of how excited she had been at all the memories it had awakened, not only of big things like friendships, but also of everyday stuff like the movies she had loved as a child. The next week her eyes gleamed as she recounted newly recovered memories of a particularly funny romantic adventure from her youth, involving a young man who had to hide in her grandmother's closet.

As she pieced together more and more puzzle pieces, she also became more aware of what was missing and more motivated and able to take steps to fill in the gaps in the picture. Two months ago, she disappeared for three weeks. When she returned it was with the triumphant news that she had been on a quest to find her father, whom she had never met and who had not known she existed. Equipped only with his nickname and the name of the town he had lived in when her parents knew each other, she had successfully tracked him down. He had welcomed her joyfully, and in addition to her father, she had found a brother her own age, with whom she has since been texting almost daily.

It was Michelle, not the LENS, who brought about these changes to her life, but as I continue to add the LENS to more and more of the work I do, I have been a participant in more and more processes like this. In these processes we see instances of the apparent catalytic effect of the LENS to which Dr. Larsen refers in his introduction to this chapter. Often it seems like the main thing required of therapists using neurofeedback is that we learn to tread more lightly, stand back, trust the brain and mind to find their own healing path, and not complain when the patient skips therapy for three weeks.

Auditory Hallucinations and TBI
MARY LEE ESTY, PH.D., L.C.S.W.

Archie was twelve years old when his new psychiatrist referred him to me for Flexyx Neurotherapy System (FNS is an early forerunner of LENS) treatment. He had recently been hospitalized by a previous psychiatrist because he was hearing voices urging him to harm others. He was put on multiple medications and diagnosed as possibly schizophrenic.

Following his release from the psychiatric unit, the family wanted a second opinion. The new psychiatrist was well-versed in the many potentially severe effects of concussion on emotional functioning. He identified a precipitating event that caused the onset of hearing voices. It was an accident in gym class, resulting in a baseball-size lump on Archie's head. In fact, the accident was the last in a series of several Grade 3 concussions whose effects accumulated to cause Archie's severe symptoms. (A grade 3 concussion in defined by the length of the unconscious period.) The horrendous peak event of Archie's struggle was being "tased" by the police as he struggled inwardly to resist the terrifying commands of the "voices" but could not respond to requests to "drop the knife."

The final concussion that tipped the scales for Archie had been preceded by three playground incidents in three years, all resulting in loss of consciousness for up to ten minutes. Combined with a Grade 2 concussion that had resulted in hearing loss in one ear after being kicked in the head during a soccer game, Archie's brain shifted into a totally different gear. He had a history of ADHD and had struggled with schoolwork, however he was a likable, very intelligent, and friendly young man. This turn of events had the entire family in emotional chaos. Fortunately his new psychiatrist was aware of the positive effects of FNS for treating head injuries and recognized that auditory hallucinations can be caused by TBI.

Archie's response to treatment was positive from the beginning. Although he had a headache after the first treatment that lasted two days (not unusual with this extreme number of concussions), he felt much better on the third day. Sleep was better and he was calmer. After two treatments, his therapist, guidance counselor, and his mother reported improvements. Archie and I had agreed that he would report to me the number of times he heard the "voices." Between the second and third sessions he had heard them only twice, and they were less powerful. He continued to be explosive at times, but there were signs of reduced irritability, even at school. His religion teacher, who did not know anything about his problems or treatments, told Archie's mother that he was now learning the material and sitting quietly. Fatigue, a major problem after TBI, was an initial problem, but after a while, energy improved. Lamictal, Effexor, and Klonopin were probably contributing to fatigue. As treatment continued, the medications were gradually reduced. Effexor was stopped after six treatments.

By the seventh treatment he had to stop and think about the number of times he had heard the voices. Very hesitantly he said "one." His unusual hesitancy led me to ask what he had actually heard and he replied, "Raid the fridge." I suspect that was a typical adolescent boy voice speaking from the stomach, and there were no more reports of voices after that.

Archie's treatment covered two years with summer and holiday breaks. Although longer than usual, two years is consistent with the preconcussion history of ADHD and the serious nature and high number of concussions. We also eventually combined FNS with traditional brain wave training neurotherapy with Dr. Michael Sitar. Archie's story underscores that neurotherapy should be a treatment of choice for even serious psychiatric diagnoses, and that taking a history of trauma is extremely important.

Archie now is in college with an academic scholarship and working toward a technical degree. He is a top athlete in a highly competitive individual sport. He excelled in honors classes and was off of medications before we stopped neurotherapy treatment. Thanks to the psychiatrist who understood the connection between auditory hallucinations and TBI, Archie's story has a very happy ending indeed!

Post TBI Fibromyalgia

*FNS Treatment—Fibromyalgia Study with Rush
Presbyterian–St. Luke's Medical Center*
MARY LEE ESTY, PH.D., L.C.S.W.

A surprise phone message to Mary Lee Esty from Phyllis, a fibromyalgia study participant, was received in April 2003. She completed her participation in the fibromyalgia study in March 2000 when she was forty-six years old.

Phyllis had been diagnosed with fibromyalgia syndrome following the onset of pain symptoms after a serious motor vehicle accident in which a cervical vertebrae was fractured. Six years later she entered the fibromyalgia study at the Neurotherapy Center of Washington (NCW), where she received Flexyx Neurotherapy System (FNS) treatment. Her research data showed significant symptom reduction. Three years after finishing the study, she left this message on Dr. Esty's voicemail.

It's probably been about two-and-a-half to three years since I was in the fibromyalgia study, and I just wanted to get your business cards to give to others. I've done so incredibly well, and I'm always being asked about the [treatment]. I'm also always being asked for your card, because I'm always recommending you.

I wanted to give you an update on my life and how things have been. I can't even begin to tell you how wonderful it is. I feel like I've been given my whole life back. Even after I left the program I slowly continued to improve. The other day I ran into an old friend who asked, "How's your stuff?" Years ago I'd automatically know what she was talking about. I had to ask what she was talking about. "You know, your pain thing." I haven't even thought of myself as having fibromyalgia in a really long time. I'm doing things in my life that I hadn't been able to do in years. This is a very long overdue thank you!

She had applied for, and received, a job promotion. In 2009 she was nearing completion of a master's degree in a health care profession. She works full time supervising a large department in a government facility and continues to enjoy good health.

Phyllis's case is illustrative of a situation in which a positive outcome in response to FNS treatment alone is likely. The critical elements are these for relatively quick resolution of major symptoms: if a person has been high functioning and then experiences a trauma that involves a mild TBI, even if from a low-speed whiplash, there are no major structural damages, and general health is stable, then one can expect a good response to FNS treatment alone. However, to increase the effect it is often recommended that surface electromyography (sEMG), or dynamic muscle biofeedback, be added to the treatment plan.

The cases below, collected and documented by Dr. Hammond, show just how extreme the injuries involved in TBI can be—and thus how amazing the benefits of neurofeedback intervention.

Post-Traumatic Anosmia

D. CORYDON HAMMOND, PH.D., ECNS, QEEG, BCIA-EEG

The brain is about the consistency of Jell-O and sits on a bony plate. During acceleration-deceleration brain injuries (e.g., during whiplashes and hard hits to the head), the brain bumps up against the insides of the skull, which can cause damage. Particularly in moderate to more severe head injuries, the sliding motion of the brain can also damage olfactory nerve fibers associated with our ability to smell. The resulting loss or partial loss of the sense of smell is referred to as *anosmia*. When a head injury results in a loss of consciousness for five or more minutes, post-traumatic anosmia is more likely to occur.

Research has shown that post-traumatic anosmia occurs in 14 to 27 percent of patients with moderate to severe head injuries, but physicians and treatment professionals often do not inquire about such a symptom. Improvements appear to occur in only about one-third of cases in the first year after injury, and close to a fifth of patients find their sense of smell growing still worse in the six to twelve months after a TBI. By two years after post-traumatic anosmia has occurred, it is widely regarded as being permanent.

A twenty-nine-year-old man we will call "Tony," with a history of post-concussion syndrome, came for treatment. He had experienced four mild head injuries. This included two mild concussions associated with water skiing and a whiplash in an automobile accident six years earlier. However, nine-and-a-half years prior to coming for treatment, he experienced a moderate-severity head injury when he was thrown from a four-wheeled recreational vehicle.

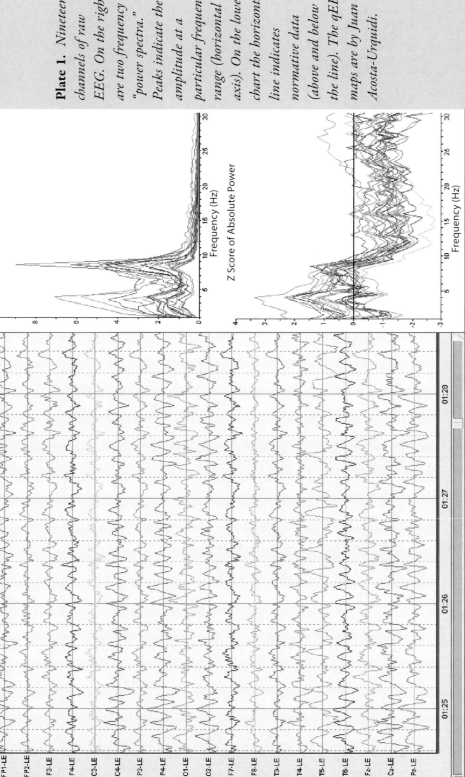

Plate 1. *Nineteen channels of raw EEG. On the right are two frequency "power spectra." Peaks indicate the amplitude at a particular frequency range (horizontal axis). On the lower chart the horizontal line indicates normative data (above and below the line). The qEEG maps are by Juan Acosta-Urquidi.*

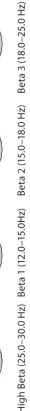

ontage: LinkEars

Z Scored FFT Absolute Power

Delta (1.0–4.0 Hz)   Theta (4.0–8.0Hz)   Alpha (8.0–12.0 Hz)   Beta (12.0–25.0 Hz)

High Beta (25.0–30.0 Hz)   Alpha 1 (4.0–8.0Hz)   Alpha (8.0–12.0 Hz)   Beta (12.0–25.0 Hz)

Beta 2 (15.0–18.0 Hz)   Beta 3 (18.0–25.0 Hz)

Plate 2. Z-scored absolute power maps derived from qEEG in typical brain wave ranges delta through high beta. On the scale, green indicates normal, whereas red and dark blue indicate SDs, standard deviations, away from normalcy.

Montage: Laplacian

Z Scored FFT Amplitude Asymmetry

Delta (1.0–4.0 Hz)   Theta (4.0–8.0Hz)   Alpha (8.0–12.0 Hz)   Beta (12.0–25.0 Hz)

High Beta (25.0–30.0 Hz)   Beta 1 (12.0–15.0Hz)   Beta 2 (15.0–18.0 Hz)   Beta 3 (18.0–25.0 Hz)

Z Score >= 1.96   Z Score >= 2.58   Z Score >= 3.09

Plate 3. Z-scored amplitude asymmetry between left and right hemispheres. The color blue indicates bad connections whereas red indicates too much connection. The thickness of the line refers to how abnormal the condition is—in other words, very thick lines are the greatest standard deviation from the norm.

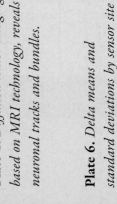

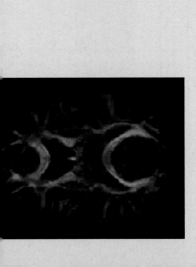

Plate 4. *Diffusion tensor imaging, based on MRI technology, reveals neuronal tracks and bundles.*

Plate 5. *Like the CAT scan, the LORETA is able to do computer-assisted tomography—that is to say, register "slices" through the brain, as these pictures of patient Michael Schacker (discussed in chapter 12), who lost most of his left hemisphere to a hemorrhagic stroke (the little triangular markers on the sides show the tomographic "slice"). The LORETA shows the deeper tissue affected and the extent of the injured areas. In effect, you can move the tomography arrows through the entire brain from different angles—sagittal, rostral, coronal, and so forth—and see what is going on in that specific geography.*

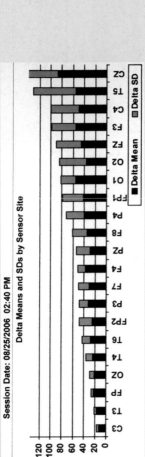

Plate 6. *Delta means and standard deviations by sensor site*

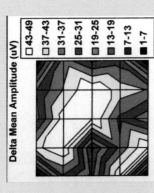

Plate 7. *Delta mean amplitude (uV)*

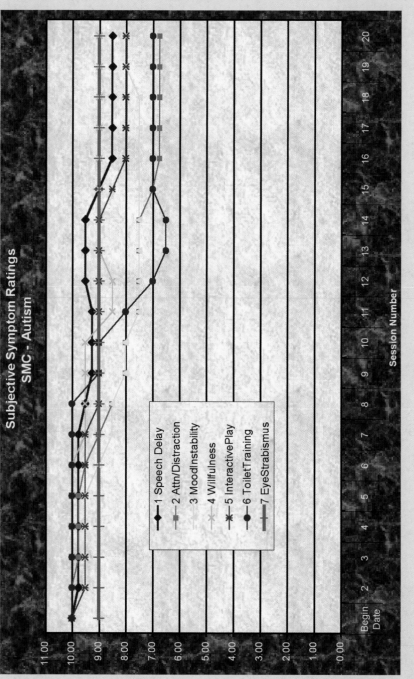

Plate 8. *The subjective symptoms rating chart for Emily, the autistic child discussed in chapter 6, reflecting her progress in 2006. Please note that the graph seems frozen until sessions 8–16, at which point things start to improve in a variety of domains. After that we have a slow plateau again until approximately twenty sessions later (as seen in plate 9).*

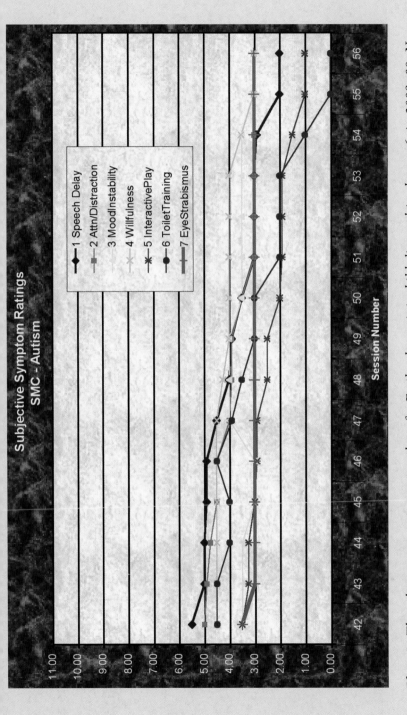

Plate 9. *The subjective symptoms rating chart for Emily, the autistic child discussed in chapter 6, in 2008–09. Note how much improvement she has displayed since 2006 (plate 8), as evidenced by this chart's lower numerical scores.*

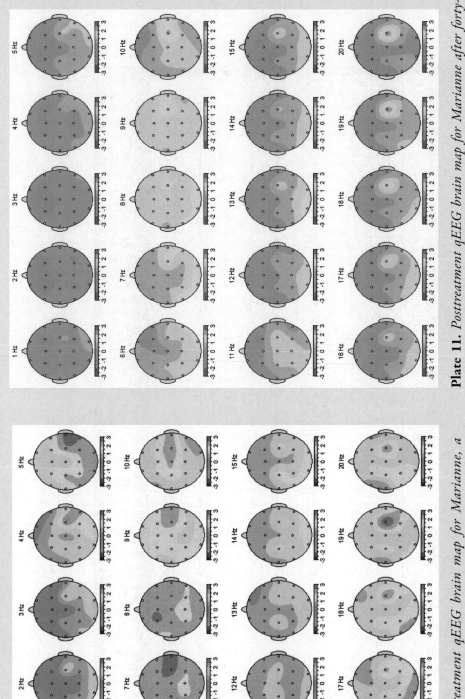

Plate 10. Pretreatment qEEG brain map for Marianne, a young woman with traumatic brain injury discussed in chapter

Plate 11. Posttreatment qEEG brain map for Marianne after forty-two treatments of LENS neurofeedback with Dr. Corydon Hammond.

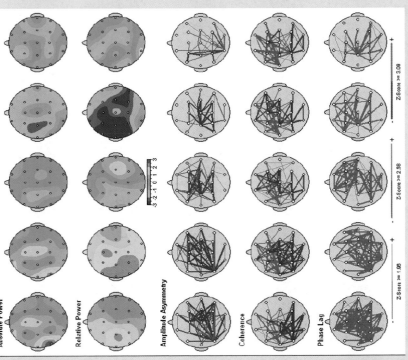

Plate 12. These qEEGs done at the Northeast Center by Dr. Victor Zelek show serious dysregulation spreading across the left hemisphere.

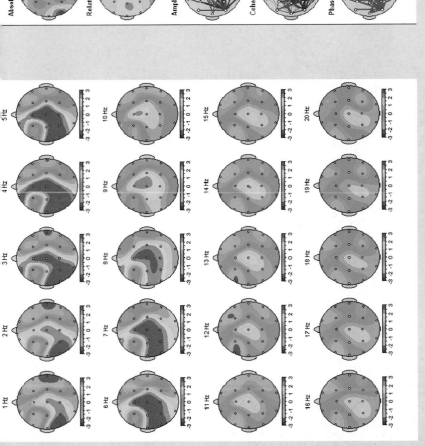

Plate 13. The impaired communication between parts of the brain is shown by the thick congested lines in the bottom half of the scans, indicating hypo- and hypercoherence and phase problems.

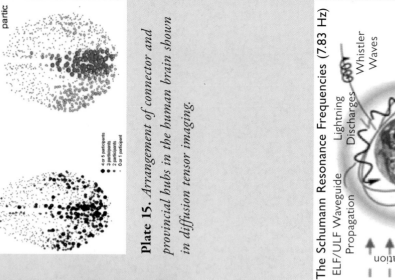

Structural connections of default mode network

RSN a

group overlap

number of subjects

>15
12
8
4
1

Plate 14. *Diffusion tensor imaging of the default mode network*

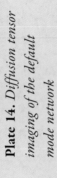

partic

● 4 or 5 participants
● 3 participants
● 2 participants
○ 0 or 1 participant

Plate 15. *Arrangement of connector and provincial hubs in the human brain shown in diffusion tensor imaging.*

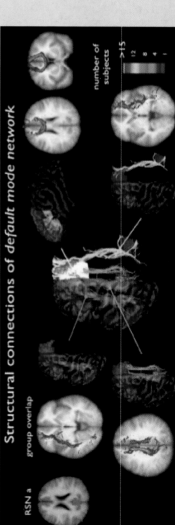

Delta (1.0 - 4.0 Hz)

Theta (4.0 - 8.0 Hz)

Alpha (8.0 - 12.0 Hz)

Beta (12.0 - 25.0 Hz)

High Beta (25.0 - 30.0 Hz)

Beta 1 (12.0 - 15.0 Hz)

Beta 2 (15.0 - 18.0 Hz)

Beta 3 (18.0 - 25.0 Hz)

Plate 16. *Different topographic brain maps showing that alpha relative power is selectively increased in a deeksha healer. Copyright Iuan Acosta-Urquidi, Ph.D.*

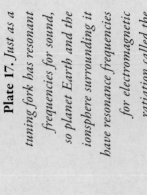

The Schumann Resonance Frequencies (7.83 Hz)

ELF/ULF Waveguide Propagation

Solar Radiation

Lightning Discharges

Whistler Waves

Schumann Resonances

Plate 17. *Just as a tuning fork has resonant frequencies for sound, so planet Earth and the ionsphere surrounding it have resonance frequencies for electromagnetic ratiation called the*

As he was riding down a mountain trail, a deer jumped across his path, its hoof hitting his head, causing him to crash his vehicle. He sustained a frontal lobe head injury, was unconscious for ten to fifteen minutes, and continued to go in and out of consciousness for some period afterward.

Tony was hospitalized for a week, and afterward reported a change in personality, increased irritability, difficulties concentrating, explosiveness, problems with short-term memory, insomnia, anxiety, and mood swings. LENS treatment began with an offset assessment (four seconds of feedback) for his first treatment session. And an offset frequency of 5 Hz faster than his dominant frequency was determined to be the most effective frequency for reducing his slowed EEG activity. His second treatment session consisted of nineteen seconds of feedback at the nineteen standard electrode sites while we gathered a LENS map. He experienced no side effects from the treatment, and after the second session he reported that he felt "clearer in the head." His subsequent treatment sessions consisted of providing one second of feedback at seven electrode sites.

At the beginning of treatment, the patient was asked to rate his eight most prominent symptoms (fatigue and lack of motivation, depression, anxiety, anger/explosiveness, insomnia, impulsiveness, short-term memory problems, poor concentration) on a 0–10 scale, where 0 represents no problem and 10 a severe problem. He was asked to provide symptom ratings at the beginning of each session. His average level of symptoms at the beginning of treatment was 9.0, and at the end of twelve LENS treatment sessions, his mean symptom rating was 5.1.

The patient had never been asked if he had anosmia. Thus it was surprising when, at his thirteenth treatment session, he indicated that after his previous treatment he had begun to smell things for the first time in nine-and-a-half years. He explained that after his more serious head injury, he had completely lost all sense of smell, and his neurologist had told him that he would never smell again. After treatment, he had first begun to notice a smell when he was outdoors on a construction site. Initially he was confused and kept thinking, "What is that?" Finally he realized that he was smelling sagebrush. It was at this interview that he also indicated for the first time that his sense of taste was also "coming back."

After fifteen treatment sessions, the patient indicated that his sense of smell was "rapidly improving now," along with his sense of taste. He had been smelling perfume, foods, and his dog. After nineteen treatment sessions he believed that most smells had now returned. He said, "I'm not used to it," and that occasionally he had been awakened in the night by a smell. It is known that olfactory input is conveyed to the hippocampus, which is part of the brain associated with memory. In this regard it was fascinating that the patient said that, as he was becoming aware of more smells, this elicited "lots of memories." For example, when he smelled the scent of pine, it evoked memories of many camping trips with his father. He also said, "Food tastes *so* good now," and it is known that impairment in smell drastically compromises one's sense of taste.

After twenty-two LENS sessions, the patient's average symptom rating had decreased from 9 to 3.75, and he indicated that his sense of smell and taste seemed completely normal. Two more treatment sessions were completed, and then the patient stopped treatment due to work demands. Contacts for up to a year after treatment verified that his symptoms continue to be rated low, and his sense of smell and taste remain normal.

The exciting results of this case were published (Hammond 2007b) because this outcome had never been reported in the medical or psychological literature. Since that time the author has had other cases in which sense of smell improved after neurofeedback, and several colleagues have reported similar improvements to me. This is exciting, because anosmia has a very severe negative effect on the quality of life, safety, and interpersonal relations, as well as eating habits and nutritional intake.

A Case of Serious TBI
D. CORYDON HAMMOND, PH.D., ECNS, QEEG, BCIA-EEG

Marianne (the patient's name has been changed) was a sixteen-year-old young woman who had experienced a serious traumatic brain injury in 2002 at the age of seven. The injury was caused by a 30,000-pound chip seal crusher that broke loose, rolled down a hill, and hit her. She was discovered unconscious and not breathing behind a tire of the crusher, with her head pinned against a wall. At the emergency room her Glasgow coma score was 8. Glasgow coma scores of 13–15 are characteristic of a mild head injury; a score of 9–12 typifies a moderate disability injury; and a score of 3–8 denotes a severe-disability injury. She had a depressed skull fracture in the right posterior temporal-central area, necessitating neurosurgery.

Before her head injury, she was a normal, happy child who always enjoyed her friends and family and was enjoying learning experiences in school. The accident seriously changed her personality, her life, and the lives of her family, as her mother described:

> The emotional battle was so hard. The doctors told us Marianne will probably either not live or not live on her own. So we tried to prepare ourselves for that. Brain injuries don't come with manuals. From the day Marianne started school again after her injury, we started seeing the full effects of the damage. Marianne would come home early from school a lot with severe headaches, frustrated because she couldn't remember things. Teachers would give her directions, and she could not follow through. We tried many different methods to no avail. She would get so frustrated over the next years because she had no friends and could not handle the emotionality of relationships, and she would feel that when someone was joking with her that they were being mean. She didn't understand.
>
> The frustration with school was equally difficult. I was in the school almost every day trying to get the schools to understand that they couldn't teach her the same way as other children. They always thought that she was not paying attention. I have fought a long, hard battle, not only at school but at home. The frustration was always worse at home because she felt safe there, and every day she would come home and vent on me. She missed so much school. I tried to find every way possible to find help from someone, to no avail. No one understood the full effect of what this brain injury had done. We have been to so many doctors and tried their suggestions. They don't work unless you have support from schools and family. We did

not have that support. Some family members turned their backs on us, believing that she was just faking most of it. Schools just didn't know what to do.

Marianne's dad also has a brain injury, so we would make trips to Salt Lake City to the university for his appointments. One day I picked up a brochure about qEEG and neurofeedback. I read it and thought, Maybe I'll try this; it sounded so good, and we had tried so many other things. I didn't know how much more I could handle. I was at a breaking point. I made the appointment with Dr. Hammond. I didn't think Marianne was going to go. She has battled with counseling and would never talk, so we gave up. She went with a fight. She did not want to go. Then he put the goo [electrode paste] in her hair. Every time we left the appointment, she was so angry she wouldn't talk to me and stormed off to the car. He had left some goo in her hair, and she hated it.

During the intake history, we learned that she had an onset of absence seizures (seizures where the sufferer "goes blank" or "disappears") approximately a year following the accident. Initially she had been on anticonvulsants, but due to side effects she had not been on medication for two years. Each day she had from three to ten absence seizures lasting one to two minutes each. In our intake interview nine years after the accident, her mother rated the following symptoms on a 0–10 scale, where 10 represented a severe problem and 0 no problem at all: overemotionality and mood swings were rated 8.5; anger and irritability 6.5; problems concentrating 9; short-term memory problems 7.5; impulsiveness 10; poor social/bonding skills 9; and problems reading 9. Although Marianne was sixteen years old, she also still struggled with cursive writing. She never smiled or laughed, displayed no sense of humor, and was flat in her affect. A quantitative EEG brain map was done on Marianne using the NeuroGuide (University of Maryland) and NxLink (NYU) databases as part of the assessment. Marianne's treatment consisted of forty-two sessions of neurofeedback utilizing the Low Energy Neurofeedback System (LENS).

We began with a LENS map using a high-efficiency LENS program, which uses a narrow-band carrier wave to provide the feedback. Dr. Len Ochs has written in his manual (for professional practitioners), "This means that there is probably a million times less energy used in the HE application. However, what energy there is occurs in a 1–kHz band rather than the usual 139 mHz–wide band." The high-efficiency map consisted of gathering four seconds of EEG data and giving one second of feedback sequentially at all nineteen standard 10–20 electrode sites.

After two LENS map sessions, we then provided treatment following a "suppression map." This procedure consists of providing feedback at electrode sites that do not have a high level of variability in the EEG, working from sites where there is less amplitude and variability toward electrode sites with more amplitude and variability. The offset frequency at which she was receiving feedback was initially 20 Hz faster than her dominant brain wave. This method of working using the suppression map and an offset frequency of 20 was chosen to approach her treatment more cautiously because of her epilepsy. By the seventh session, she was receiving twenty-eight seconds of feedback, and no side effects had been noted (she never experienced any side effects during the entire course of treatment). Therefore, after the seventh session, we followed a regular LENS map sequence, providing feedback at seven electrode sites in a session and rotating through all nineteen electrode sites during treatment. By the tenth session, we were providing her with thirty-five seconds of feedback with an offset frequency of 2 Hz. She was having two treatment sessions weekly, and we continued systematically to increase the amount of feedback every couple of sessions because we were seeing only positive progress and no side effects.

We saw symptom improvements very quickly, and we tracked symptoms by asking her mother to provide weekly symptom ratings in consultation with Marianne. After fourteen sessions, her seizure frequency had declined to only once a week, and she was now laughing. After fifteen sessions, she never experienced another seizure. After forty-two sessions, her average symptom rating had decreased from 8.5 to only 0.29. All her symptoms were now being rated a 0 except for problems with reading, which was rated 2. She made much progress in her symptom ratings (apart from seizure activity) for mood swings and emotionality, irritability/anger, focus (problems concentrating), memory problems, poor social/bonding skills, impulsiveness, and problems reading.

In the final interview, Marianne's mother tearfully said, "Thank you for giving me my daughter back." She later wrote the following to describe the treatment progress:

After a few weeks the changes started. The trip became my and her time. We could actually talk, and communication was becoming easier. As the weeks went by, you could see a change in Marianne. Initially she would never give Dr. Hammond the time of day. No smile, no nothing. Then one day she smiled. Then she joked and quit being angry about the goo. She would laugh about it. She was bonding with others as well. She would sit and watch TV or have a conversation with a complete stranger. I was in shock. This was not Marianne as we had come to know her after her injury. She has become so mellow, talkative, and a social butterfly. The school has commented on what a change they have seen. She is willing to try instead of just giving up and not understanding. She has made new friends this year with great choices. Last year the choices were not so good. She can see now why they were bad choices. Her learning has improved so much that in most of her classes she is getting As and Bs, because she tries.

She has also learned how to control her emotions. She has learned how to problem-solve, instead of storming out of a room or yelling. She has learned how to let someone know she is frustrated, and so she goes for a walk or somewhere to calm down. Then she talks about it. She knows how to take a joke, and she can give it right back to you.

We started in therapy in May of 2009. By July 2009 Marianne became seizure-free. Her reading is improved. She can now follow directions and understand them. Marianne is so happy now, as well as the rest of the family. We finally have peace of mind, and Marianne will live on her own as they predicted she never would. She has the most amazing personality and strength, and she is so caring of others. Thank you for giving us our life back and proving the doctors and other people wrong. Oh, she drives now!

The week after Marianne completed the forty-two LENS treatment sessions, another quantitative EEG brain map was done. Please refer to plates 10 and 11 of the color insert to see her before-treatment and after-treatment summary results from the NxLink database and the changes that occurred in 1–20 cycles-per-second maps from the NeuroGuide database. The qEEG evaluation provides us with additional scientifically objective data on how Marianne's brain functioning changed.

When Marianne was sitting with her eyes closed, the EEG—as you can see in the color plates—showed a reduction in slow delta brain wave activity in the back and central areas of the brain, a dramatic reduction in inefficient excess theta activity throughout her brain, and a decrease in the excess alpha, beta, and high-beta brain wave activity. Similar positive changes were documented in the brain map done with her eyes open. The place on the graphs in the right central area that continues to show more amplitude is an artifact, because this is where a burr hole was drilled in her skull to relieve pressure on the brain shortly after her head injury.

One of the tragedies in current brain-injury care is that physicians commonly believe and tell their patients that by eighteen months after the head injury they have attained as much improvement as they can expect. They counsel, therefore, that the patient must simply adjust to the disabling symptoms that still exist. The case just cited clearly demonstrates the fallacy of this thinking.

Conclusions

From Michelle to Marianne, we have seen examples of how neurofeedback helps the head-injured, whether the injury is from a fall into a cement foundation or being pinned under a runaway chipper-crusher. From closed-head injury, where there is little in the way of external mark on the head, to cases where the skull is cracked or removed, neurofeedback seems to help because it signals the plastic brain to rebuild itself. Sometimes it has been likened to "breaking up the logjam" or "pouring Drano" into a clogged drain. The neurofeedback ameliorates the *functional* impasse and signals the brain to repair its *structure*. (It seems if you talk to the brain nicely, it will oblige.)

In the next chapter, we discuss a comparable mechanism with athletes; and then in the chapter after that with a stroke victim, whose hemorrhagic stroke was so serious that it literally "took out" half his brain.

ELEVEN

HEAD GAMES

SPORTS INJURIES AND BRAIN TRAUMA

With Elsa Baehr, Ph.D., and Lynn Brayton, Psy.D.

W e now move to a topic that probably merits a whole book in itself: head injuries, and the recovery therefrom, among athletes. A considerable literature already exists in scholarly journals and on the Internet. This chapter is a contribution pointing to an intervention for these life-occluding insults seldom mentioned in the literature: neurofeedback.

As I wrote in my book *The Mythic Imagination,* there is a perennial urge to see the human being behave as if it were a bodiless spirit—incapable of injury. The cartoons children watch have characters who fly or who, if they fall off a cliff, catch themselves, turn around, and climb back on again. Superheroes in comics or video games exhibit extreme risk-taking behaviors of all kinds and clobber each other, only to leap up and fight another day. Unfortunately, the real children exposed to such unrealistic scenarios are extremely vulnerable. Their large and brainy heads ride atop still relatively weak and uncoordinated bodies. They run when they should walk and often act without thinking first. Becoming teenagers, their misled imaginations outstrip their capabilities, leading them to pop wheelies or ski or snowboard beyond their abilities, right into the nonmythical land of TBI.

And let's face it, even when boys grow up, the rough games don't stop. In fact, the kinetic forces escalate with increased muscular strength and coordination. These head-injury-promoting activities have been going on a long, long time (and only in the last few decades have neuroscience and medicine developed the tools to measure the extent of the injuries). Could the madness of Ajax in the Trojan Wars (immortalized in *The Iliad*) have been due to TBI, or PTSD—or both?

In my book *The Fundamentalist Mind,* published in 2007, I hypothesized that there is a fairly good chance that much of the confused history of the Middle Ages was enacted by people (okay, let's face it, *men*) with TBIs. (Think about it for a minute; do you think it is harmless to be hit over the head by a sword or a mace, even if you are wearing an iron helmet?) Jousting, that favorite sport of the time, looks pretty wicked, especially when you consider the momenta of force involved—TBI and whiplash injuries, here we come—and with a flourish of trumpets, fantastic costumes, and the attention of the royalty!

Unfortunately, as I relate it to the theme of that book, post-TBI cognition is often marred by concretistic, black-and-white thinking—fueled, in fact, by powerful emotions that urge: "Act now! Confront the enemy! Take back Jerusalem from the infidels, start something—maybe a crusade!"

The romance of war, jousting, and fights to the death has by now (mostly) been sublimated into spectator sports, which thrill and excite audiences—themselves safely munching popcorn—but invite serious consequences for the actual antagonists. Injuries from boxing, called *dementia pugilistica,* were among the first to be recognized.

Down our country road near New Paltz, New York, lived the well-loved boxer Floyd Patterson. His boxing students, formidable-looking heavyweights, would chug up and down the road or the adjacent rail trail. Over many years I would run into Floyd in a repair shop, or the local Sears, and chat. Unfortunately, he always seemed to have forgotten the last encounter, but he masked the memory lapse with his geniality and warmth. The disorder among boxers is so significant that it has become one of the best-studied areas of sports-related TBI. Some recent studies have proposed that there are genetic susceptibilities that mark those likely to have lasting consequences from the injuries.

"The ultimate fate of the neuron," writes G. I. Iverson, in *The Little Black Book of Neuropsychology*, "is related to the extent of traumatic axonal injury: High intracellular Ca2+ levels, combined with stretch injury, can initiate an irreversible process of destruction of microtubules within axons. The disruption of the microtubular and neurofilament components contributes to axonal swelling and detachment (i.e., secondary axotomy)." In layperson's language this means that neurons, and their connections, can be destroyed by an excess of calcium in the cells.

According to Iverson and as stated in *The Little Black Book of Neuropsychology*, features of complex neurometabolic cascade following a concussion include:

• Influx of calcium
• Efflux of potassium
• Cerebrovascular blood flow subtly decreases
• Neurons enter state of hypermetabolism
• Anaerobic energy production and build-up of intracellular lactate
• Intracellular magnesium levels remain low for days after concussion
• In general, most injured cells (1) do not undergo secondary axotomy and (2) appear to recover normal cellular function

Athletes can recover rather easily from routine injuries on the microbiological level (Schoenberger and Scott 2011). Recovery time is between about two and twenty-eight days. They say, however, that many concussions may not involve loss of consciousness but may still involve a "neurometabolic cascade."

To simplify the technical details as much as possible: calcium coming into the cell and potassium going out results in a state of depolarization, or depletion. The ion pumps shift into high gear, requiring more glucose and oxygen to restore functionality, but decreased blood flow impairs that emergency measure. (This is probably reflected in the EEG by high beta. We will return to that topic shortly as we speculate how neurofeedback can help this stasis.) The continued calcium influx leads to mitochondrial dysfunction (mitochondria are the little energy-producing organelles of the cell). More emergency measures have the cell overutilizing anaerobic (non-oxygen-requiring) pathways, which increase lactate as a by-product (just like athletically-fatigued muscles become saturated with lactic acid). The same process depletes magnesium required to maintain membrane potential through the ion pumps and allow the mitochondria to produce adenosine triphosphate (ATP), which is necessary for energy. (Hence the energy depletion so often found with TBI, which neurofeedback sometimes helps rather quickly.)

The question then becomes whether the cell dies through *apoptosis* (cell death) or *axotomy* (the axon is cut off), or whether it can recover. The disruption of ions and energy production is *functional injury*—that is to say, a system that once worked well has all its parts in place and can be coaxed back into operation—versus *structural injury,* in which stretching or tearing of axons and cell mutilation or death takes place.

When people marvel at how quickly neurofeedback or other forms of stimulation, including acupuncture, hyperbaric oxygen, or CES (cranioelectrical stimulation) devices, work sometimes, it is because they affect change on the first, the functional, level.

Here also repeated injuries complicate the picture, in which you have partial or incomplete kinds of recovery only to have the tissues retraumatized in a new mix of functional and structural impairment. Then the trajectory of improvement might move by fits and starts (a bumpy road) if it is not traumatically frozen and unable to move at all. In these cases, stimulation, injudiciously applied, could backfire and work against recovery.

The Sports Concussion Crisis

Fortunately, public and media attention is now open to covering the effects of athletically induced TBI. As the Brain Injury Resource Center estimates (www.headinjury.com/sports.htm), in the United States alone there are an estimated 300,000 sports-related traumatic brain injuries per year. The same web page mentions the truism that vastly complicates the picture: *Once you have had one head injury, you are (exponentially) inclined to have more.* Why? (Sounds really mean and unfair.) Because the compromised brain makes "kinesthetic" judgment errors—call them "mistakes" if that makes you feel any better—and they accumulate until repeated, seemingly mild brain injuries occurring in a short space of time (hours, days, weeks) can be catastrophic or fatal.

Heretofore, to the zealous coach fixed on glory, the (invisible) injuries seemed dismissable. It was far more important to get that prime athlete back on the playing field. But public awareness has been inflamed by the sudden death of athletes who were put back into play after a recent injury and then sustained a second injury. With that awareness, there are now restrictions on how quickly a player can return to the field after any of the other markers of concussion: loss of consciousness for a period of time, dizziness, and disorientation.

This phenomenon is called *second impact syndrome,* first named only in 1984 but studied more intensively since then. Its primary cause is believed to be retraumatization of an already swollen or inflamed brain. Websites are studded with "in memoriams" to young athletes (mostly football players) who died between ages seventeen and twenty-four from the above-described syndrome. One theory is that there is a sudden demand for glucose in the injured area, combined with "inexplicable reduction in cerebral blood flow." The combination, obviously, can be deadly.

That is the short-term and acute peril that the athlete faces if he brings his already compromised brain back onto the playing field. But then there is the longer-term consequence, less dramatic, but far more insidious. It is called *chronic traumatic encephalopathy* (CTE), and it is regarded as a degenerative brain disease based on repeated "concussive and subconcussive brain injuries."

The CDC has now formed its own agency for injury prevention involving TBI, especially among high school students (www.cdc.gov/concussion/headsup/high_school.html). Then there is the Sports Legacy Institute (SLI), the mission of which, according to its website, "is to advance the study, treatment and prevention of the effects of brain trauma in athletes and other at-risk groups." SLI was founded in 2007 to "solve" the "sports injury crisis."

Major conferences at Ivy League institutions—long the strongholds of football followings—have begun to take a long, hard look at what such rough play takes from players for the rest of their lives. Conferences on the neurobiological dimensions (comprehension, prevention, and repair) have been held in the past five years in Vienna, Prague, and, more recently, Zurich.

Dr. Ann McKee, professor of neurology and pathology at Boston University, examined slices of the brains of professional football players who were provident enough, before their deaths, to bequeath their brains to science. The famous players she was examining usually died demented or with premature senility, as had their counterparts, the professional boxers. The disease is not even that subtle; it announces itself under 100× magnification of the slices, in the form of "a brownish protein called *tau*, which along with TDP-43, a protein known to cause neuron degeneration, chokes off cellular life in the brain." (See also http://sportsillustrated .cnn.com/vault/article/magazine/MGG11; search on Ann McKee.)

Dr. McKee and her group identified fourteen former National Football League players since 1960 who had been given diagnoses of amyotrophic lateral sclerosis (ALS), a total about eight times higher than what would be expected among men in the United States of similar ages. ALS is a frightening disease that involves loss of control of all the muscles in the body, which whither away, leaving the person conscious inside a body that cannot move. It is sometimes called "Lou Gehrig's disease" after the baseball legend.

Some recent scientific papers, however, have disputed whether Gehrig really had ALS, or the very similar-appearing CTE (chronic traumatic encephalopathy). (See the *Journal of Neuropathology and Experimental Neurology*.) For head injury experts, the case is quite plausible. Gehrig, the Iron Horse, as he was called, was known for multiple injuries and for playing even while seriously injured, logging 2,130 consecutive games in his baseball career. What is less well known is that Gehrig had a prior football career as a halfback, first in high school, then at Columbia, where he was known as a "battering ram" (the kind of specific injury acquisition being studied in football TBIs). Subsequently, during his stellar baseball career as a first baseman, his injuries included being "beaned" several times (no baseball hardhats in those days). A pitcher throwing an errant ninety-plus-miles-per-hour hardball hit him in the forehead, almost knocking him out cold. Then there was a stadium scuffle with rival Ty Cobb, in which Gehrig slipped and hit his head on a concrete curb.

Subsequent X-rays would reveal multiple skull fractures for the Iron Horse. By the end of 1938, his batting average had dropped from the .340s to .143, and it was evident that he was "losing it." James Kahn, a reporter who regularly covered Gehrig, said, "There is something wrong with him. . . . I have known ballplayers to 'go' overnight, as Gehrig seems to have done. . . . It's something deeper than that in this case, though. I have seem him time a ball perfectly . . . and drive a soft looping fly over the infield. . . . He's meeting the ball, time after time, and it isn't going anywhere." Gehrig would slip and fall while running the bases, and he began tripping in the street and falling.

Gehrig's decline at only thirty-six years of age was swift and terrible. He died three years later, in 1941, from a disease that may or may not have been ALS (http://moregehrig.tripod.com/id29.html).

Treating Athletic Injuries at Stone Mountain Center

For a number of years now, we have treated the injured equestrians of the Hudson Valley—sometimes victims of multiple injuries: "eventing" or steeplechase falls, occasional kicks, the scary "ride" when one falls off with a foot still stuck in the stirrup and is dragged by the galloping horse. One injury was merely from a startled horse swinging around its eighty-pound head and knocking a woman handler unconscious.

Near our property are the legendary "Gunks," the *Shawangunk* rock-climbing area. Only recently has it been common for most climbers to wear helmets. And even with helmets, leader falls or rockfalls can injure heads or spinal columns. Without helmets, of course, the injuries are far worse—as in one instance I am treating currently of a fairly low fall as such things go—only twenty feet. (Of course it doesn't help if you land on your head!) The nearby Catskills are a winter ski and snowboarding desti-nation, and just south of us in Gardiner is a major sky-diving area. At our center we have also treated football players, soccer players, rugby players, lacrosse players, gymnasts, circus performers, dancers, trapeze artists, even yogis who fell out of a headstand and fractured their cervical vertebrae.

People often come to us when they have exhausted conventional treatments. Only among discerning neurologists and neurofeedback providers is the full complexity of treating such multiply overlaid TBI cases appreciated. General practitioners might just prescribe for the most salient symptom: say cognitive impairment, putting the person on Concerta or Adderall. Not infrequently, since TBI patients react atypically, the stimulants evoke insomnia and explosive irritability. TBI is not only the "chameleon" of *DSM IV,* it can reveal underlying genealogical faultlines in the constitution, so that a bipolar episode is triggered, or delusions begin to manifest. Benzodiazapines to calm the overexcited brain may then have the person sleeping sixteen hours a day and only emerging to go to the bathroom.

Such was the case for Tom, an early patient who came our way and was of great concern to his family. He had been in a slow and steady decline for a number of years. He was foggy, stumbled over his words, and had had to leave his job, even though he was only in his forties. He couldn't get up in the morning and would often sleep twelve to sixteen hours a day. Even when he appeared to be up and about, he was narcoleptic and could be asleep in seconds. His topographic brain map indicated extensive damage in the form of several focal high-delta areas. This man was literally asleep all the time. Probing for a causal injury, there seemed to be no decisive concussion. All we could elicit was a successful high school and college career playing football. He had been good enough to try out for professional play, but "something," he said, intuitively stopped him. Thorough medical examinations did not reveal a thyroid problem. All the evidence we could put together seemed to indicate that no single injury was afflicting him but an accumulation and overlay of them. The problems persisted even after about twenty LENS treatments, and he discontinued.

A couple of years later Tom returned for more treatments. He had had a round of craniosacral adjustments and some hormone therapy in between. This time the neurofeedback treatment seemed to work much better, and the patient was restored to better functionality. He took a renewed interest in his growing boys, coached the soccer team, worked part-time, and managed to save his marriage. (More on hormone therapy for TBI in just a few pages.)

EEGs of such people may reveal focal areas of delta, theta, or high beta, and not infrequently, if the injury is due to physical trauma, a bullseye of activity at the site, or perhaps its "contra-coup" site rebounds around in its cranial cavity. The older injuries may not even surface in the EEG until much later, or may be indicated by a "rug" of spread-out coherence. Multiple injuries lead to longer courses of treatment and may be characterized by a bumpy road of improvements followed by many regressions as well.

Invictus

Out of the night that covers me,
Black as the pit from pole to pole,
I thank whatever gods may be,
For my unconquerable soul.

FROM "INVICTUS"
BY WILLIAM ERNEST HENLEY

Anyone who has seen the extraordinary film *Invictus,* based on the life of Nelson Mandela, knows the central part that the popular sport of rugby (that is, in the U.K., Australia, New Zealand, and South Africa) plays in the story. The moving film is directed by Clint Eastwood and stars Morgan Freeman as Mandela and Matt Damon as François Pienaar, the white rugby team captain, who comes to love and respect Mandela. The 1995 World Cup victory of the team, against all odds, parallels Mandela's consolidation of his popularity, after emerging from twenty-eight years of Robben Island prison into the presidency of South Africa; it is a testament to how sport can quell prejudice and unite a divided land.

"Matt" (our patient—not the actor—whose story is told below) acknowledges that for many years rugby was his life, and Pienaar was his personal hero. Matt was small for a rugby player but very fast and tough (he looks a little like Matt Damon), and he still loves the sport that injured him (you can see why watching the film or any live rugby match; it is sort of a cross between soccer and American football, played without helmets; very fast and very rough!).

Here Matt tells his own bittersweet story of love for a sport and the injury that helped his own personal courage develop.

Matt's Own Story

I was always told as I was growing up that I was "tough," "resilient," "hard-nosed," "tenacious," but little did I know that those labels would someday come to haunt me.

I grew up like any other middle-class American boy in the West. I attended school and played sports, both organized and unorganized. The sports I played were mainly full-contact sports including football, wrestling, and rugby. I was always a bit smaller than the other boys, so I had learned to become more aggressive in my play in order to keep up with them. Unfortunately, this led to the many injuries I received, including concussions (around eight, give or take a few). I incurred the first one as a freshman in high school, the second as a senior in high school, and the rest as a rugby player in college. The last four were inflicted on me in games during consecutive weeks in 2000.

We played on Saturdays, and my symptoms would always clear by the following Wednesday, so I would always participate in the next week's game. Back then, no one understood the long-term ramifications of getting multiple concussions; so if your symptoms cleared up, the doctor would clear you to play. *After the last one, the symptoms never went away, and my life was changed forever.*

I spent the next few years in college struggling to get by. I had what the doctors termed postconcussive syndrome, or PCS for short. My main symptoms included short-term memory loss, lack of impulse control, lack of focus, insomnia, word searching, and depression. Before the concussions, I was a premedical student with a solid 3.5 GPA, and I was the captain and president of the rugby team. After the concussions, I was still able to get through school, but my GPA dropped to a 3.0. I also began drinking and partying excessively to escape from the symptoms that the PCS was causing. I managed to graduate and took employment at a molecular biology research laboratory. I was fired from that job a year later and spent the next several years repeating that pattern.

In 2007, I discovered a therapy technique called "neurofeedback," and I tried it for about a year. Unfortunately, it didn't work that time. In 2009, I had managed to get into graduate school, but I was soon forced to

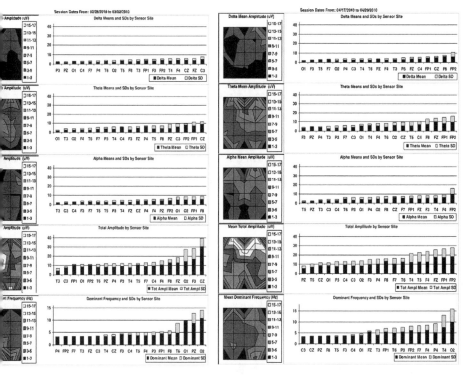

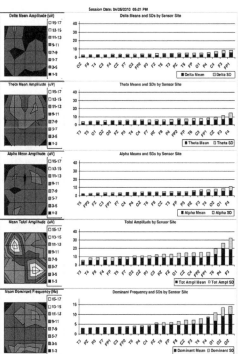

Fig. 11.1. Three maps a few months apart from Matt, indicating the principle of "peeling back the layers of an onion" to show successive injuries—bright-colored areas are "hot spots," the focus of an injury (in one of the six cortical layers, where the cortex is compromised and hence does not inhibit subcortical rhythms). At this point Matt was doing three to four LENS sessions a week at home (under Dr. Larsen's supervision), so the changes are rapid.

take a medical leave of absence due to the stressors imposed by graduate study. At this juncture in my life, I had had enough of the way my life was going, and I decided to do something about it. Luckily, I had a science background, so I went back to the Internet and revisited my search on brain injuries. I discovered that in many cases, hormones become imbalanced from single and multiple brain injuries. So I then sought out a health care practitioner who was experienced in hormone replacement therapy. After seeing four doctors, I finally found one with the knowledge and experience to treat me. Through blood tests, I had discovered that I was deficient in testosterone, cortisol, human growth hormone, and thyroid hormone. The treatment for this was to replace these hormones to their optimal physiological levels with bioidentical hormones.

After that, I was still convinced that neurofeedback was a viable therapy for my brain injuries, so I began a search to find a neurofeedback practitioner who was experienced in treating head injuries. Not long after I began my search I ran across the Low Energy Neurofeedback System, or LENS for short. I soon also discovered Dr. Larsen's website and book. I read his book and decided to make the trip out to New Paltz to see him. He set me up with some protocols using the LENS and also Z-score neurofeedback, and he has been monitoring my home training ever since then.

I also came across a study that used hyperbaric oxygen therapy (HBOT) to treat brain injuries, and I decided to give that a try as well. So I found a local HBOT clinic and began my therapy, which entails eighty treatments.

So far I am about nine months into my treatment, and things are progressing slowly but in a positive direction. It definitely has been a very bumpy road, but it is a road worth traveling. One thing I noticed is that after I got on hormone replacement therapy, the neurofeedback and other therapies began working and having a greater impact. After almost ten years of suffering, I can finally see the "light at the end of the tunnel," and I am very hopeful for my future—so much so that I plan on reentering graduate school in the fall of 2011.

Conclusions

I really like Matt's story, not only because he was our patient, but because of its basic honesty and the ultimately good outcome—or at least good "work in progress," moving in the right direction. He is a tireless researcher on his own behalf; it doesn't hurt that his parents and friends have been immensely supportive. And, best of all, it shows that neurofeedback is far from a sorcerer's wand that works under all circumstances. Rather it is one tool among many in a neurological magician's toolkit.

Note that neurofeedback by itself may not work—especially in chronic and complex cases—until some other things have happened. Attached as I was to the LENS when I first started treating Matt, and though it undeniably helped, his was one of the first cases that showed me (the author as a clinician) that it also slowed overall progress and almost ground things to a halt, until Matt began getting the hormone replacement, craniosacral, and homeopathic treatments and made some lifestyle changes. (Now, it is increasingly regarded as something resembling neurological malpractice not to make the patient aware of the importance of hormone treatments immediately after injury—something important enough that the military is now taking it seriously; Urban et al. 2011.)

Then came a time when Z-scores seemed to work better than the LENS. Matt came and got a qEEG at our center and fine-tuned his self-administered Z-score treatments. Z-score addresses connectivity and phase problems the LENS may miss. The hyperbaric oxygen kicked everything back into high gear at one point (remember that the TBI brain may starve itself of oxygen through constriction of the blood vessels). Every treatment he tried seemed to do a little, making its own contribution, but the whole package worked a whole lot for this resourceful, invincible soul!

The following case is from the office of a senior clinician in the neurofeedback field. Elsa Baehr and her husband, Rufus, have been practicing for more than thirty years in the Chicago area. The treatment is very complete in that it combines the LENS with other methods of conventional neurofeedback, with targeted areas and ranges of training, along with Z-score training (of which we will learn more in chapter 13), as well as breathing and HRV training.

Neurofeedback Treatment of a Forty-Year-Old Man with Multiple Head Injuries

ELSA BAEHR, PH.D.

The Presenting Problem

Bob Winter was a forty-year-old single man at the time of his initial interview. He was referred for a quantitative electroencephalogram evaluation (qEEG) by his psychiatrist to rule out head injury as a factor in his behavioral issues. His low self-esteem prevented him from dating, and he had never engaged in a serious relationship with a woman, although he had many male friends. For the past thirteen years he had worked in a highly stressful situation in the world of finance. His job included advising clients and making decisions regarding financial investments.

Bob was unhappy. His job was very demanding, and he felt that he could not perform up to par. He complained of memory problems that affected his ability to recall numbers. He had difficulty spelling, and he stammered when he spoke. It was difficult for him to sustain his attention while on the job. He had restless sleep and could not recall his dreams.

History

Bob was born in the Midwest and was raised by an intact family. Early developmental history was normal. When he was six years old he sustained the first of many head injuries. He recalls being hit by a baseball bat in the right temporal region of his head. About the same time he also remembered playing hard with friends and hitting his head on a cement floor. He attended a parochial school and was demoted in the second grade because he "wasn't focused." He had developed speech problems and began hating himself for "being dumb." *Apparently no one related his head injuries to the difficulties he was experiencing in school.* He was always interested in athletics, and he developed his skills in swimming and in soccer. Being very bright, he was able to overcome some of his learning difficulties and went on to college after graduating high school. He earned a bachelor's degree and then went into the military for two years.

After his time in the service, he played professional soccer for thirteen years. During that time he sustained more head injuries, including being stepped on the head by a person wearing cleats, colliding heads with another player, and falling and hitting the back of his head. He recalls the experience of this concussion as seeing "yellow and brown" colors and feeling "cloudy." He noted that he "spaced in and out" when he was in school and at work. He occasionally felt mildly depressed.

Diagnosis

Bob was diagnosed as having an attentional deficit disorder most likely related to his head injuries. A quantitative EEG (qEEG) was done in April 2007. The results of this test showed excessive slow-wave activity in the delta, and theta brain wave frequencies in the frontal, temporal, and central regions, with average peak frequencies ranging in the theta range. Theta and low-alpha frequencies peaked in the parietal and occipital regions. There were asymmetries at almost all the homologous sites. The most prominent qEEG deviations were found in beta and delta coherence in the eyes-closed position. The Minimal Traumatic Brain Injury Index (MTBI) showed a probability of 99.5 percent of closed-head injury.

Treatment Recommendations

1. Reduce stress by teaching Bob to control his autonomic nervous system using techniques to control heart-rate variability and to increase parasympathetic functioning with regulated breathing.
2. Reduce hypercoherence in delta and beta brain wave frequencies.
3. Reduce slow-wave activity by using focus protocols designed to decrease frontal and central slow-wave activity (theta) and to increase fast-wave activity (beta in these same brain wave regions).
4. Repeat qEEG during therapy to assess progress.

Course of Therapy

Bob began treatment in May 2007 and ended in December 2008. There were a total of 115 sessions. Bob initially came four days a week, gradually cutting back to one session a week during the last month of therapy. Each session began with stress-reduction techniques. The LENS was used as

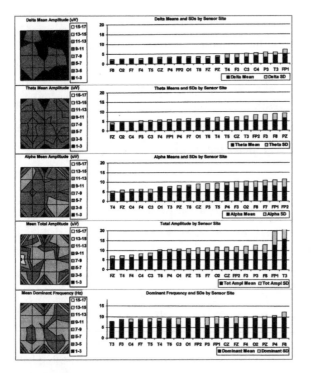

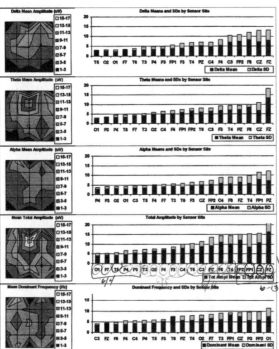

Fig. 11.2. Bob's maps also show hot spots appearing and disappearing under intensive LENS treatments

part of his daily sessions from May 2007 to September 2008. Focus protocols, coherence training, and Z-score training were also included.

Stress Reduction
Coherent breathing techniques designed to regulate heart-rate variability and increase parasympathetic activity were part of every session. The Em Wave Stress Relief System software was used in conjunction with Respire, a CD developed to train coherent breathing. (These are used in conjunction to develop stability in the autonomic nervous system.)

Low-Energy Neurofeedback (LENS)
Over the course of therapy there were twenty-three LENS maps. Treatment followed the site assortment produced by the maps by treating four to five sites in one session. The total number of sessions was approximately eighty-one (not including the maps). This traditional LENS treatment was followed until June 2008, when Rocking protocols and 9–12 Hz protocols were added. LENS was termininated in September 2008. Five patient goals were defined and ranked at the initial session and reevaluated again in October 2007.

Focus Protocols
Focus training was done concurrently with the LENS training. A total of eighty-two focus sessions were completed at frontal, central, temporal, and occipital sites, with the emphases on decreasing delta and theta brain wave frequencies and increasing alpha and beta brain wave frequencies.

Coherence Protocols
There were seventeen sessions designed to reduce bilateral beta and delta coherences between frontal and temporal hemispheric sites.

Z-Score Training
There were twenty-four Z-score training sessions at frontal, temporal, and occipital sites designed to further normalize brain wave activity after the completion of the LENS therapy.

COHERENCE:

Ia. LEFT INTRAHEMISPHERIC (Z)

	DELTA	THETA	ALPHA	BETA
F1F7	1.75	1.00	0.47	1.58
F1F3	1.46	1.25	0.97	1.63
F1T3	2.05	2.27	0.62	3.30
F1C3	1.86	1.76	0.87	2.20
F1T5	2.87	2.14	-1.19	4.12
F1P3	2.16	1.53	0.20	3.35
F1O1	3.49	1.49	-0.69	3.02
F7F3	0.31	-0.30	-0.15	0.82
F7T3	1.01	1.46	0.65	2.15
F7C3	0.96	0.59	0.62	1.51
F7T5	1.69	1.10	0.10	3.99
F7P3	1.35	0.52	0.57	2.73
F7O1	2.03	-0.12	-0.78	4.26
F3T3	0.86	1.15	-0.02	1.58
F3C3	0.98	1.14	0.46	0.79
F3T5	1.22	1.22	-0.56	2.94
F3P3	1.08	0.91	0.24	1.55
F3O1	1.42	0.91	-0.80	3.07
T3C3	0.88	0.84	0.54	1.42
T3T5	1.25	0.84	0.94	2.13
T3P3	1.07	0.67	0.67	1.97
T3O1	1.74	0.93	0.23	2.88
C3T5	0.98	0.79	0.52	2.37
C3P3	0.75	0.42	0.32	1.01
C3O1	0.94	0.68	-0.15	2.48
T5P3	0.76	0.82	0.74	1.48
T5O1	0.56	0.50	0.08	1.09
P3O1	0.24	0.60	0.02	1.50

Ib. RIGHT INTRAHEMISPHERIC (Z)

	DELTA	THETA	ALPHA	BETA
F2F8	1.42	0.91	0.67	0.12
F2F4	1.01	0.67	0.64	1.33
F2T4	1.76	1.47	0.63	1.50
F2C4	1.29	0.96	0.71	1.35
F2T6	2.26	0.59	0.48	2.30
F2P4	2.06	1.15	-0.45	1.55
F2O2	2.51	1.09	0.31	1.75
F8F4	1.71	0.72	0.77	0.43
F8T4	1.37	0.74	0.50	0.11
F8C4	1.33	0.54	0.66	-0.04
F8T6	1.42	-0.18	0.51	0.67
F8P4	1.66	0.42	-0.39	0.11
F8O2	1.90	0.20	1.12	0.78
F4T4	2.00	1.64	0.72	1.28
F4C4	1.29	1.11	0.74	1.08
F4T6	1.57	1.05	-0.04	1.93
F4P4	1.45	1.08	-0.39	0.88
F4O2	1.36	0.97	0.17	2.28
T4C4	1.90	1.69	0.78	0.96
T4T6	0.62	0.12	-1.48	0.51
T4P4	1.86	1.42	0.20	1.50
T4O2	1.33	-0.07	-1.74	1.25
C4T6	1.22	0.89	-0.02	1.39
C4P4	0.91	0.71	0.12	0.60
C4O2	1.07	0.77	-0.61	1.66
T6P4	1.51	1.79	1.40	2.05
T6O2	0.92	1.11	0.60	1.59
P4O2	1.30	1.54	1.02	1.65

Ic. HOMOLOGOUS (Z)

	DELTA	THETA	ALPHA	BETA
F1F2	0.71	0.82	0.47	0.98
F7F8	0.70	1.02	0.33	0.85
F3F4	1.81	1.66	0.97	1.77
T3T4	1.53	1.00	-0.14	3.86
C3C4	1.43	1.22	0.85	1.17
T5T6	1.36	1.56	0.76	3.67
P3P4	1.08	1.13	0.88	1.63
O1O2	0.63	0.97	1.00	2.02

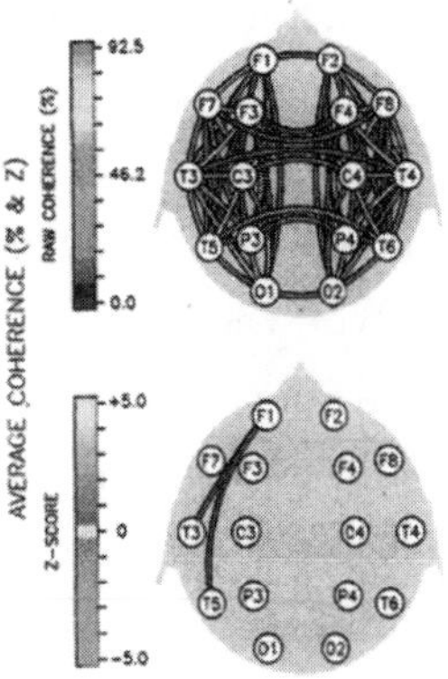

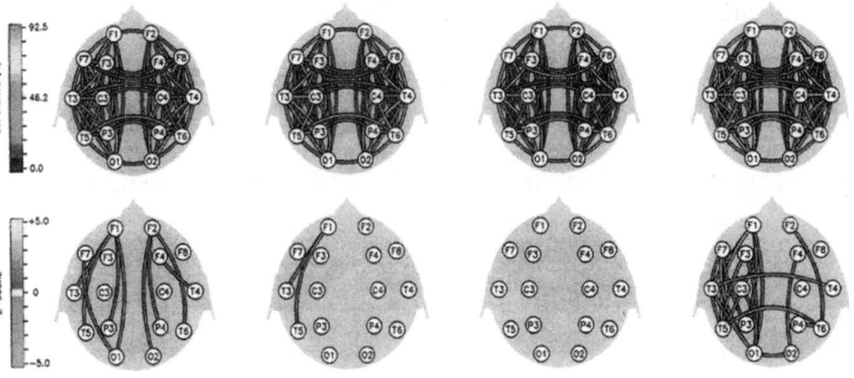

DELTA (0.5-3.5 Hz)   THETA (3.5-7 Hz)   ALPHA (7-13 Hz)   BETA (13-22 Hz)

Fig. 11.3. Bob's qEEG (SKIL) maps

Cognitive Fitness

Memory training and cognitive fitness training began in September 2008 using the game Think Fast and the Brain Train software.

Quantitative EEG

There were a total of seven qEEG evaluations during the course of therapy that were used to diagnose brain wave activity and to measure progress in therapy.

Results

Subjective Reports

Bob responded well to the LENS after experiencing dizziness during the first two sessions. With the exception of the RTS protocol, which he claimed affected his speech in a negative way (he preferred the protocol that focused on 9–12 Hz), he handled all interventions without a problem. By June he reported feeling better and more focused. In September he said his thinking was clearer and his speech had gotten better.

In spite of the fact that he incurred two additional head injuries during treatment, Bob continued to improve, and his self-esteem was better. By the end of the first year he had started a relationship with a woman, whom he married in December of the following year. Treatment goals on a subjective scale with rankings from 1 to 10 (10 being the worst) were recorded initially in May 2007. Issues and ranking were as follows: more control over eating (10), reduce fatigue (10), be more organized (7), follow through on tasks (8), less procrastination (8). On a follow-up evaluation in October 2007, all scores were half of the initial scores, showing progress. While there were no additional follow-up evaluations on the initial treatment goals, there was an assessment in June 2008. Bob reported that his listening skills improved and he had a better capacity to remember numbers. Typing skills and reading were greatly improved, he was better organized, and he procrastinated less. For better efficiency he made lists of things to do because he "couldn't leave things undone." His speech had improved, and he was more effective interacting with his clients.

In a telephone interview in July 2010, he stated that he was "doing great." He continued to maintain the improvement he had gained during therapy. He was doing well at work and in his marriage. He was happy to inform us that he and his wife were expecting their first baby in a matter of weeks.

Clinical Findings

The quantitative EEG (qEEG) was repeated numerous times during his therapy to assess progress. Data from the first of these evaluations, dated April 23, 2007, showed significant deviations in measures of coherence in the delta and beta brain wave frequencies. The final qEEG, dated September 30, 2008, showed remarkable improvement in both delta and beta coherence. (A clinican's note in November indicated that the remaining temporal deviations had been normalized during Z-score training.) The average peak frequencies on the first qEEG were basically in the theta to low alpha (except at the right occipital site). There were asymmetries at almost all the homologous sites, indicating left and right hemisphere differences. The average peak frequencies on the final qEEG were basically to the alpha brain wave frequencies. There were no longer significant asymmetries at the homologous sites. These findings were consistent with the first LENS map, dated May 30, 2007, and the last map, dated September 23, 2008. Observation of these maps shows that there was a shift in dominant frequencies from theta to alpha, with alpha means increasing at the end of treatment, and theta means decreasing.

This case study is an example of how the dedication of the client, over a period of a year and a half, was critical to his successful neurotherapy treatment. This was particularly apparent in the improvements in coherence, which can be seen by comparing the coherence data on the first and last qEEG maps dated April 2007 and June 2008. Even though there were seventeen sessions of coherence training in addition to the LENS training, it was felt that the LENS was most important in reducing the delta and beta coherences. This finding is consistent with findings of numerous other clients who improved on measures of coherence as a result of LENS therapy. In addition, the focus training and Z-score training also contributed in the reduction of slow-wave activity and the increase in alpha and beta brain wave frequencies, and in general normalized his measurable brain wave functioning.

The techniques used to control stress (the Em Wave and the coherent breathing techniques) seemed to have an impact on his speech as well as on his anxiety. He continues to use these methods in his daily life.

In this beautifully presented, complex case, we see all the elements that have been introduced in this chapter, resolved with a variety of treatment and evaluational tools. The LENS breaks up entrenched neuroprotective mechanisms and galvanizes the process. The often repeated qEEGs give an ongoing and reliable way of evaluating progress—in reference to the normative database, and studying the connectivity, coherence, and phase lock or lag in the frequency domain (alongside the amplitudes and frequencies of the LENS maps). The qEEGs also are preparation for the Z-score training and establish the sites and the protocols to be used in the training. In the background, the improved respiration afforded by the EM Wave (a HeartMath device) delivers maximum oxygen to the brain, which is trying to repair itself. The further use of cognitive therapy exercises (Brain Gym) is also helpful (especially when the other brain stimulation and balancing techniques have been used).

The LENS and Sports Enhancement

This section may seem almost an afterthought in this chapter, but although it is brief, it actually has profound implications for athletes. If neurofeedback can help athletes who sustain injuries, can it also help athletes in their performance—maybe, in some measure, sparing them from injuries (at least the self-induced kind) where they make repetitive mistakes and incur repetitive injuries? The below cases by Lynn Brayton seem to indicate they can, as well as avoiding the more stupid excesses of injuries compounding upon injuries.

The Case of Eddie
LYNN BRAYTON, PSY.D.

Eddie is a retired firefighter in his early sixties. He was referred for neurofeedback from his psychotherapist, who had successfully assisted him in his recovery from alcohol and gambling addictions. Although it had been years since he had a relapse from either addiction, he had frequent problems with his temper. He reported he was easily stressed and provoked into anger, which was a significant problem in his marriage. He reported no other problems and felt he had a very strong relationship with his therapist, whom he saw on a monthly basis.

Eddie had an immediate response to treatment. From the first session, he noticed he did not have his typical angry response to stressful situations. This was a change his wife also noticed and appreciated. However, the most welcome change was in his golf game. Since he was retired, he spent much of his free time golfing, reading about golf, and vacationing at golfing tournaments. He reported his golf game was the best it had been in the more than twenty-five years he had played. His golfing buddies had noticed the change and were very puzzled as to how he had made such a remarkable improvement overnight. Eddie had a total of four sessions before he felt his temper was gone and his game was at its peak. He is scheduled for another tournament this fall, which may bring him in for a refresher.

In working with a numerous patients, there are two things that almost always improve as a result of using LENS. They are a bad temper and sports performance. Although I have never seen a single patient with the presenting issue of sports performance, I have seen improvement in performance in almost every single patient who is involved in any type of sport. I have had runners report longer running distances and faster times, sharpshooters improve their accuracy, even more wins by Ping-Pong players. The results are typically noticeable very early in treatment and are easily recognized by patients because they are objective and measurable. Changes in mood and cognitive performance are often influenced by external circumstances (e.g., I was in a better mood because my wife was out of town; I did better on the test this week because it was easier than it usually is; I read the book faster because it was more interesting). With sports, patients often have a very clear sense of their ability, and they own it (e.g., I couldn't hit a decent shot today; I'm low on energy; This was my best game ever).

Perhaps the most dramatic case that I've seen of sports enhancement was that of a sixteen-year-old boy whose mother sought treatment for his poor grades and stuttering. He left his first LENS session and went immediately to basketball practice, where he made forty free-throw shots in a row. After a few sessions, the father started bringing his son for a LENS session before his games because he noticed such a remarkable improvement in his sports performance. His father confessed he always thought his son wasn't hustling enough but realized that it was his timing that had improved. "It was that split second where he was behind that made all the difference in his game," reported his father.

I expect most LENS practitioners have experienced similar results; however, many may not have queried in this area, since it is unlikely to be the patient's presenting problem. I expect it to be some time before LENS is used in college or professional sports, since it is utilized almost exclusively in the field of mental health. When some coach does get the idea of using it on all his or her team members, I believe the results will be remarkable.

TWELVE

STROKE FAMILY

With Barbara Dean Schacker, M.A., Victor Zelek, Ph.D.,
and Mary Lee Esty, Ph.D., L.C.S.W.

I have borrowed for this chapter title, with Barbara Dean Schacker's permission, the name of her website, Stroke Family, because when a loved
person is "stroked," the whole family is "stroked" or traumatized. Barbara is
also my coauthor for this chapter, and we begin with her narrative of how
she developed the wonderful method called the Sensory Trigger that she
has evolved to help other families—for much longer than I've been researching the subject. As well as Michael's dramatic recovery, along with detailed
brain maps, this chapter brings in the backstory of a remarkable, loving,
and resourceful spouse, and it introduces the reader to an excellent facility
for rehabilitating serious head injuries of all sorts: the Northeast Center for
Special Care. My other collaborator on this chapter is Dr. Victor Zelek, the
neuropsychologist at the Northeast Center who first mapped Michael and
saw to his care during Michael's year and a half at the facility.

In 2010, Dr. Zelek and I presented Michael's case at the ISNR, the
International Society for Neurofeedback and Research's annual confer-
ence in Denver. The presentation (also given at the national LENS confer-
ence in Los Gatos, California, in a preliminary form) is called "Turning
On the Lights: How Neurofeedback Helped a Cultural Genius Do Soul
Retrieval." The "Cultural Genius" part is really true, because Michael is

indeed a Rennaissance man: writer, environmentalist, musician, and composer. With a little help from his friends (including neurofeedback), he may win his way back to the richly brilliant cognition he had with a whole brain instead of half.

My third collaborator on this chapter is Mary Lee Esty, one of the first therapists to begin using neurofeedback. Since 1994 Dr. Esty has used LENS/FNS to treat more than two thousand people diagnosed with various disorders including TBI, ADHD, depression, anxiety, Asperger's Syndrome, pain, and other central nervous system problems. In this chapter she documents her work with "Paul," a fifty-five-year-old stroke victim with a myriad of problems to overcome.

Barbara's Story: Prisoner of Silence
BARBARA DEAN SCHACKER, M.A.

That day, I had no idea that my life was about to change forever. I remember standing in left field playing softball during recess on a beautiful spring day in Nebraska when my teacher suddenly appeared and motioned me off the field. "You have permission to leave school immediately," she said gravely. "Your sister is waiting for you in her car." Climbing into the car, I immediately knew something terrible had happened. My sister said, her voice trembling, "Daddy has had a stroke. They don't know if he will live. He is in the hospital with Mom."

When we arrived at the hospital in Lincoln, my sister and I rushed to the entrance. At the door, I was asked, "How old are you?" "I am thirteen," I replied. The nuns declared, "She is under age, she can't come in. You have to be fifteen to enter the hospital. That is the rule." My sister took me back to the car to wait while she rushed inside. It was midday. I waited and waited, but no one came for me. I moved into the back seat to lie down. It was late at night, about twelve hours later, when my sister returned to find me hysterically whimpering in a fetal position—curled up in the back seat. She had finally gained permission to bring me in.

I remember walking down the clean, echoing halls to my father's room to see him in a coma. My mother seemed to be in a trance, until we went to the women's room where she broke down and sobbed, "What will I do without him?" All the things my father was to me, all the things he had done with me—flooded into my mind. The times he let me drive sitting on his lap around our plowed wheat field even though I was only six years old. Because of this early training, I already knew how to drive, even though I was only thirteen. The time there was a tornado that raged right over our house, taking the chimney and a beloved weeping willow tree, while we huddled together in the basement, his strong hand holding mine and reassuring me to "have faith—all will be well." Teaching me to hammer and saw so I could build a tree house—all by myself. This kind, intelligent, affectionate father, a robust forty-eight years old, now lay crushed by a massive stroke that had come out of nowhere. It didn't seem possible; it was completely unreal.

Coming out of the coma, he was in the hospital three months before returning home to be taken care of by my mother. We were told he would never walk or talk again. He didn't understand anything we said and was totally silent. The neurologist told us he had "global aphasia." As a young woman, I liked books and wanted to know the answers to my questions, so I looked this up in the Encyclopedia Britannica—it said that this condition was "incurable." Yet something just didn't fit, even though I couldn't explain my discomfort at the time. I remember mother telling me, "Barbara, you have to just accept it. He will never talk again." But something in me didn't believe her, didn't believe the speech therapists, and didn't believe the Mayo Clinic that declared him "untreatable."

About a year later, something was wrong with the car, and he couldn't tell us what it was, although he knew what was broken. He took a pencil and piece of paper and with his left hand (his right hand was paralyzed by the stroke) drew a complete diagram of the car engine with one area circled. Everyone was amazed he could do this. Obviously he had all his memory, but he just couldn't talk! I took the piece of paper with this drawing to the mechanic who confirmed that it was, indeed, the clutch plate—the part that he had repaired. The fact that he could draw this diagram struck me, and I thought, "There is a way I can help him. There must be some way he can talk again." Although I didn't know it at the time, this was the beginning of a whole life's journey and the discovery of what I would later call the Sensory Trigger Method.

Years later, at twenty-one, I was working in the Lincoln Public Library as head of the printing department. I had a young daughter, Jennifer, who at age two was learning to talk. I became fascinated with the work of Maria Montessori. Montessori, a French woman, was one of the first women to receive a medical degree. She was to become famous for discovering a way to teach brain-damaged children in the asylum how to talk, read, and write using the sense of touch. Her theory that children can be guided to master their senses, even with learning disabilities and brain damage—that they could master fine motor coordination and develop abilities that may at first not be apparent, or may be lacking in their development, but are the very basis and foundation of adult intellectual and verbal abilities—made a deep impression. Hungrily, I went on to devour books on the evolution of language and the history of writing. There was something more there than just wanting to know how to help my two-year-old express herself!

Then one day, while I was clearing off my desk, it suddenly came to me—of course! The drawing that my father had made . . . it must have to do with that. He could communicate with pictures—pictograms . . . like the cave drawings at Lascaux, France. The recovery of language could follow an evolutionary pattern. He could communicate with pictures—that is the starting point! Being an artist, I quickly took card stock and cut it up into small cards and drew pictures on each one. "Vernon"—a picture of my father—"point to"—a hand pointing—"cup"—a picture of a cup. I made one for myself and other objects: a door, a chair, a hammer, and an apple. The opinion of the speech therapist who had asked my father to "Point to the cup" and then diagnosed him "untreatable" because he couldn't do that—suddenly became unimportant. But this new way I had discovered became my new challenge.

Armed with my set of cards and a few objects, I duplicated the speech therapist's test, only this time it would be nonverbal—we would be communicating with pictures and with touch! I laid the cards down in sequence on the desk before my father. "Vernon"—"point to"—"cup." Avoiding body cues, I didn't give it away by looking at the cup. I waited. Silently, I placed my finger down to touch each card in sequence. I showed him how to do the same with the index finger of his left hand.

He followed my demonstration, touching each one in sequence, left to right. Then his eyes lit up and he pointed to the cup! And even though when I asked him to point to the door or the chair he looked at me blankly, when I used the cards, he understood and could answer by pointing to the correct object from the group of objects that were on the table or in the room.

I then launched into intensive research. I had the library at my disposal and could access research that was unavailable even to college grads, who were only reading the curricula but not the most recent studies. Yet the real revelation came when by chance I picked up a *Psychology Today* magazine on my break at the library. In it was an article about the "split brain operation" and the findings of Michael Gazzaniga, Norman Geshwin, and Roger Sperry about the dominant speech center and the passive speech center. They had found a direct developmental and neurological link between the dominant hand and the dominant speech center.

When I wrote to Dr. Michael Gazzaniga and told him I had invented a picture language for global aphasia, he was so intrigued he invited me to visit him where he was researching at the State University of New York at Stonybrook. There, I might consider a degree in the new field of neurolinguistic psychology and find out more about his research. I traveled to New York City and had lunch with him. We had a very exciting conversation. He took me back to his office at the school and introduced me to Norman Geshwin and Roger Sperry. After a few months, however, I decided that I didn't want to do pure research. Rather, I wanted to find a way to apply the knowledge and make a system that could directly help stroke patients communicate and maybe even recover their speech.

Further clinical studies showed the right hemisphere could only say three or perhaps four words in sequence. It appeared there was a limit to sequential memory in the right hemisphere. It is still generally believed that due to the specialization of the adult brain, the right hemisphere speech center is incapable of initiating fluid speech. This was before the current concept of brain plasticity—the ability of the brain to change and learn, even an aged brain. No one considered that the reason why the right hemisphere couldn't talk after brain injury was not because of some innate characteristic but because it had not *learned to be the active talker.*

A few years later, studies revealed that we talk with both sides of our brains as young children, before the brain specializes. More studies came out that indicated that the right hemisphere could learn to talk. As I continued to research, I found a study that showed that aphasia is rare in Asian populations. Because their writing is pictographic, their brain symmetry develops differently, and active speech is probably stored in both hemispheres. It has also been found that bilingual people who have a stroke or brain injury on the left side can often speak their second language, but not their native tongue—especially if they learned it after the age of seven. Their brain stored the new language on the other side of the brain. I wondered, what if we can make a new dominant hand? What if we can access the passive speech center through its corresponding hand, and get it to talk again?

Later clinical studies showed the right hemisphere could only say three words, perhaps four words together. It appeared there was a limit to sequential memory in the right hemisphere, and that, due to the specialization of the adult brain, the right hemisphere speech center was incapable of initiating fluid speech.

So, after eighteen months of working with my picture-language cards, mostly independently with the help of my devoted mother, my father said his first spontaneous word—it was nine years poststroke. It was the first and only documented recovery from global aphasia.

He had progressed from being able to say only about nine words to being able to repeat words and copy them, writing the letters under the picture. As the long months passed, it seemed hopeless that he would ever be able to talk spontaneously, however. But then about eighteen months later, watching a report on TV on the Mars Explorer expedition, he drew a picture of the solar system and near the fourth planet wrote the word "Mars," and then, pointing to it, said "Mars." He then found that he could say "Mars" whenever he wanted to. That was the beginning.

In 1973, I moved to California to find employment and left my father to work on his own. I remember coming back home to visit him;

he looked up at me and said, "Amazing." Tearfully, I told him it truly was amazing! As his speaking vocabulary increased to over 700 words, he was able to go downtown on the bus by himself, go to the grocery store and the post office, even the bank. He became an artist with his left hand and showed his works in the state capitol building.

I went on to create the first talking software for aphasia recovery in 1988. It ran on an Apple IIe computer with an Echo Speech device. My husband, Michael, helped me design and produce the program, while speech pathologists reviewed the plan and tested it at the University of California at Davis Medical Center. In 1991, *Reader's Digest* published "Prisoner of Silence," written by Geeta Dardick—one of those "amazing stories." Also, in 1991 Johns Hopkins University awarded me a Certificate of Achievement as the creator of the first talking software for speech therapy and aphasia recovery—I had won over 2,000 other entries in the competition. The program, called Breakthrough to Language, sold to the speech therapy field, as well as to special education, and by now has been sent to over 50,000 adults to help them recover their speech.

This success was to be short-lived, however. Computer technology was advancing so rapidly that we were forced to upgrade. But the investors didn't understand the need to upgrade the software to high-resolution graphics. It would cost a half-million dollars to duplicate the program—it would be too costly. Without the upgrade, the program became obsolete. Sadly we closed the company and retired the program.

Michael's Story
BARBARA DEAN SCHACKER, M.A.

My husband, Michael, and I decided to move to Woodstock, New York, in 1995 to start over. There we would be close to writers and publishers as well as old family networks that could us help us. After about a year, I realized that a whole new program could be created as an online program. I learned to program in HTML and created, with Michael's help, the first online talking software for speech recovery in 1998. I focused more on self-help for stroke and brain-injury survivors and added different Sensory Trigger programs and techniques that were not computer based. I created

StrokeFamily.org, a website devoted to helping stroke and head injury survivors recover their speech, rebuild their bodies, and prevent stroke. The
Let's Talk software program sold well and helped many people recover
their speech. I continued my research and wrote guides and paper programs to make the Whole Speech Practice Kit. We didn't know then how
important this work would be to our own family—that catastrophic traumatic brain damage would strike again.

In the spring of 2008, Michael had just finished the last edit on
his book *A Spring Without Bees: How Colony Collapse Disorder Has
Endangered Our Food Supply*—a book that the publisher realized was so
important, it had to be rushed to publication. After overworking under
unusually high stress for nine months, Michael did not look or feel well.
His complexion was ashen, even though he ate well, and he had been falling asleep in the middle of the day, sometimes sleeping for hours. The way
he walked was almost lopsided and weak. Michael shrugged this off as
exhaustion and the fact that he had not had time to exercise for months.
Melissa, our daughter, and I were worried about him—our premonitions
told us there was something quite wrong with him. When we pleaded
with him to see a doctor, he dismissed us. "No, that's not necessary," he
said. "I'll just get back in shape now that the book is finished."

Then on the evening of April 2, 2008, Michael developed a sudden severe backache. He said he wanted to lie down for a while and
went upstairs. For some reason I followed him, deciding to work on my
computer near him while he rested. Suddenly he said, "Barbara, I've got
this terrible pain in my back—it's getting worse. I don't know what's
going on."

"Is it like a spasm?" I asked. He groaned: "No, it's a like a knife ripping
into me!" Instantly, I was on the search engine, typing in "heart attack,
back pain." It came up as a symptom. "Does your shoulder hurt?" "Yes."
"Do your fingers tingle or feel numb?" "Yeah, a little." He struggled to sit
up but fell back on the bed. "It's getting worse—I can . . . I . . . I . . . can
. . . feel . . . it—my chest." Now he was having trouble getting the words
out. Suddenly I remembered the nightmare I had three nights earlier. In
the dream I had come home to find Michael dead on the floor in a pool of
blood with a hole in his heart that looked like a bullet wound. A strange

feeling came over me that this was not just a bad backache. "You're going to the ER right now!" "Why?" he asked in disbelief. "Because you're having a heart attack, and you have clear signs of impending stroke. There isn't time for the ambulance—we live too far away, and it might take an ambulance a half an hour to get here." I knew from my research that there is usually only a twenty- to twenty-five-minute window of opportunity to get to the hospital to receive lifesaving treatment. "Melissa!" I called as we rushed out the door, "Call the hospital—the number is on the computer screen. Tell them a heart attack and possible stroke will be in the ER within twenty minutes. Tell them to have the stroke team and expert cardiologist ready and the CAT scan scheduled for use."

Michael now was noticeably limping and leaning heavily toward his right side as he quickly got to the car. "I'll have to speed to get there in time," I said. Now Michael wasn't talking but making struggling sounds next to me in the front seat. I drove at seventy miles an hour with my hazard lights flashing. "What am I doing?" I thought to myself.

"You know this is the only way to save his life," was the answer I heard in my head. "You're going to be okay, Michael," I said, as I reached over to hold his hand. Miraculously, there happened to be no one on the highway as we sped toward Kingston, and strangely there were no patrol cars to pull me over—and all the lights turned green. No one was even in our lane as we streaked down Broadway and turned into the hospital ER at 8:30 p.m.

As it turned out, we made it just in time. If we had been ten minutes later, he would have died. When the CAT scan revealed a problem with the aorta (an artery that feeds the brain) and not the heart, Michael was immediately airlifted to Albany Medical Center, where he was rushed into a seven-hour high-risk operation to install an artificial artery before it burst and he bled to death.

He survived the operation, but the next day it was clear he had massive brain damage to his left hemisphere, and even some to his right hemisphere. The neurologist showed me the scan, and my heart sank. Almost his entire left hemisphere was gone. I knew what I was looking at. The area of damage looked like it was about 20 percent greater than the amount that would wipe out his speech and comprehension. The doctors said, "There will be no speech." "What about speech therapy?" I asked. The top neurologist shook his head and paused. "It's not possible . . . there will be no speech."

Numbly, I walked away, wondering, "Is he one of those I can't help?" Then, trying to reassure myself: "Well, I have helped my father, who was declared untreatable, and I have helped countless other 'hopeless' cases . . . maybe. He is an expert musician—maybe he has mixed dominance . . . his right hemisphere was virtually untouched . . . I have to believe! I just have to believe in him, in God . . . in myself. And if I don't know how to help him, even if I don't know the answer, I promise, I'll find it!"

Holding Michael's left hand and leaning close to him, I started at once with the Sensory Trigger Method. He was still in his coma. I talked to him and told him not to give up, that he knew that I would help him recover and that one day he would walk and talk again. I talked to him for at least thirty minutes each day while stimulating his left hand. My mind raced with all the things I needed to do . . . with all the things I *had* to do and all the things I *could* do.

Michael had to relearn how to breathe. His lungs had been shut down so long that when the heart was restarted, they were collapsed and no longer worked. He spent the first month connected to life support with an artificial breathing machine that made horrifying sounds as the air was sucked in and then was forced out through the plastic-rimmed tube in his throat. There were all kinds of tubes; feeding tubes and drainage tubes sprouted from all parts of his body. A large piece of his skull on the left side had to be removed to relieve the pressure from the swelling of his brain. His head bulged out grotesquely on that side for a few weeks, and then, as the swelling went down, it caved in.

His left brain had collapsed, and he couldn't make any sounds at all. But he could nod his head for yes and no if I held his left hand. I showed this to the nurses, who were flabbergasted. They couldn't get answers out of him . . . but I could. I could, because I was using the Sensory Trigger Method that was going to the undamaged right hemisphere, while normal speech without the touch signal only went to the damaged side.

It was the end of April, and he had just been moved out of critical care at Albany Medical Center and into an acute care program at Sunnyview

Rehabilitation Hospital in Schenectady, when the publisher sent the prepublication copy of his book. Melissa and I drove there to visit him almost every day, and this day we had his book in hand. When we arrived in his room I brought out the book and placed it in his hands. He wept as he realized he had lived to see his book published. I put the book in his left hand and held the book for him on the right side as Melissa turned a few pages. He looked hard at the print and I noticed his eyes scanning from left to right. "I think he is trying to read," I said. After a while I noticed the light of recognition in his eyes as they efficiently moved from left to right, and he broke out in a huge smile. "I think he is reading! Are you reading, Michael? Can you read?" He looked at me and made a little sound. "You can read, Michael, can't you? You can still read!" and he nodded slightly, his eyes shining!

After he put the book down and we had all taken a break, the thought came to me to try to get him to say the word "read." So I went back in, took up his left hand, and told him, "I believe you can say 'read'. Let's try it!" I let him watch my face. I said softly, "read"—exaggerating my facial expression. "Uh," he responded. "Read," I repeated. "You can do it—rrrrr—eee—d." "Uh, ruh . . . dah," he said. "Good! You made the R sound!" Over and over again we tried. I held his left hand while working with him. Finally, in about an hour—it seemed like eternity—he said the word . . . "Read." "READ! Yes! Read! You said the word 'read'!" I exclaimed. Melissa and I hugged him and cried, and he cried too—he had said his first word. The doctors and nurses were so amazed—no one could believe it. "It's very unusual—so early on," one physician said blandly. But for me it was a sign—he *could* recover his speech.

Months passed, and all he could say was "read." "Read—read— read." He would say it for "I love you." "Read," he would say for "Yes," and "Read" he would say for "No." It was his all-purpose word. He said "Read" for everything. This is because he not only had aphasia, the loss of speech, he also had apraxia and dyspraxia—repetitious speech not tied to meaning, unintelligible speech, and partially intelligible speech. He even had left-hand motor apraxia, which meant that he could not gesture to something that he wanted. He would reach over and pick up a pencil when he meant to pick up his spoon. He was far more damaged

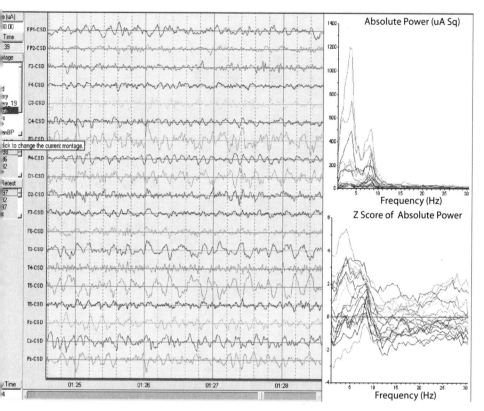

Fig. 12.1. A qEEG done at the Northeast Center by Dr. Victor Zelek

than my father had been. He would have to overcome all these different speech disorders.

Speech therapy was not really successful at Sunnyview. He could repeat the days of the week after the therapist and repeat numbers. He then could recite the numbers from memory in order up to ten, but he could not say them, or verbally identify them, on his own. Yet, with the Sensory Trigger Method, words were popping out spontaneously—infrequently, but "there" all the same. When this happened, they came out perfectly clear—though often they were not retained and were seemingly never used again. He progressed to being able to repeat more and more words spoken to him. I challenged him and got him to say—much to his delight—"regeneration," "synchronicity"—the words he had talked and written about in his book *Global Awakening: New Science and the*

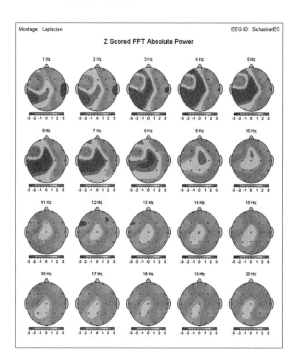

Fig. 12.2. These qEEGs done at the Northeast Center by Dr. Victor Zelek show serious dysregulation spreading across the left hemisphere. (See plate 12 for a color version.)

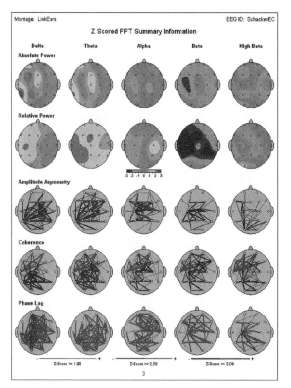

Fig. 12.3. The impaired communication between parts of the brain is shown by the thick congested lines in the bottom half of the scans, indicating hypo- and hypercoherence and phase problems. (See plate 13 for a color version.)

21st-Century Enlightenment. We gave him all kinds of books to read. One day he said, "Sentient beings" spontaneously! And then, excited by the change in political climate in the country, "Obama!" (With great enthusiasm.) This was after he had moved into the Northeast Center for Special Care with their traumatic brain injury recovery program.

The Northeast Center, or NCSE as it is affectionately called, is an innovative, skilled nursing facility—perhaps one of the most innovative in the country. The idea here is that traumatic brain injuries take a long time to recover from, and that most severe brain injuries don't recover fully because the brain is not stimulated in creative ways. The center features an extensive and extraordinarily successful art therapy program and music therapy program. Michael, being an amazing musician, not only performed as lead singer, he composed and recorded his own original music, playing the violin, guitar, and mandolin with virtuosity. In their music program he was allowed to be the "star" and could sing the words

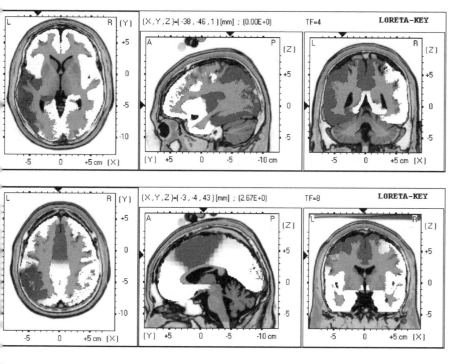

Fig. 12.4. *LORETA images show the deeper penetration of the damage from the cortex into and a small distance across the corpus callosum. (See plate 5 for a color version.)*

to his songs clearly, while the center's band learned and performed the music complete with musicians and backup singers who were also recovering from strokes and brain injuries.

I petitioned the center to have a computer placed in Michael's room so he could run my Let's Talk program alongside their speech therapy program. It was an informal adjunct speech therapy program. This, at first, raised eyebrows, but as he progressed more rapidly with the Sensory Trigger Method and the programs in the kit, the speech therapist was allowed to include it in her therapy sessions with him. As predicted, in six weeks his brain had grown new connections, and now more spontaneous words were coming back every day. His tendency to say the word "Read" for everything slowly faded away into the background. I started sentence practice with him, beginning with three-word sentences. And then six months later, he began to say spontaneous phrases and some sentences on his own . . . words that were not practiced, but words and sentences coming from the right hemisphere speech center's ability to grow new connections in the brain.

Around this time we gained permission to take Michael out of the center to receive special treatment given by Dr. Stephen Larsen. Ironically, we had been great friends of Stephen and his wife, Robin. Here it was: miraculously—"synchronistically," you might say—our friend Stephen, who had successfully treated the severely brain-injured with LENS neurofeedback and other neuroregenerative therapies!

When Michael started with LENS, he couldn't walk more than a very short distance, and he was still bound to his wheelchair. A few short months after treatment at Stone Mountain, he was walking with assistance into the office with a hemi-walker cane, sitting down in a regular chair, and walking back out to the car! And now, at almost three years poststroke, he walked into the office without his cane with just a little assistance from his aide and me to help him get up the steps and steady his balance.

Dr. Larsen mapped Michael's brain and has kept careful records—charting the increase in brain wave activity that is now traveling through of its own accord in the previously dead zones of the left hemisphere. It appears that the two therapies have a synergistic effect when it comes to speech, as both methods make new pathways in the brain. Both confirm

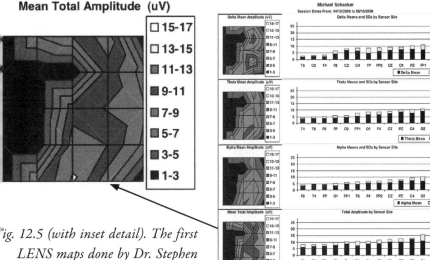

Fig. 12.5 (with inset detail). The first LENS maps done by Dr. Stephen Larsen at Stone Mountain Center in July 2009. No electrodes were placed above the area where there was no skull (black area at far left).

the new paradigm of brain function—the plasticity or learning capability of the injured brain—the brain that can heal itself.

Today, almost three years later, Michael speaks in short, clear sentences and continues to say new words and phrases every day, entirely on his own. His writing lags behind his speech, but we are now working on that in earnest, as I design and develop new more advanced Sensory Trigger programs that can break through the iron walls of apraxia and dyspraxia in both speech and writing.

Now, I often think of the thousands—perhaps hundreds of thousands—of stroke and head-injury survivors who have not been so fortunate to have the Sensory Trigger Method or neurofeedback therapy and are still trapped in the silence of aphasia or the repetitive meaningless speech of apraxia and dyspraxia.

I have videotaped Michael's progress at each step, each breakthrough in his recovery, and I have published these clips on Strokefamily.org for others to get a sense of what real speech recovery looks and sounds like. He still has dyspraxia and makes some mistakes in his speech. He still works to break through the blocks to what he is trying to say. Yet he continues to recover with brain-regenerative approaches like LENS neurofeedback and the Sensory Trigger Method and, remarkably, more and more independently.

Michael becomes more like himself every day.

Stephen Larsen Describes His Treatment of Michael Schacker

When I first visited my friend in the Northeast Center, I was overwhelmed with sensations; the open, inviting lobby was flanked by two lofty atria, filled with plants—and with the art work of patients. A woman played respectable jazz piano on an electronic keyboard in the lobby. But even to get to the elevators, one passed dozens of patients who were extremely compromised by their injuries: wheelchairs, irregular locomotion. A few people seemed caught in a private conversation with themselves; some others shouted and gesticulated. A few were high-functioning enough to engage in personal conversations. One man told me quite lucidly of his accident that had left him wheelchair bound and with a complicated brain injury.

Michael was on the second floor, in a large room with his own bathroom and a window. All around was tangible evidence of his political and environmental affiliation; a picture of Barack Obama, nature scenes, lots of books, a computer and a keyboard. Not bad for a hospital! Michael wore a purple football helmet because of his open skull. One false move in the bathroom, one lunge from his bed to the wall, and the brain damage could be incalculable. Day and night, he had to wear that helmet. But he seemed to remember me and greeted me warmly. His smile was lopsided, but very genuine. The only words he could say were: "Read read read!" But he smiled with great warmth and enthusiasm as he said it. Barbara had already been working with the Sensory Trigger and the imagery work that she had developed to help her father. There were cards around, and she could start up a computer program. Michael was working cheerfully and willingly every day.

I was in the process of negotiating a professional agreement to come into the center and treat Michael when the founding director, Anthony Salerno, died, and there were major administrative shifts. Barbara decided to schedule weekly appointments for LENS sessions at our center, about

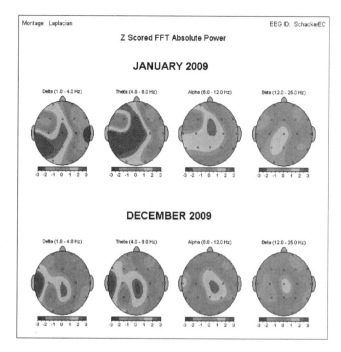

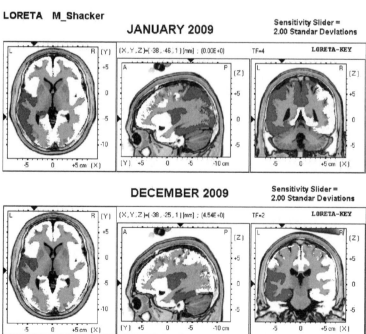

Fig. 12.6. The two sets of maps show Michael's brain a year apart and after about twenty-five LENS treatments. Note the size of the dark gray injury areas in both the qEEG images (above) and the LORETA (below).

fifteen miles away from the Northeast Center, on an outpatient basis.

Michael arrived in a wheelchair wearing his purple helmet and smiling broadly at the outing. Dr. Zelek had already done a qEEG on Michael at the Northeast Center. He confessed to me that he was "trepidatious" because the q requires a cap, and the cap covered the place where Michael had no protective skull. But the map was completed and confirmed the extent of the damage that the CAT scan had also showed (see above).

I was thrilled when Michael's skull plate was restored in November 2009 after about twenty-five neurofeedback treatments, because it meant the retraumatization caused by the restorative surgery was now behind us. And we could begin to treat the area underneath it (where theoretically there was no brain) in earnest.

Michael is now able to walk into the center with a cane and has a vocabulary of several hundred words. The LORETA map also shows profound differences.

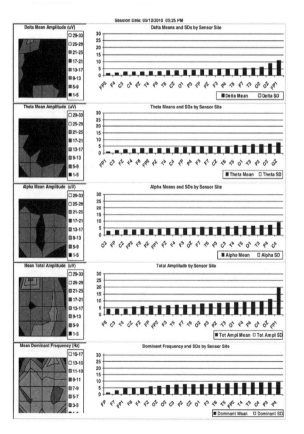

Fig. 12.7. These are the most recent LENS maps done on Michael in May 2010, after about forty-five treatments.

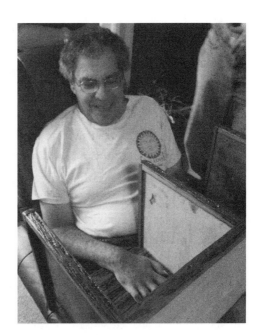

Fig. 12.8. Michael Schacker using the Ramachandran box

As of this writing, Michael Schacker has been living in his own apartment on disability, with caretakers coming in to help him, on a schedule. He is growing stronger every day. He was recently able to walk into the center without his cane and with a little assistance. The man who would never talk now has a vocabulary of between 700 and 1,000 words. He is able to read and use the computer and is practicing to regain control of his right hand with the Ramachandran box we have had built for him.

For more information on the Sensory Trigger, visit Strokefamily.org. The PowerPoint of Michael's recovery is being posted on www.stonemountaincenter .com.

Integrating FNS, sEMG, Acupuncture, and Interactive Metronome for Recovery of Movement after Stroke: A Truly Comprehensive Treatment Plan
MARY LEE ESTY, PH.D., L.C.S.W.

In 2005, "Paul," fifty-five, had a stroke with several infarcts in the vertebral, middle cerebral, and internal carotid arteries, leaving him with left-sided paralysis, left neglect in the visual field, working memory problems, severe depression, and fatigue.

Paul had completed physical therapy (PT) and occupational therapy (OT) and was receiving vision therapy, massage, and acupuncture in 2009 when he began Flexyx Neurotherapy System (FNS) treatment four years after the stroke. Paul could walk only by swinging the left leg from the hip while being held to prevent falling. He had fallen many times after leaving the rehabilitation center because he could not lift his left leg. He usually used a wheelchair. His psychiatrist referred Paul for FNS treatment of depression and crying spells.

After twenty-six FNS treatments, vision testing showed improvement in the left neglect field of vision, his energy improved, he was able to socialize longer, and he required fewer naps. Crying spells were rare, and significant recovery in his cognitive and emotional functioning improved quality of life for him and his wife. As his reading speed increased, it was much more enjoyable to talk to him about books and current events, discussions enlivened by his wicked sense of humor, which had returned. His balance and reflexes also improved, which made his life easier and prevented further injury through falls. He could walk longer distances, and he was able to turn onto his left side by himself for the first time in four years. Because his cognitive and mood problems were resolved and the subtle physical sensations were more frequent, Dr. Esty thought that with surface electromyography (sEMG) training he might be able to control movement.

In March 2010, sEMG treatment began, in addition to acupuncture and Interactive Metronome,* which began in September 2009. The sEMG evaluation used surface electrodes to determine if there was any electrical activity generated by muscle contractions in his left leg. As Paul watched the computer screen, he was excited to see that his leg was actually responding to his efforts to make it move. Seeing real-time activity coming from inside one's muscles is strong motivation for learning and working with exercises at home to speed progress. In each sEMG session he was able to increase his ability to move the leg. Watching the sEMG screen, he could see exactly how much power is in the electrical signal that

---

*The Interactive Metronome or IM is a biofeedback device originally developed by jazz musician James Cassily. It measures response times to stimuli in thousandths of a second. It is used to help recover the "timing mechanisms" in the brain (www.interactivemetronome .com).

shows the strength of the muscle contraction. Paul responded vigorously to this process and practiced faithfully at home.

One of the first benefits of sEMG treatment was that he could isolate activity to the leg muscles. This allowed him to position his left foot flat on the floor to move from a sitting to standing position and smoothly move his leg back and place his foot down with control. It was a *My Fair Lady* moment: "I think he's got it! I think he's got it!" And he did! He could then get in and out of the car without hitting the gearshift, and it was easier to put on his brace and shoe. His additional movement capabilities also made getting in and out of the tub chair less difficult. All in all, he was bruising himself much less than previously because of better leg movement and control.

Incredibly, in only nine sEMG sessions Paul was able to raise his left leg and place the ankle on the right knee and lower it again with total control! Only two months before this, he had been unable to move his foot without assistance when preparing to stand. He could also stand longer without help. All this has occurred four years after the stroke and after completing PT and OT.

Coordination of sEMG treatment between Emily Perlman, the acupuncturist, and the IM therapist focused all efforts in a synergistic plan. For example, to enhance the sEMG work with Paul's left leg, the IM therapist had him lift his knee in response to the IM signal instead of extending his foot. This strengthened the signal to the muscles that were relearning correct function with sEMG. In May 2010 Paul was able to stand for ten minutes without holding on to anything during an IM session. The acupuncturist changed her treatment by working on the specific muscles that are the target of the sEMG for continued leg function and also prepared to begin on the left arm treatment. FNS treatment continued weekly along with sEMG, acupuncture, and IM. These combined therapies have resulted in Paul being able to stand on his right leg, with some support, and extend his left leg forward. All four of his therapists are excited about the results.

Expectations for significant recovery of function tend to be lowered as time passes after a stroke with extensive loss of function. Paul's case is an excellent example of using neurofeedback to enhance neural plasticity, then using sEMG to determine if the muscles are capable of being made functional again. This allowed new use of existing therapies, specifically

Interactive Metronome in Paul's case, to build on the newfound abilities. Combining these therapies strengthened the often unappreciated capacity for change that is inherent in the human system. Biofeedback therapies may be sufficient in some cases to create a return of function. When combined with other therapies, the synergistic effect is powerful and should always be considered whenever these resources are available.

THIRTEEN

New Directions in Neurofeedback

With Hershel Toomim, Ph.D., Jeffrey Carmen, Ph.D.,
Henry Mann, M.D., Nicholas Dogris, Ph.D., BCIA-EEG,
Victor Mcgregor, Ph.D., A.N.P., N.P.P., Mark Smith, L.C.S.W., QEEG,
Siegfried Othmer, Ph.D., Martin Wuttke, C.N.P.,
Michael Gismondi, M.A., L.M.H.C., and Thomas Collura, Ph.D.

What is the cutting edge of this cutting-edge healing technology? Unlike mainstream medical or imaging developments, neurofeedback does not have much in the way of institutional backing, nor big, well-funded labs. A lot of it has been done by clinicians with a technical flair, in home laboratories—some call them "Mom and Pop shops." One thinks of Siegfried and Susan Othmer, who founded the company now called EEG Spectrum; Hershel and Marjorie Toomim, whose company still bears the Toomim name; Tom and Terri Collura of BrainMaster; Mary-Jo and Ron Sabo of the Rockland Health and Wellness Center; Nancy White and Leonard Richards of the Enhancement Institute; Helen and Tom Budzynski, Len Ochs, and Cathy Wills of Ochslabs; Les and Susan Fehmi of Princeton Biofeedback; Tom Brownback and Linda Mason and Lynda and Michael Thompson of the ADD Centre and the Biofeedback Institute of Toronto. And come to think of it, my wife,

Robin, and I pioneered new directions in LENS neurofeedback for animals, and even though she is not a clinical biofeedback practitioner at our center, she helps keep our computers running at Stone Mountain Center and gives me wonderful support in all other ways. So I not only approve of couples partnering their biofeedback enterprises, I personally feel the benefit of working together and mutual support. (Hey, is a successful partnership itself not some kind of "feedback" system, do you think?)

I say it is a sign of vitality, that this is truly a healthy grassroots industry, hatched out of loving and mutually supportive relationships. (In chapter 4, we also peered into the heart of how people become neurofeedback providers—to help a loved one, often a child, who is in distress.) In the couples businesses in the best cases, one member of the partnership is a clinician, the other the technical person, innovator, or maybe business manager. We will shortly see a beautiful dance of how innovation and long-term love story go together with Hershel and Marjorie Toomim.

About two decades ago, when I started to look at what it would be like to become a clinical biofeedback provider instead of just a college professor and psychotherapist, I asked Dr. Mary Jo Sabo, who already had a successful biofeedback center established, what she thought.

"This business is full of wonderful, heartful people—who are really open to new directions and ideas," she said. "Talk to as many of them as you can about how they run their businesses." And I found she was right. I started attending many more conferences and professional trainings. Biofeedback people mostly get along with each other—except when they don't. And it is true that over the years one has only to attend a professional meeting or two to experience some wicked infighting. People get very invested in their own method, and then, it seems, they must be in competition with everyone else—except when they're not, and a beautiful synergy can take place. In this book we've already discussed complex cases, best helped not just by single but by multiple or integrative modalities, such as HRV, the LENS, NeuroField, and Z-score; and maybe even photonic stimulation, Scenar, Interactive Metronome, and Brain Training. Because each of these modalities addresses different systems that may be out of balance in the person's overall body/mind/energy, they can often work beautifully together.

When I first started presenting studies on the LENS (or its predecessors EDS or FNS, since the method had *preprandial acronym dyslexia*) at the Winter Brain Conference, later at the Association for Applied Psychophysiology and Biofeedback (AAPB) and the International Society for Neurofeedback and Research (ISNR), I felt like a bit of a weirdo because of how controversial the LENS was. It didn't use operant conditioning or reward-based training and yet Len Ochs was claiming it worked twice as fast as regular neurofeedback. He claimed some courses of treatment were only a few sessions—and then the person was better and didn't need any more. (At one point the AAPB challenged him professionally and ethically for these claims.)

It wasn't until a number of early practitioners replicated his results and presented them at professional conferences—isn't that the stuff that science is made of?—that the LENS won more acceptance in the field. When in 2007 Kristen Harrington and I published our 100-person study in *The Journal of Neurotherapy*, the field really sat up and took notice. That, along with Robin's and my publication of "The LENS with Animals" in that same journal (also presented at a 2005 AAPB conference), has moved the LENS more squarely onto the neurofeedback map. Even though it doesn't use reward-contingency-based training, more practitioners than ever consider it a legitimate form of EEG biofeedback—because consciously or unconsciously, something is still fed back. And as we've seen, individual situations seem to invite uniquely designed treatment protocols, using a variety of modalities to help people find inner balance and relief from their symptoms.

Dr. Dogris's NeuroField also hovers between the categories of biofeedback and energy medicine, because while there is no feedback per se in the pulsed electromagnetic field (pEMF) emissions of the NeuroField, he has now wisely introduced EEG and HRV feedback, as the machine feeds back the result of each pEMF treatment from the brain and heart. (Here, though, in an interesting variant on the model, the feedback is for the clinician to see the efficacy of the energy that has already been administered to the patient.)

Dr. Robert Thatcher paved the way for Mark Smith and Tom Collura to develop Z-score training, in which the feedback principle is not something determined by a preset clinical protocol but by comparison to a carefully constructed database, the NeuroGuide database, *for which the person trains at statistical approximations of a normal brain.*

One of the modalities, presented briefly in this chapter—infra-low biofeedback—has been a controversial area in the field. Once again, some say, "This is not real or believable biofeedback!" Others wonder if DC slow cortical potentials (SCP) or very slow EEG—because the waveforms are so long, and their movements so slow—can even *be* trained. (You will learn a rationale for why this might be an extremely important area from Jay Gunkelman in chapter 14.)

These are really quite different modalities, all weaving in and out of the feedback principle: to deliver therapeutically useful information—or stimulation—to the subject (or patient). Throughout the years of attending professional conferences, I have heard again and again that each person is his or her own worst enemy when it comes to succeeding at biofeedback training. It is usually trying too hard or having a rigid or fixed idea about results that causes treatment to freeze up. This is another reason to support the idea of multiple modalities for a more comprehensive balancing of the nervous system. You try something, and if it doesn't work you try something else, and so on—and guess what? Often self-regulation goes on by itself, day in and day out, as we sleep and wake, work and play. Sometimes our intervention is merely to jump-start our own intrinsic ability to regulate ourselves.

Hemoencephalography

STEPHEN LARSEN INTERVIEWS
DRS. HERSHEL TOOMIM AND JEFFREY CARMEN

*When I first started doing this, everyone got better,
everything I touched turned to gold.*

HERSHEL TOOMIM

About fifteen years ago, in the mid-1990s, there emerged another brain-based biofeedback technology that was totally unexpected. The major focus of the field seemed to have been on the dynamics of the EEG, problem areas reflected in the waveforms and on retraining them (something that conventional medical science still seems to disallow).

Hemoencephalography, in contrast, is defined as "near-infrared spectroscopy to control cerebral blood flow changes through increasing blood oxygen levels." Its developer, Hershel Toomim, had a long history of technical accomplishments, beginning with some genuine innovations in adding new controls to remote-controlled airplanes (he was honored for his work in this area not so long ago). In the '70s and '80s Toomim designed and marketed some of the first affordable stand-alone biofeedback electromyographs, temperature trainers, and GSRs.

Intrigued by the scientific impact of MRI studies, which image the brain by measuring cerebral blood flow, Hershel Toomim envisioned that a parallel kind of technology could be harnessed with a far less complex and expensive technology, and adapted to the methodology of biofeedback. Toomim would irradiate the brain with light in the red and near-infrared (blood-colored) wavelengths, instead of the very high magnetic fields used by the MRI. Toomim's inexpensive, noninvasive contribution would be called nirHEG, or near-infrared hemoencephalography.

On a parallel track, New York state psychologist Jeffrey Carmen developed a similar, but not identical, technology that measured temperatures (the "thermal decay" of endogenous brain processes, he called it) but did not use an external light source, as did Toomim's. Still, it read infrared light. Dr. Carmen's approach would be called pirHEG, for passive infrared hemoencephalography. Both methods make sense because even though the brain is a small organ physiologically, it uses disproportionate amounts of glucose and oxygen to do its (admittedly complex and important) work. Regardless of the measurement technique, the brain's consumption of nutrients (or lack of it) now emerges as a major parameter to be trained using biofeedback techniques.

In 2010, at the ISNR (International Society for Neurofeedback and Research) national meeting in Denver in early October, I was lucky enough to get both innovators to sit down to lunch with me so I could interview them together. You see, the really remarkable story is that rather than seeing each other as competitors, these two innovators have become fast friends. When I had phoned Jeffrey Carmen during the summer and mentioned that I might like to interview him at the conference, he said, flatly: "You must talk to Hershel!"

Why? I knew the answer before he said it. Hershel would be ninety-five that year and had not only watched but greatly contributed to the development of both the broader field of biofeedback and the kind based only on the brain, called neurofeedback.

"The world deserves to hear Hershel's story," Jeffrey said. And he was right. Beyond the biofeedback community, Hershel and Marjorie Toomim were major contributors to our field, and their contributions range up and down the scale of innovation, verging on genius. What you will read below was well beyond my expectations in terms of vividness, emotional color, and historical significance for the field of biofeedback.

Interview with Hershel Toomim

STEPHEN: Hershel, I want you to take me back to the beginnings of your interest in biofeedback.

HERSHEL: During the '70s and '80s, I devised a series of instruments for my wife, Marjorie, who was a skilled psychotherapist. It was a kind of pioneering thing in those days to use instruments as an aid to psychotherapy. In the beginning, I think it was feedback more for Marjorie, for the therapist, than for the patient. She was treating a young lady who had been a child in Nazi Germany and had terrible anxiety, especially around men. Now the lady was, I think, in her thirties, with a very flat affect, so that even Marjorie was unable to reach her. We tried to use GSR or skin conductance (the heart of the classic lie detector) to elicit her blocked emotions. It didn't do much, but in conversing with her, it came out that she would perspire on her bottom whenever she sat down.

Marjorie elected to put the electrodes on her bottom, under her skirt. There it was: the conductance began to go up when she was reminded of a tune from *Hansel and Gretel*—"Lost in the Woods." That song also reminded her of a nurse's cap. As she reminisced about her childhood in Germany, she remembered a nurse who took her to the woods every day. Then a gentleman joined them. He was an SS officer. Her nurse and the young man in uniform would have sex while the young girl looked on with a kind of horror, knowing she was witnessing something forbidden and that she shouldn't be there; neither was the potential threat of what the uniform represented lost on her, Jewish or not.

Regaining the memory elicited a recovery of more detailed memories and the traumatic feelings that went with them. It was a major therapeutic breakthrough for the patient and changed her life. We felt like we were at the beginning of something: biofeedback-assisted psychotherapy.

STEPHEN: I genuinely believe you were. And what a concept. You combine a human interaction with a little robot, and you have a unique formula for self-disclosure and healing.

HERSHEL: The HEG was born in 1994. We were working on eighteen possible instruments. [Dr.] Victoria Ibric was working with us as a therapist. We were working with the Othmer EEG, but I didn't believe in it. There was a paper by Raichle correlating the beta and alpha ranges with the fMRI. I was also aware of the work of F. F. Jobsis, who had learned to read the oxygen of the brain. I was aware of SPECT [single-photon emission computed tomography]. You could do SPECT first, then EEG training, then SPECT. I had two bright young graduate students at the State University of New York and the University of Maryland at Baltimore. A young M.D. replaced the Ph.D. psychologist, and he refused to inject a radioactive dye (SPECT) for no medical purpose. One of the graduate students, Julie, had a research paper on infrared spectroscopy. I looked it over and said: "Hell, I can build this one."

After I did, I put the sensor on my own head. I discovered I had voluntary control of brain oxygenation, a different thing than thermistry [head sensing] per se. If I could do it, others could too. That was the beginning of hemoencephalography.

STEPHEN: I like it that you tried it out on yourself, and then reasoned that others could do it.

HERSHEL: They could. Marjorie and I presented it at AAPB in 1995. Another biofeedback innovator, Jon Cowan, said, "You're lying to people; you can't really do that." I said, "I beg your pardon?"

Then along came Jeffrey Carmen, who had been using infrared thermisters to help with migraines.

Jeffrey: I was working with an intense pain disorder called RSD (short for reflex sympathetic dystrophy) in those days (now renamed complex regional pain syndrome, because it turned out that it didn't have much to do with the sympathetic nervous system). Nothing helped these unfortunate people, so I was getting referrals to try biofeedback. The referring physicians didn't even have a clear idea what biofeedback was, but they thought it would not hurt and might help. One of the prevailing theories was that if you could train someone to warm the affected area, the increased blood flow would help the pain. It was a very logical although incorrect assumption. This presented a problem because touching anything to the skin generated intense pain. That got me started experimenting with infrared heat measurement, because you could measure heat without touching the skin. This was an extremely powerful procedure. People easily learned to control blood flow to the affected area with the noncontact sensor. The problem was that the theory was wrong. Increased blood flow made the pain dramatically worse. A great idea without such a great outcome.

Once I had the system established to monitor and train temperature using a noncontact infrared sensor, I began thinking about migraines. Back then, the theory of migraine pathophysiology was that it was caused by excessively dilated blood vessels in the scalp and brain. This made intuitive sense, because migraine headaches tend to pound in synchronization with the pulse. So I figured if I could train people to reduce cerebral blood flow, it would help the migraines. Wrong! Another good idea with a bad outcome.

Back then, the theory of migraine was that it was all vascular. Then I heard about Hershel's work teaching people to increase brain activity in the front of the brain. I thought it would make the migraines worse and just kind of set the whole idea aside. But I had a couple of colleagues who kept bugging me to pursue the whole idea of training the brain through temperature monitoring. One day I had a chance to try it out. I had just developed a very primitive prototype. Very primitive. The sensor was actually buried inside a kitchen sponge and held in place on the head by a cloth strap. One of these two colleagues, named Ed S., was visiting me and tried it out. He discovered that if he placed it on his forehead, he could control the thermal emissions from the front of his brain to change the signal on a digital readout. We didn't think much more about it, and he left.

It was wintertime. After our session, Ed had to drive some distance home. He stopped for a cup of coffee, and while he sat there warming up, the battery in his car died. Now you have to understand, Ed was never much of a mechanic. He did have jumper cables but never seemed to use them correctly. He called me and told me that he had a problem but had solved it effectively. Someone who had parked next to him let him jump the two batteries. The thing that surprised Ed was that the process went smoothly. Nothing he ever did with a car went smoothly. He got the right cables on the right terminals almost without thinking about it. It was the smooth precision that struck him, which is why he called me with the observation. It turns out now that everyone understands the role of the prefrontal cortex, but back then this was a surprising observation. I began thinking: "Something went on in the front of his brain!"

At some point, I got brave enough to try it on a migraine. I was shocked to find that increasing prefrontal brain activity was both prophylactic and abortive of migraines. This was counterintuitive, but it worked. Eventually I collected enough cases to publish my "100 Migraines" study using pirHEG. This study showed that over 90 percent of the people who completed six sessions experienced significant headache improvement.

I met up with Hershel at the annual ISNR meeting, maybe in 1999. We just hit it off and have been friends ever since. Everything from that point on is history. Hershel and I have been working in the prefrontal region of the brain ever since. In retrospect, this was not so surprising. The prefrontal cortex has a huge regulating function on the rest of the brain. It's not surprising that if you train someone to increase brain activity there, it will help with all kinds of problems related to excess rate and magnitude of response.

We found we are doing the same thing with different hardware. He is measuring the color of the blood through oxygenation. He's measuring the fuel and I'm measuring the exhaust—I suppose you could call it "thermal urine." The brain needs to get rid of the thermal excess so it doesn't overheat. Humans have hair on the head, which is a thermal insulator, and don't have hair on the forehead for a good reason. The hair on the head insulates from the sun, and the bare forehead helps cool the very active prefrontal cortex.

HERSHEL: I got to treat everything that Marjorie would send my way involving the brain: memory loss, paralysis, stroke, depression, TBI, toxic encephalopathy, neurological blindness.

There was the case of a young lady affected by asphalt paving in the atrium of her building. She and her roommate both had sudden onset symptoms: skin cracking, tunnel vision to the point of blindness, cognitive confusion, fibromyalgia. Along with blindness, my patient had a total dysregulation of her thermal balance. She had to take off her clothes and jump in the shower every few minutes, it seemed. She joked it was so often, and so spontaneous, that she didn't know who she would find in there with her.

I told her it was the toxic equivalent of a TBI. I got the idea hyperbaric oxygen would be good for her. She went off to a rehabilitation place in New Mexico, and when she came back, she could get around with a cane. I gave her more treatment with lots of visualization exercises, as if she could really see. Finally she went on a vacation to the seashore, and while sitting on a rock and listening to the surf, she found herself visualizing one of those big *Hokusai* waves. When it knocked her over and got her really wet, she realized she had actually seen the wave. After that, her improvement was steady until she reached 20/20, and she is now driving a car.

JEFFREY: One of my first migraine patients, I came to realize later, had familial hemiplegic migraine. One half of her body would become paralyzed, and then on would come a whopper headache. After training, she reported long periods with no symptoms. No migraines, but a new symptom: "My eyes are killing me." Her blink rate had slowed or stopped.

If you activate the frontal cortex, the blinking rate slows. I did a research study in 2004. A lot of women of childbearing years didn't want to take the antiseizure meds [Depacote, Dilantin] prescribed for them because of the danger of birth defects. We had a variety of responses: frequency down, intensity up; intensity down, frequency up. When the cure is well along, they can sense the headache coming—maybe at intense times: under stress, or combined with a menstrual cycle. You teach people to calibrate their symptoms. In my experience, even that one proprioceptive exercise has people getting better.

HERSHEL: When I first started doing this, everyone got better, everything I touched turned to gold. I got back letters from these first people, and they described how everything got better, how memory improved, how they could remember phone numbers. I found myself changing emotionally negative memories so they were no longer so destructive. I would occupy the limbic system with the HEG task so the brain couldn't put the traumatic memory back in its original place in the brain. It's a little like Roger Callahan's or Gary Craig's tapping procedures, where you reroute a memory to different places.

You know, one important insight that can't be overstressed is that memory, probably all memory, is stored in multiple places in the brain. If you can change that order, you can achieve amazing things. This understanding brings a lot with it.

JEFFREY: That's so true.

HERSHEL: In the beginning, the neurofeedback community wasn't so thrilled about the results I was presenting, but I tried to keep a low profile. I disagreed from the first about thresholds in biofeedback, arguing that incremental training was far better. [Instead of a reward for being in the zone, or no reward if you're not in the zone, Toomim is talking about an incremental approach: as your hands warm, a tone rises, following the warming with its pitch.]

STEPHEN: That really is a big issue in biofeedback or neurofeedback, isn't it?

HERSHEL: Joe Kamiya supported me and said he understood what I was saying. Still, I don't think we affected the field very much [which still predominantly uses thresholds], but Joe and I became good friends.

STEPHEN: I do like it when that happens. Was it Blake who said, "Opposition is true friendship"? But working through misunderstanding to commonality is something I appreciate. I have a great deal of love for Joe myself; we've shared a few high-quality sake-and-sushi occasions. It was he who said—and I never forgot it—"Conventional, reward-based training is only one kind of application of biofeedback,but there are lots of others. This field is in its infancy!—and there is so much more to learn."

Dr. Henry "Hank" Mann on HEG and NeuroField

This summer, as I was interviewing people out at Hank Mann's place in Stonington, Connecticut, sitting on his back deck, resplendent with flowers of every color and sort, the venerable psychiatrist and gourmet chef spontaneously began talking about his HEG experience. Fortunately, I had my notebook and recorder right nearby.

Interview with Hank Mann, M.D.

STEPHEN: You were going to tell me about your experience with the HEG, which you said was pretty pivotal.

HANK: As you can imagine, I've done many, many things over the years, but I think the HEG can be life-transformative—it was for me.

I'm in my early seventies. Way back when I was a child, my mother was pretty explosive and abusive. Thus I've always been concrete and removed; every little human situation I had to understand, as it were, bit by bit. I've had a long professional life as a psychiatrist, but I always felt a little detached. If I was separated from my patient's experience, I was also separated from my own. But I had been in therapy for years—done biofeedback, neurofeedback, the LENS, but never had anything like what happened with the HEG.

If you want to train in this stuff, try Jeffrey Carmen. He knows what he's doing. You're watching the movie on Bio-Era. It's great. The movie comes off and goes on, like you expect. The prefrontal cortex and the deeper structures engage and disengage. The equipment measures hundredths of a degree temperature. Mine drops a tenth and then goes up again. The movie goes off and comes on. You're learning to take it off and put it back on line every minute and a half. You're engaging and disengaging the prefrontal cortex.

Back to my life: I'm married to a delightful person and have a great kid. But I told you I'm kind of concrete. My life itself was a little like a movie, like an abstraction. Then, bang! I get it. I have a family! I don't know how else to say it. It's really there, the support, the love, the reality of it. I knew it and felt it beyond shadow of a doubt. How real, how precious this family is . . .

A little later, I'm in the therapeutic situation. I'm working with a foster mother; helping her deal with her frustration, pain. I say, "Everyone needs a foster mother like you." And then I notice that I'm crying.

STEPHEN: Every time I've managed to be transparent in that way to a patient, it has been really transformative. It's like you're trained not to do that and it's the wrong thing.

HANK: I love being that open and in touch. It's like a veil is taken away, and there you are. I was able to be there for my patient and work on myself as well. I realized how sad my own childhood had been. I feel these procedures have been enormously helpful.

STEPHEN: You said that the NeuroField was also helpful to you.

HANK: Oh, yes, I work in a very high-pressure private psychiatric setting. I work with psychoses, bipolar and schizophrenia. It's very easy to get cut off. One day I realize my depressive patients have been getting to me. I'm depressed.

I tried one of Mike Beasley's NeuroField protocols for depression.

I tried it three times—they're really quite short, you know. The depression was gone. But I was still right there and empathetic with my patients. In fact, work had been burdensome for me before the treatments I'm talking to you about. I mean, hard to face the day, the patients. Now it's not effortful. Curious and engaged—and warm, I guess.

STEPHEN: I love it; curious, engaged, and warm. You still keep working. And I think I feel your warmth right now—especially after the gourmet meals and the generosity you've poured out the last few days.

NeuroField—Nicholas Dogris, Ph.D.

We could now take three giant steps back to chapter 4 and the amazing story of AJ and how Dr. Dogris both discovered and added to the LENS, and then, to complete his son's healing, developed a device called the NeuroField. As Jay Gunkelman says in his interview in the next chapter, "If anything has an effect physically, you can measure it physically." (In the same paragraph he calls for a conversation between neurofeedback and energy medicine—we have things in common, and our knowledge bases can complement each other. Mysticism does not need to hide behind inscrutability.)

Nick Dogris has to have a bit of the tough mountain man in him to live in Bishop, California, on the eastern flank of the Sierra Nevada, and conduct a practice. To treat hardy clients, he has to be hardy himself. This comes across in the story about how he moved mountains and invented totally new treatment modalities in order to help his son. So the most important part of his story is already told (you might want to look it over before reading this brief description of how the NeuroField works and what it does).

My mind goes back to the 2010 LENS conference in Los Gatos, California. Two of the plenary speakers were people I had already met and studied closely, before encountering them in the quality time we enjoyed together at the conference. Dr. Beverly Rubik, a serious scientist, spoke of "living dynamical systems," and because of the principle of dynamic resonance, how little it takes to tweak them toward homeostasis, or really allostasis when you consider the organism in its own environment, as well as the outer environment. Homeodynamics, said Dr. Rubik, count on very small, accurate interventions applied at intervals. It's a very different thing, she said, than allopathic medicines, which blunt the "responseability" of the system with massive chemical blockades.

She acknowledged she didn't yet know for sure, but she thought it possible that "the LENS speaks the language of the brain." Instead of invasive chemistry, we have tiny tweaks of energy—physics—working on the same homeodynamic level as the brain itself.

James Oschmann, true to form, delivered an erudite tour-de-force, ranging up and down the archives of physics and chemistry. All molecules above the temperature of absolute zero, he said, vibrate. What, then, are the vibratory frequencies of substances, of pathologies, of states of consciousness? He mentioned that *Borrelia burgdorferi,* the pathogen of Lyme disease, was the first pathogen to be sequenced: 636 Hz—in fact, a Rife frequency*—emerged as important for treating Lyme disease. Having had Lyme—as have two-thirds of our rural farm community in the Hudson Valley of New York—I stopped in my tracks. I remembered that Nick Dogris had inserted a Lyme protocol as one of his NeuroField frequencies. Oschman helped me make sense of Dogris.

He spoke of the "human antenna" theory: that all our molecules, healthy or pathological, vibrate at knowable and measurable frequencies. Our cells, he said, are probably not bound by "neuron time" at all (only about 18' per second) but by the almost instantaneous connection of polymers in the connective tissue around the body—in the brain it is not just neurons, but microglia that are involved in a "crystalline lattice." We function more like "wireless radio sets"—picking up energies from ourselves as well as others—than old-fashioned electrical machines requiring wires (the neurons).

Nick Dogris wisely puts in his biofeedback measures of changes in the HRV and EEG as he applies the NeuroField treatments. Do they

---

*A Rife frequency is one of the many frequencies studied by Royal Rife, an energy-medicine innovator, whose work was regarded by the FDA as very "controversial."

move in the direction of health and vitality, or against it? If they move the wrong way, you're using the wrong frequency, or at the wrong intensity, so that the living dynamical system freezes up! We also use feedback measures that are simply unavailable to the unaware. As you treat (with NeuroField or LENS, or psychotherapy, for that matter), do you see physiological changes—skin tone, the delicate muscles of the face changing, softening of the eyes? What about changes in breathing? Sighing, sitting more—or less—erectly? (Does the person laugh or smile easily, even at my bad jokes?)

While on the quest to help his son—by definition a "path with heart"—Nick Dogris, already knowing how the LENS works, asked the universe for some help in designing a new instrument. If only he could find a radio engineer! A few days later the talented, just out of work, RF engineer Brad Wiitala came into his life and helped him solve some of the technical and engineering problems of the NeuroField. Rather than describe it succinctly in my language, I quote from the NeuroField website (http://cns-wellness.com/brain-based-intervention/photonic-stimulator/69-neurofield).

The NeuroField system is a variable DC stimulation device that is designed to reduce stress, and energetically balance the human body. NeuroField is designed to deliver small electrical pulses to the energy field that is generated by the human brain. It is theorized that the energy field created by the brain can absorb energy and deliver it to damaged molecular systems in the body. When the molecular systems are repaired they allow the natural wisdom of the body to engage its regenerative systems so as to promote stress reduction and healing.

NeuroField stimulation acts to replenish cellular energy and results in reduced stress. NeuroField theory is based on the premise that the human brain emits a field of energy that extends outside the skull. This field of energy is theorized to be an interactive conduit that can travel to any region in the body. The natural healing wisdom of the human body is complex, adaptive, fluid and intelligent. When a person becomes imbalanced they become susceptible to many different types of illness. NeuroField was designed to strengthen the body and promote healthy, balanced states, and allows the body to engage its own restorative systems so as to return to a balanced, homeostatic state. NeuroField was designed after years of study, searching and research by Nick Dogris.

I was originally skeptical of the NeuroField, even though I like Nick Dogris and use his advanced LENS protocols all the time. Then one of my clinicians, Alexandra Linardakis, trained with Dogris and acquired an early machine. At first, very cautiously, we tried it out on ourselves, and then, with notice that it was an experimental modality, on patients. Word began to come back that people were really feeling relieved of insomnia, Lyme arthritis, gastrointestinal distress, depression, and anxiety. We were off and running!

The following is a single example from Victor McGregor, a colleague whom I trust and know rather well.

BV Reports to Victor McGregor
VICTOR MCGREGOR, PH.D., A.N.P., N.P.P.

BV is a sixty-three-year-old white Caucasian man, divorced, who lives with "his best friend," a black Lab (dog). He was born to a superhigh-achieving, very dysfunctional, alcoholic family and says he has been depressed most of his life. He told me he had been on high doses of MAO inhibitors most of his adult life. Now he is still on Wellbutrin and a little Adderall.

He attended four years of medical school, then went into chemical engineering research. A few years ago, he went on disability for his memory problems. He also has chronic diabetes, anxiety, insomnia, a bad rage problem, and erectile dysfunction from the diabetes. At the time he began to see me, there were amazing stressors: loss of the family estate, and then the illness and death of his brother.

Amazingly, he drives every week from New York City to Saugerties, New York, to see me. I don't think he'd do that if something wasn't working.

I decided to use a composite approach. I use Nick Dogris's and also Jackie deVries's protocols for improving circulation, inflammation reduction, and anxiety reduction. I have also used the "de-habituator," alpha-omega balance, and "smoothing the field."

BV seemed motivated to really get better, and by agreement he kept in e-mail touch. He sent this on October 15, 2010:

> Victor, it is now six days since the treatment, and I still have a relatively stable emotional plane, not depressed, facts as facts, and still separated from intense feelings. Not so attached to these (which normally occurs with me); a feeling of clarity. I also have faint traces of memory improvement.
>
> Two days ago my brother was told that the chemotherapy and radiation were being stopped as ineffectual, and I am okay about this.
>
> Everyone in group [BV goes to group therapy with a well-known New York therapist] instantly experienced me as stable (not calm), still emotional, including Stan M. [the therapist]. I do not seem to feel the panic reaction or find severe avoidance. There are no more sensory experiences in the areas of the brain since I left the treatment. I "normally" feel EVERYTHING is personal, and therefore I had no experience of "strictly business." Everything was PERSONAL. The separation has given me a new freedom to look at things and people. See you tomorrow noon?
>
> BV

A week later, he wrote:

> Hi, Victor!
> The [NeuroField] effect continues to create some improvement in my mental functions and state of mind. I still have the enhanced feeling of clarity in spite of medications that have been giving me a sensation of being drugged. This is clear now.
>
> My mood is better. By this I mean that the same facts and perceptions that were integrated in the depression type of thoughts are still there, but the despair and "judgmental" link ("No, I never had kids") is a statement of fact, without the linkage of the feeling of me

not existing in life—no footprint in the sand of time (a complete failure—not even there). I feel okay!

At night I have some ice cream (raising my blood sugar over 160–200) or Advil PM with a relative of Benadryl to knock me out, but last night I was clear even after the Advil PM. I did feel somewhat hung over from it, although this sometimes happens based on how late I take it. The curiosity about, and instantaneous design of, problem solutions and devices [a creative feature] is now five days present, although faint, but present for the first time in over two years.

I am hopeful in a calm way—for the first time in my life, in that there is no feeling of wishing, no anxiety about whether this or that is perfect and/or permanent, no fear of failure.

In mid-January, BV had a flare-up of gastrointestinal problems after the treatment—which involved the "dehabituator," a very strong treatment, done for ten to fifteen minutes. He wrote:

I have had ulcers since the age of thirteen. I have had (the last ten years) two simultaneously, plus acid reflux, requiring two Aciphex/day, so I would doubt that it is the protocols. I'm much better, only it's just too early for Vietnamese food (spicy) (my test).

He reported on treatment on January 15, 2011:

Improvement continues, with specific reference to my stomach ulcer medications and reflux. The usual (more than six years) two Aciphex/day have been reduced to one a day. I no longer get sick and nauseous after every meal. At most I get uncomfortable. Erectile dysfunction continues to improve. The stimulant "cap" has been utilized by placement on my lap over the genital area and under the prostate area [for the erectile dysfunction]. After a four-week lapse in treatment from Thanksgiving to New Year's (January 8?), there is continuing improvement without backsliding. Sleep improves to one or two (nonbladder) wakeups during the night.

January 22, 2011: Memory seems stable, and improvement may

be occurring, but I am unable to calibrate the improvement. There is no backsliding. This session there is maximum voltage as waves in maximum cycles of antihabituation. My stomach has backslid as to acid reflux, so two generic Aciphex per day are restored. I may have overstrained the stomach state with my food tests two day in a row.

There is less obsessive thought and behavior now, but the lack of force usually tied to recurrent obsessive thoughts is new, without emotional force/hammer. Sleep slowly improves.

Neurofield Protocols below Developed by Nick Dogris, Mike Beasley, and Jackie deVries

- Glandular and organ tune-up: adrenals, endocrine general, pancreas, parathyroid, thyroid, pineal, pituitary, hypothalamus, geriatric
- Body function normalization
- Sweep: 12 cycles at 5 volts, for 5 sec stim, frequencies from 1 to 1335
- Circulation protocol: Blood pressure balance and support, blood strengthener, capillary healing, circulation
- Balance, circulation sluggish, heart function balance, intermittent claudication, Raynaud's, *Mucor racemosus fresen*
- 49 cycles frequencies from 1 to 10,000
- With cap on head (NeuroField is administered through a traditional qEEG "cap," through a specially designed helmet, or through "coils")
- 1st: STF smoothing field, followed by inflammation reduction, brain fog reduction, memory improvement, cell regeneration, and CNS repair
- Dehabituation: Addiction protocols (1 and 2) up to 44 plus TrueFocus addiction frequencies, frequencies 953, 551–34; 50 cycles 5 volts 100 millisecond stim
- Emotional well-being (J. deVries)
- Ended with ultra-slow-wave frequencies

Conclusions

I am quite impressed by this course of treatment in a chronic, complex case. Dr. McGregor put the NeuroField through its (versatile) paces to help this high-risk patient make these gains. Underneath it all, I believe, BV is pretty robust and hardy to have responded so well—and not to have backslidden during the month and a little more of no treatment. In addition to being motivated to get well, he is also responsible in his reports, allowing his clinician to regulate the treatment accordingly.

BV is a bright and discerning client. He does not distinguish between physiological and psychological conditions; he gives equally nice reports on the condition of stomach, phallus, and psyche.

The Evolution of Z-Score Training

It seems the stuff of science fiction, especially if the patient has gothic tattoos and is watching *The Matrix* with electrodes all over his head, grinning fiendishly. Our patient, once suicidally depressed, and with whom we have used combined LENS and psychotherapy for four years now, only began Z-score training about six months ago. But he says he notices big changes: He is more organized, more proactive. He recently traveled out of the country for the first time in his life—and is actually thinking of attending college.

While the LENS uses little bumps and jostles to open pathways and help the brain balance and repair itself, Z-score training takes on the task of making sure that the lines of interconnection *are not too open—* not so wide as to cause chaos or information overload but also not shut down. Rather there is a healthy, clean connection in which Central Communication Headquarters in the body is in touch—with the inside world, and the outside world.

Z-score technology is science-fictiony because it couldn't really get started at all until solid-state circuitry and microchip technology reached a certain high level of speed and sophistication. EEG processors, and the computers that talk to them, may sample information about the brain at 256 times a second—or even much faster. Now imagine this being done from nineteen channels simultaneously—as in the cutting-edge nineteen-channel Z-score training—and the relationships between them compared almost instantaneously. This information then has to be rendered into displays the clinician can read, feedback the client can respond to, and memory, so we can really see afterward what went on in a given training session. It does this blindingly quickly and accurately, and the brain—also kind of amazing—is usually able to make use of what it has gotten. Brain-computer interface, cybermind. It is indeed the stuff of science fiction, and let's hope we evolve enough along the way to use it wisely—for helping to heal our wayward, confused species.

Background: The NeuroGuide Database and Robert Thatcher

The NeuroGuide Database is the brainchild of a very brainy man: Dr. Robert Thatcher. A student of biology, psychology (his Ph.D. is in psychology), and mathematics, he has also mastered computers—to the extent that he bends their architecture to his neurological purposes. To meet him in person is to think you're meeting a middle-aged movie star or celebrity—he lives on his own sailboat in Florida, looks tanned and healthy, and dresses elegantly. Then he starts to talk, and a hush falls on the room; even the feisty neurofeedback nerds and savants listen up. His academic portfolio can be read on line, and it is exceptional, even for a professional academician. He has published in many a peer-reviewed and pub-med* journal. His topics combine MRI and EEG analysis of traumatic brain injury; a severity index of TBI based on the EEG; forensic articles on the admissibility of EEG-based evidence in court; EEG and IQ (yes, there is a strong correlation); EEG and sensory scanning speed; and, with others, the mathematics of the "inverse solution," which allows for elegant and noninvasive maps of deeper brain structures (LORETA) to be created from the EEG. He developed life span normative databases for the EEG. His presentations at professional conferences are too numerous to list, as he is a popular and often-invited speaker. You can read all this

---

*Pub-med is a service of the U.S. National Library of Medicine, with over nineteen million citations.

in Dr. Thatcher's CV online, the first eight pages of which can be found here: www.scientificartsfoundation.org/page/page/3529693.htm.

For a number of years Professor Thatcher was part of the neurological "dream team," the Brain Research Laboratories of the Department of Psychiatry at New York University, people who largely defined—in one way or another—the field we call neurofeedback or EEG-based biofeedback: E. Roy John, whose recent passing saddened the international community; his friend and companion Prof. Leslie Prichep, with whom he published papers on EEG correlates of pathological states and responses to medication; and Rodolfo Llinas, the distinguished Colombian neuroscientist and protégé of Sir John Eccles. Following, as we discussed in chapter 3, the development and availability of the low-cost (compared to most biomedical research instruments) Lexicor, it became possible to do lots of comparatively inexpensive quantitative EEGs in a variety of settings. The generation of databases—statistical compilations of lots of data from individual subjects—to form statistical ideas of what is normal or normative from making mathematical distributions of the data comes from this pioneering work.

One of the oldest, the classical X-R database, as it was called, began under the direction of E. Roy John, assisted by the able Robert Thatcher—to examine, for a large starter project, the EEGs of children with ADD and ADHD.

During its thirty years of existence, the mission of the Brain Research Laboratory (www.med.nyu.edu/brl/aboutus) included (I use their own description):

1. Study of brain processes mediating learning, memory and cognition;
2. Development of new mathematical methods and biomedical computing systems to analyze QEEG and ERP [event-related potential] data;
3. Studying the effects of drugs on brain electrical activity and integrating this approach with the design of optimized interventions which move the brain toward the normal space.
4. Building the largest quantitative electrophysiological (QEEG and ERP) database in the world;

5. Developing algorithms using QEEG for objective classification as an adjunct to diagnoses of psychiatric patients.

6. Performing cluster analyses for sub-typing within psychiatric diagnoses; and demonstrating the relationship between such subtypes and treatment response;

7. Development of New Technology, including Neurobiological Computer Systems for Intraoperative Monitoring of Depth of Anesthesia, Neurosurgical or Cardiovascular Surgical Monitoring or Assessment of Brain Functions in ADHD, Dementia, Chronic and acute Pain, Traumatic Brain Injury or Cerebrovascular Accidents, and methods for 3-Dimensional QEEG-based Source Localization and Brain Imaging;

8. Construction of theories of the physiological bases of anesthetic action and of neural processes mediating the construction of subjective experience and consciousness. Based upon such theories, innovative methods of aggressive treatment for disorders of consciousness [sic]. These methods are being applied to patients in persistent vegetative state, minimal conscious state and to children with autisic spectrum disorders.

9. Operating the Neurometric Evaluation Service to provide clinical EEG, QEEG and multimodal ERP examinations;

10. Publication of scientific papers.

Robert Thatcher was most involved with, as he puts it, the "assembling of the world's largest 'quantitative' electrophysiological database." He began by assembling information on the EEGs of ADD and ADHD children in the New York area; it has since that time expanded considerably to include all kinds of ages and diagnostic categories. The value, again, of a database is that it allows us to form an idea of what is "normal."

As with any normative database, a Gaussian analysis (bell curve) places an individual, as measured, within a population, so that we can see the normalcy on a distribution. This is social science at its best: measuring populations statistically and then measuring the individual to place him or her in an age- and gender-matched cohort. All subjective opinions are wiped aside by the power of statistical analysis, which can't be argued with. (It was such analyses that finally, during the sixties and seventies, allowed the American Psychological Association to stand alongside the American Psychiatric Association in Congress, where vital legislation concerning mental health care is made, and say, "You say your diagnostic and your pharmaceutical interventions are superior, so you are entitled to a kind of primacy: preferred standards of care, higher rank, and higher salaries in health care establishments. Now prove it!")

Part of Thatcher's contribution, by the way, consists not only of using EEG to screen for diagnosis or likely responsiveness to psychopharmacology, but also courtroom probity of whether or not someone is legitimately brain injured (TBI) or disabled by some other neurological diagnosis—or simply faking it. He has done something dozens of times that the author (Stephen Larsen) has only done twice: legally testified, in depositions or in jury trial, using EEG-based brain maps, as to just how seriously someone was damaged, in case 1, by a blast of high-voltage electricity, and, in case 2, of a New York artist and celebrity who was head-injured in a bike accident. It wasn't really much fun, and the opposing lawyers were vicious in cross-examination, but the jury's eyes got wide and attentive as they saw the incontrovertible visual evidence of the brain maps, and winning the cases netted the clients a million dollars each.

Whether physical or social scientists are examining evidence of whether something is true or not, the probability factor plays a very large part. Significance, for example, means that something found in a controlled experiment could only have happened one time in a hundred by chance (significance at the 0.01 level; or one time in a thousand, the 0.001 level; or ten thousand, the 0.001 level). The mathematics of significance does not pretend to absolute knowledge, only the probabilities that an event is due to a causal factor (the independent variable, or the active factor being examined).

Thus there is immense power, for the scientist, in numbers. The greater the number of subjects in a controlled experiment, for example, the higher the validity or significance attributed to a positive outcome. Originally, all the work at the NYU laboratory was statistical and analytical rather than therapeutic. Is something normal or abnormal? If it's abnormal, what will it take to fix it (bring it back to normal)?

Mark Smith Finds a Solution for His Son's Epilepsy: The Evolution of Z-Score Training

By now the reader is familiar with the idea that much invention and dis-covery in neurofeedback has been done by people wanting to help a family member or a loved one. It was no different for Mark Smith, a licensed clinical social worker with an epileptic son—and a fortunate background as an electrician and a mathematician (Smith 2008).

The gist of the story is that Mark's son Jack, at three years old, sud-denly developed atonic drop seizures. This well-coordinated and very active boy would suddenly lose all muscle tone and fall to the floor wher-ever he was—schoolyard, playing field, concrete sidewalk. A few moments later, such was his vitality, he would be up again running around. But the bruises and injuries began to accumulate; and living in New York City, as the family did, both parents were really alarmed at the potential for a much more serious injury. A pediatric neurologist gave the name "crypto-genic, benign Rolandic epilepsy," which means, in short, that they don't know the cause, that it is expected not to worsen (the benign part), and that it happens at the Rolandic fissure in the brain where sensory and motor capabilities are organized—hence the sudden loss of control.

But the disorder wasn't exactly "benign"; it got much worse. The frequency increased, and Jack developed "absence" ("no one home" for a while) and myoclonic (muscle spasm) seizures. His coordination deterio-rated and his personality changed, from sunny and cheerful to labile and violent. Doses of anticonvulsant medication seemed ineffective to slow the progress of the disorder. Jack's mother was against allowing Mark to try neurofeedback, but she was finally persuaded when Mark used it to help her with terrible menstrual pain. But the technology was not yet there. Mark worked with an experienced neurofeedback therapist, using coherence training. Jack was "hypocoherent," but the training worked in one direction only. There were some improvements, and Jack got his athleticism back—enough to get a second head injury in the orbital area while diving onto furniture in the house.

Now nothing seemed to avail. His EEG recording showed interictal spikes of 300–400 microvolts (very high). Jack was up to about a hundred neurofeedback treatments, and Mark was using bribery, or anything, to get Jack to continue. He turned to the qEEG and neurofeedback-savvy neurologist Jonathan Walker, who recommended a two-channel "inhibit" protocol. Mark wrote, "I was astonished to observe an EEG without inter-ictal discharges" (Smith 2008). The seizures ceased, only to return when coherence training was begun. (The inhibit training did not hold, and the coherence seemed to trigger seizures.) The neurologist wanted to try new medications, and the family was now desperate.

It was at this point that Tom Collura of BrainMaster introduced Z-score training, and Mark immediately bought the equipment. It still was not a linear process, but, working with Collura, Thatcher, Bill Lambos, Rick Stark, and others, an idea began to emerge of training coherence within the limits of positive and negative standard deviation, "a floor and a ceiling."

Mark told me in a recent interview that he credits other clinicians for developing this approach: Robert Thatcher for the databases that made the normative comparisons possible at all, and Tom Collura, president and founder of BrainMaster, for programming a range function into the computer software for the BrainMaster system. (Mark has built a cross-word puzzle in the *NeuroConnections* article mentioned above that shows, in a truly humble way, how it takes a technical and clinical community to save a child.) When the prototypic "Mark Smith Z-score ok" protocols were first used, the daytime seizures stopped (there were still delta, slow-wave sleep discharges, for a while, but then these also discontinued).

Mark writes, "Thanks to neurofeedback, Jack is thriving today (2008). He has been seizure free for over a year and one half. His renewed ebul-lience has brought many friends and much social activity. We are working on eliminating his anticonvulsant medications. Most important, Jack has not suffered cognitive decline from his disorder. He is doing well after being selected for a gifted and talented program in his school" (Smith 2008).

Mark knew the method worked because of Jack's life-changing response, and he became one of the first teachers of the Z-score method. Other clinicians began climbing on board. But the problem was that the elders in the field had a real attitude. They just couldn't get their minds around it. Bob Thatcher, on the other hand, thought Z-score was the next new thing in neurofeedback. Most serious practitioners said that the method shouldn't even be used without a qEEG beforehand, which would suggest the pattern of sites to be treated and their relationship and/or lack of relationship to each other described at the outset. The qEEG would show coherence or lack of coherence, connectivity or comodulation, or its lack, and phase advance or retardation. Based on the qEEG, the Z-score protocol would be devised that trained the abnormalities toward normalcy. The statistical outliers—real anomalies in the EEG—would be brought into relationship and communication with each other. In general, this practice is now followed: qEEG first, then a Z-score protocol, starting with just a few sites, and gradually working up.

Most conventional Z-score training is done with two or four sites in relationship—easily done with a BrainMaster *Atlantis* 2×2, or 4×4. With the *Discovery* 24, however, a much more ambitious program of nineteen-channel Z-score training may be assayed. It requires a very high-performance computer to do all the number-crunching (say an *Asus* G-5 or G-7 with 64 bits and at least 8 gigabytes of RAM) and a full nineteen-channel EEG cap, so that all sites can be read simultaneously—and compared.

As the client sits in the treatment chair, a movie of his or her choice ("interesting, but hopefully not too violent") is put on, and the client's only task is to watch the movie. As criteria set by the clinician are met, the movie fades or brightens; the process is effortless and kind of automatic—most people like to watch the movie in a satisfactory manner. (Alternatively, just turning on music or animation can be used. After a certain number of training sessions, say ten or twenty, another qEEG is administered, which will usually show the extensive modifications of the brain in the parameters—coherence, connectivity, phase.) It is important to note, however, that, as in the LENS, no brain modification by itself is taken as significant of progress without concomitant clinical changes in the patient's mood, cognition, sleep, energy, and so forth.

Mark said it was when he began doing regular presentations at the professional organizations (the AAPB and the ISNR) that the climate really began to change. By now there are somewhere between three hundred and five hundred practitioners using this method all over the world.

At our own clinic, Z-score has become a part of our clinical offerings.

After a course of the LENS to loosen things up and break up dysfunctional and habitual patterns, we might suggest a qEEG to see how the normative dimensions of this client are progressing. The qEEG itself will suggest a pattern of site placements, although the default, if a qEEG has not been done, is called F3/F4 and P3/P4, a kind of rectangle designed to pull the anomalies or "outliers" toward the center. To be more precise, irregularities in the idiosyncratic brain map will be addressed. In our clinical experience of about a year of using this method, patients suddenly find that they are becoming more organized, proactive, and able to solve certain kinds of problems that before seemed out of reach for them (as in the case presented at the beginning of this section).

Z-score is a little closer to operant conditioning than the LENS, in that it requires conscious attention, involvement, and something like "the will," whether that is conscious or unconscious. Based on our experience so far, Z-score may anchor the amazing changes initially facilitated by the LENS and make them more permanent and more available to the will or intention of the client. Our next new direction in neurofeedback seems to anchor these changes still further.

Slow Cortical Potentials and Infra-Low Frequencies

It is very easy to get these two: SCPs or Slow Cortical Potentials, and ILF or Infra-Low Frequencies, confused. That is because they resemble each other, and seem to morph in and out of each other. The issue, as we shall see in the remainder of this chapter and the next, is that the subject studied most in neurofeedback has traditionally been "brain waves," usually measured in Hertz or cycles per second, all the way from 1 Hz up to about 40, and sometimes even up to 100. The "ranges" of these waves are given Greek letter names: Alpha, Beta, Delta, and so on. If languaging and naming things guides thought, and it certainly seems to, then these provide the vocabulary, the "memes," and the grammar— or syntax of discourse—in the EEG field.

In this section we move to talking about DC, or direct current "potentials," or AC so slow that it looks like DC: the ILFs. Hence the controversy in the field; we have to change not only some parts of our vocabulary, but perhaps the very syntax, and our ways of talking and thinking about how to do neurofeedback.

Slow cortical potentials (SCPs) have been the subject of study for years at Nils Birbaumer's lab in Tübingen, Germany. Only in the past decade, and even more recently, has it attracted the attention of American clinicians, whose results have also been impressive—and controversial, as were HEG, the LENS, and Z-score when they were first introduced. First, the classical research from Tübingen:

Several studies have found a consistent relationship between cortical negativity and reaction time, signal detection, and short-term memory performance (review, see Birbaumer et al. 1990). Therefore, slow corticol potentials (SCPs) have been conceptualized as a tuning mechanism in attentional regulation and the self-regulation of SCPs hypothesized as a plausible treatment for disorders characterized by impaired excitation thresholds. In a series of experiments, the ability to self-regulate SCP shifts was investigated. Findings indicated that both healthy and clinical patient populations were able to learn self-regulation of negative and positive SCP shifts over central electrode sites (Birbaumer et al. 1992; Holzapfel et al. 1998; Coben et al. 2011).

Training is often done at Cz, the "vertex," also Lubar's favorite spot for determining the theta/beta ratio. Unlike operant conditioning methods, where the brain is asked to move in a certain direction, say raising the frequency or lowering the amplitudes of something, SCP training rewards bidirectional regulation of two tasks, negative or positive shifts. Patients seem to have an easier time producing a positive shift if the baseline is negative, and a negative shift if the baseline is positive; that is to say, there is an intrinsic balancing aspect to the SCP training. The distribution of negative and positive shifts the brain is asked to make is selected randomly. There are also no-feedback trials that are thought to simulate and transfer to everyday life in some protocols.

In some ways, SCP training proves the principle I have long held, that in a dynamical living system, it is not just telling the system what to do ("Produce more alpha, suppress that theta . . .") but rather, "Flex, relax, stretch and flex again, relax again . . ." and so forth, just like Pilates or yoga. In effect, what we are training is the flexibility and elasticity of the system.

SCPs belong to the family of event-related potentials (ERPs), meaning that they are time-locked to a specific event (a stimulus), whether external or internal. They last from the range of the classic ERP, the P-300 wave—about 300 milliseconds—to several seconds in length. They also vary from amplitudes of a few μv (microvolts) to more than 100μv (during seizures). But I have seen similar huge microvolt changes from psychotropic drugs (*Salvia divinorum* is an example) or yoga breathing practices. The classical wiggle (AC) of the EEG rises and soars through the other records, or drops, as massive DC voltages surge and sweep through the record.

Birbaumer's theory is that negative shifts increase the firing probabilities of a given cell assembly, while positive shifts decrease them. This is probably accomplished through coordination of glial and neural cell assemblies and is known to change throughout the diurnal cycle. The *Bereitschafts potential,* or "potential for movement," can be either voluntary (internal stimulus) or external (outer stimulus). It was first identified over forty years ago and is one of the most researched of brain potentials.

We are now moving close to topics that are addressed in the next chapter: namely consciousness, awareness, intentionality. If you are like me, these are topics that might arouse your interest or wake you up, because they hover close to the essential mysteries of being alive and the very mysterious cusp between consciousness and the unconscious. We experience ourselves being alive and aware, and having intention or volition—that is, "conscious" and yet, as we all know, the very processes that keep us self-regulated, viable, and alive are all "unconsciously" regulated. Where is the interface? Where does the soul live?

Infra-Low-Frequency Neurofeedback (ILF)

As mentioned, slow cortical potentials (SCP) and infra-low frequency (ILF) are very closely related and may at times be indistinguishable. For the sake of theory, SCP belongs to true DC or direct current shifts, always present in some measure in the EEG (and many other bodily functions, being the essential movement of energy through the organs and the acupuncture meridians—including through the brain).

Infra-low frequency, by definition, has "frequency," hence conceptually

belongs to the AC, or alternating current domain, even though its alterations are so slow as to resemble DC. ILF lies below delta, so that its frequencies are measured in decimal places: tenths, hundredths, or thousandths of
a Hz, oscillations so slow as to be difficult to measure without special or
sensitive equipment.

ILF manages to be one of the most controversial areas in neurofeedback as of this writing. Proponents say that it is dramatically effective
for regulating conditions such as post-traumatic stress disorder (PTSD),
attachment disorder, and asthma, which are unresponsive to other
approaches. Critics are suspicious that you can even train anyone's brain
to decimal points of a Hertz (the wavelengths are too long and too slow,
they say).

The Othmer Approach to ILF, with a Focus on PTSD

Siegfried and Susan Othmer have been doing neurofeedback for a long,
long time. They have probably taught more clinicians than any single
"school" in the field. Their own pioneering work in neurofeedback could
easily fit into chapter 4, "The Compassionate Healer"—they evolved their
protocols while healing their own children. Siegfried is the research scientist, and his wife, Susan, the clinician. Their synergy has moved our
field forward in an optimal way: the scientific and the human journeys
entwined—or married, so to speak.

This part of their story begins around 2001. With the rest of the
EEG biofeedback field, the Othmers had come to accept that neurofeedback is not aimed at particular symptoms, but at overall brain regulation.
"The promotion of CNS stability is the first objective of brain training,"
writes Siegfried Othmer. Over the years, the Othmers had tried all of
the ranges for training: beta, Sterman's SMR, alpha and theta; but the
quest for an "optimal reward frequency" (or ORF) for each person seemed
to lead them lower and lower into the frequency ranges. Here they were
held back by "hardware" problems; EEG processors weren't made to go as
low as they seemed to be finding optimal training frequencies required.
"By 2006," writes Othmer," a gradual trend toward lower frequencies had
already been underway for some five years. The training of mid-range

EEG frequencies had mandated the use of a 3-Hz signal bandwidth and with this limitation the lowest available setting of the filters was 0-3 Hz, for a center frequency of 1.5." (Othmer Othmer and Legarda 2010) Most EEG evaluations stopped at .5 or "half a Hertz," considered very low delta.

Hardware was deliberately designed by the Othmers and their technical associates to extend this range. Initially it was dropped to .05Hz ". . . as more clinical data were acquired, ultimately to .01 Hz, then to .001Hz, and finally to .0001 Hz, or .1 milliHertz (mHz)" wrote Siegfried. The way to find this ORF is by clinical trial and error—the frequencies are brought up and down until the person feels a clinical sense of well-being or comfort: "The reward frequency is adjusted during the first session," he wrote, "to the state in which the person is as maximally calm, alert and 'euthymic,' as the nervous system is capable of being at that moment" (Othmer 2009). ("Euthymia" was first described by Democritus as a "gladness, good mood, or serenity." It is to be distinguished both from "dysthymia," low grade depression, or "euphoria"—giddiness, unrealistic happiness.) That is to say, while the client is training, the clinician is constantly checking into his or her proprioceptive or "interoceptive" state— known only to the person him- or her-self. In this process, giddy is no better than mild depression or fatigue. The therapist will be constantly changing the settings, until the client feels optimal well-being, or "euthymia."

In effect, this process relies on a theory of *state* as opposed to *symptom*. Though it relies on how the client feels, it aims at more broadly based regulatory mechanisms rather than temporary conditions. The Othmers hypothesize that the process depends on the resonant property of brain waves, because such an optimal frequency can be found, but it is different for each person. The question may then be raised whether ILF actually is training the brain, or is more similar to peripheral biofeedback— which measures things like skin conductivity or hand temperature, gradients which move more slowly than those produced by the familiar rapidly oscillating AC brainwaves. (In summoning scientific support that ILF is actually a type of EEG, though, Othmer cites a publication by Kelly, Uddin, Biswall, Castellanos, and Milham, which claims that EEG rhythmicity in the brain has been measured by independent researchers, down to 0.01 Hz.)

In 2009 I chaired a symposium at ISNR on Soldier Return Syndrome (Indianapolis, annual ISNR meeting). Dr. Siegfried Othmer was one of the invited speakers, and he presented a case that was truly impressive. This was a soldier with multiple problems, including flashbacks, insomnia, nightmares, night sweats, anxiety, fatigue, mood swings, alcoholism, and cognitive problems (a not unusual litany of symptoms for traumatized wartime vets). Dr. Othmer presented clinical evidence using a *Likert scale,* 10→1, symptom checklists, before and after neuropsych testing, and, most impressively, a filmed interview in which the vet claimed that the training (a mixture of the ILF and Peniston-type alpha-theta training) had literally "saved his life," that most of his symptoms were "decreased" or down to "nonexistent," that his medicines had been discontinued, and that his quality of life was much improved.

The following is an abbreviated and edited recital of therapeutic improvements:

After the first session he was able to go to grocery store where he was previously disoriented. He came to the second session with neck pain, which was reduced during the session. During session three, a trash bag elicited a "flashback"; by session five he had no reaction to same. After alpha-theta training was introduced (in session eight), he was "strangely calm," saw traumatic images "dissolve in water." He had a visit from a deceased grandfather and a reactivated pain in the right leg, but he also enjoyed sleeping through the night for the first time since beginning treatment.

- More alpha-theta: reduced muscle pain and recovery of memories.
- After session eleven, smoking less.
- After session thirteen, "felt like a million bucks."
- After session fourteen, able to talk about the war (in Bosnia); less OCD.
- Continuous performance test given and showed normalized attention (TOVA).

Most impressive of all was the video interview in which this wounded warrior talks about how his life has changed. It is available from the Othmers at EEGInfo.com.

In my estimation, it was the best presentation in the symposium, which means that it was systematic, well-documented, and held out the most hope for the men and women who have become grievously injured in the defense of their country.

More recently I have seen hopeful work for returned soldiers come from the LENS, a variety of other neurofeedback approaches, a new technique developed by Dr. Ronald Ruden called "Havening" (see *The Past is Always Present*) and some excellent work for larger groups developed by Drs. Richard Brown and Patricia Gerbarg (see www.haveahealthymind.com).

Mark Smith's Approach to ILF

Mark Smith, one of the developers of Z-score training, as detailed above, says he originally learned about ILF by studying one of Susan Othmer's protocols in 2008. He says he was impressed by what he heard about the Othmers' success with the machine they developed to train at the ultra-low levels: the *Cygnet*. Thereafter, he set about developing his own approach. Working with Tom Collura at BrainMaster, they developed Infra-low protocols for the Atlantis. He felt that the Atlantis/Discovery machines at 0.002 Hz were filtering lower energy than the Cygnet at 0.01 (Siegfried Othmer disagrees). Mark said he was in search of a lower signal-to-noise ratio, and that there was no "corner frequency" (the lowest frequency the amplifier can read)—with the signal going down into DC, so he went with the BrainMaster.

In his tightly structured weekend training workshops for professionals, which some of my staff and I have taken, Mark is thorough about detailing both the benefits and the risks of ILF. He does not quibble about the fact that not paying careful enough attention to the client as you attempt to find the optimal reward frequency (ORF) can do the opposite of what is intended: give the client a headache, or worsen the one he or she already has, or occasion a bout of depression or a bad mood.

The training is not so different from the Z-score in that the client watches a movie that dims and brightens, but there is a low thrumming sound in the background that reflects the client making and losing the goals. Once again, this kind of training exercises the brain as the client goes into and out of the desired range. It is a "bipolar treatment" in which the electrodes or "sensors" are placed either on both hemispheres (T3 and T4) or one, say T4 and P4 sites (based on the International 10–20 system). T means Temporal, P Parietal, and odd numbers indicate the left or even the right hemispheres. The ground is on the top of the head, not the ears, and it rewards an increase in the difference between the two signals, both amplitude and phase, and also trains the phase relationship.

Smith says the training is neither "operant" nor "classical" conditioning, but it provides the brain a "window on its own functioning" as it moves toward the optimal reward frequency and the "still point" where the client is the most calm and yet most alert. He hypothesizes that the ILF may be addressing the basic timing mechanism of the thalamocortical networks.

Three categories of its action include:

1. Instabilities (including migraines, vertigo, seizures, mood swings, asthma, panic attacks, fibromyalgia, and parasomnias)
2. Developmental disorders or trauma (including autism, attachment disorders, personality disorders, addictions, and PTSD)
3. Arousal and activation deficits (attentional problems, ADD and ADHD, depression, anxiety, tics, and OCD) (Smith 2010)

This discussion does not allow us to go into further details of the treatment method; that is knowledge for the professional, who in my opinion should be a licensed mental health professional of some sort, because of the risks and volatility possible to evoke in this kind of approach. It requires subtle and skillful monitoring of the outcome of treatment—in each individual session and as the treatment effects unfold and accumulate.

In the training sessions that I attended, some people had negative reactions. One went into a funk, another got a headache, some had insomnia; most of these were corrected by skillful tweaking in the second session the following day. (Smith insists that especially in the beginning, people should train twice a week under careful supervision of the professional to "get it right.") For myself, I noticed an immediate euthymia bordering on euphoria. I drove skillfully in challenging New York City traffic and parallel parked effortlessly, but later, after a meal and a couple of glasses of wine, I felt exhausted. On going to bed I fell into a deep sleep. (But I was up at 5:00 a.m. with plenty of energy, attended the workshop the next day in a euthymic state, and drove two hours in an alert state to get home again, before falling into a restful sleep.)

Smith takes this method seriously enough to offer weekly online or phone-counseling sessions for his trainees. He is currently reporting extremely positive results with autistic children at a school for children with spectrum disorders. He is able to present impressive-looking before-and-after qEEGs, along with positive clinical reports of outcomes. A colleague, Jackie deVries, who uses both the LENS and Z-score as well as ILF, says they all are effective, each in its own way. But she feels that the ILF can "anchor in" previously attained benefits so that they do not dissipate over time.

Critics of ILF claim the method can cause abreactions, overstimulations, and adverse reactions—thus giving neurofeedback a bad name (Hammond 2010b; Hammond and Kirk 2008). Hammond also points out that in the intense questioning that goes on with this method, which is clinically or symptom-driven, rather than protocol-driven, it is possible hypnotically to influence negative reactions or "nocebo" responses as opposed to positive "placebo" responses (Hammond 2010).

To me, it would be wonderful if the innovators of this marvelous new method would extensively train themselves, their friends and staff, and get expert supervision, before trying it out on patients. The exception would be with patients who one knows are fairly hardy, have tried extensive neurofeedback already, and still are looking for changes.

Z-Scored LORETA (Low-Resolution EEG-based Tomography) Neurofeedback

Neurofeedback is clearly a moving target—for anyone hoping to circumscribe or interpret it. The most recent clinical development based on Robert Thatcher's work is Z-scored LORETA neurofeedback. LORETA Z-scored diagnostics represent the ultimate noninvasive dynamic brain imaging technique, based on qEEG data, and using a mathematical process called "the inverse solution," to infer what is happening in the deeper, less accessible structures beneath the cortex. Thatcher has provided abundant evidence about the validity of LORETA imaging for subcortical conditions, including comparisons to other, more conventional imaging techniques such as MRI, PET, or SPECT (as discussed in chapter 3). (Please also see LORETA images in the color insert, plate 5.)

LORETA Z-scored neurofeedback takes this imaging into the realm of therapy. If through LORETA imaging we find *a subcortical area that is instigating the problem,* say the legendary "hot" anterior *cingulate gyrus,* imagine training *not just the adjacent areas in the cortex* (outer layer of the brain), as in most forms of neurofeedback, but the deep-down *instigator itself.*

Could this "cut to the chase" technique explain why the preliminary reports about this method are so startlingly positive? While we have learned to expect fast results with just a few sessions with the LENS (in less complicated conditions), I have not heard of results like those veteran clinician Marty Wuttke (interviewed herein) told me about in a recent phone conversation. A desperate woman patient from an alcoholic family, with thirty years of her own chronic alcoholism, resolving the problem in a single session! From years of treating addictions and other deep-seated familial problems with neurofeedback, Marty told me he was "blown away." He is now teaching the method internationally.

As of 2011, there are only preliminary reports on this new development, but they are very encouraging, so I am happy to include a brief section: an interview—by experienced neurofeedback practitioner, Michael Gismondi—with LORETA biofeedback trainer Marty Wuttke.

Michael Gismondi, L.M.H.C., Interviews Martin Wuttke, C.N.P., about LORETA Neurofeedback

[Note: This interview was originally prepared for NeuroConnections, *the* ISNR Newsletter, *but deferred to a future edition. —Ed.]*

Marty Wuttke's latest project documents the remarkable clinical power of NeuroGuide's Z-score guided LORETA neurofeedback (and related tools) with an eye toward its clear, comprehensive instruction and appropriate integration into clinical practice.

MICHAEL: What excites you about LORETA Z-scored neurofeedback (LZN) and what does it add to your existing tool bag?

MARTY: What excites me is it appears that LZN is able to produce very significant changes in clients, very rapidly. It cuts back the neurofeedback treatment process from the typical forty to sixty sessions, down to a fraction of that . . . usually ten visits *or less*. I was not prepared for that! So, to have a tool that can allow us to take on difficult clinical conditions, and have clients feel profound changes almost immediately, and feel "done" in so few sessions, can revolutionize both the economics and common perception of NFB. The other thing that excites me is it produces some very strong psychological or perhaps more precisely *psychodynamic* changes in clients . . . changes in core identities, defenses, interpersonal strategies, and the sense of one's life narrative. These changes are very important, often transformational.

For example, clients who have been addicted to alcohol or drugs start to lose their compulsions. We have chronic PTSD clients who suddenly start facing their demons, with insight and a depth of self-perception they said they never possessed before, often in just a few sessions. I've seen OCD clients very quickly get relief from those symptoms, in a timeframe I have never seen before. *These are very consistent responses that we're having, and I have been doing this long enough to know just how out of the ordinary this is when compared to traditional surface neurofeedback.*

It is also exciting to me to see how the NeuroGuide NFB software allows relatively novice practitioners, who don't yet possess a strong command of clinical neurophysiology, to be able to select target symptoms and see how the neuroscience literature would link it up with which circuits in the brain, and from there, how a Z-scored normative database would target EEG values for training. This clear, step-by-step process can eliminate a lot of practitioner error. You know: overtraining, undertraining, training compensatory structures and getting adverse reactions, and so on. And yet, at the same time, for someone like me who has a good working knowledge of neurophysiology, it's fascinating to be able to target deeper brain structures and systems and see how the EEG, and the client, will respond.

MICHAEL: OK, not to be difficult, but I know we both realize that your observations must be compared to what has been experienced by experts in traditional surface NFB who branched out into using newer "power tools" like the LENS, NeuroField, infra-low frequency techniques, and BrainMaster's four—or even nineteen—channel Live Z-Score techniques.

MARTY: Absolutely, and as I start training clinicians who are versed in some or even most of the techniques just mentioned, things will quickly come into focus.

MICHAEL: I spoke just the other day with Mark Smith, who is getting remarkable results with his version of infra-low frequency techniques, and is a master of Live Z-Score Training, and he was commenting on the power of LZN in a manner very similar . . . almost identical to your descriptions. I hear through the grapevine Bob McCarthy in South Carolina is seeing similar things as well.

MARTY: So it's not just me!

MICHAEL: But let me ask you this; how do you suppose LORETA NFB works? In various conversations I have heard you and Joel Lubar talk about LZN working on entire networks or areas of the brain at once, and deeper or more inclusive networks, moreso than any form of surface NFB. What exactly are we talking about here? Entire Brodman areas, Hagman "connectivity hubs" [see chapter 14 for a description of how these "hubs" revealed by the latest imaging techniques are the functional "organs" of the brain—Ed.] . . . or something in addition?

MARTY: Really, all of the above and then some. But what really sticks out for me is the impact LZN has on enhancing connectivity . . . coherence and phase lag, surprisingly enough. We are seeing much bigger, faster effects that last longer. The advantage of using a full nineteen-channel cap for training vs. one-, two-, or four-channel NFB is *huge*. We are getting a whole brain trained at once, on multiple levels of brain architecture. We are seeing how changes in one area, in one set of EEG metrics, ripple through and affect the rest of the brain and it's EEG *in real time*, and the training is modified accordingly.

MICHAEL: You can do some of that with Tom Collura and Mark Smith's "Percent Z-OK" and "Z-Plus Multichannel Training," but not with the same deep grounding in neuroanatomy and Brodman's functional brain architecture. I would think that with whole cap LORETA training, you can target precise structures and functional circuits in the brain to a far greater extent.

MARTY: I agree, but it depends where you are training. Even with one or two channels, if you are training the supplemental motor areas, for instance, you will be covering a lot of territory in the brain and other structures and functions that are far more challenging to recruit and affect. But that's the power of training Hagman hubs with LZN!

MICHAEL: Why do you believe that LORETA NFB changes connectivities more rapidly than other approaches?

MARTY: For the most part, the rate of change in clients' connectivities has been fairly measurable and consistent . . . Z-score standard deviations going from 4 or 5 down to 1 or less. Now perhaps that's the strength of whole head, nineteen-channel Live Z-Score Training in general, it is so profoundly self-documenting. (Because it is done with a full cap, a complete database-referenced qEEG can be done every time.) To press that a little further, I think the proponents of the other "power tools" emerging have yet to step up to the challenge of documenting *the process* of their outcomes so well. And as Bob Thatcher likes to point out, it's building software that supports, seamlessly, the tight coupling between client symptoms, the neuroanatomical symptom correlates, and the EEG values you target . . . that is key.

MICHAEL: In your experience, what advantage does LZN have over surface Z-scored NFB?

MARTY: What stands out for me is the profound and rapid, almost immediate, impact LZN has on the *cingulate gyrus* (anterior and posterior), the *cuneus* and *precuneus,* the *insula*—these are really critical areas, clinically. You see client complaints change very quickly when those areas are causally involved. I've worked with some addicts that lost their compulsion to use in one or two sessions. It isn't the precision of localization that matters, it's the engagement of the right network in its entirety. [Again, see chapter 14 for a description of the "default mode network" and the "hubs."]

MICHAEL: I was sort of indoctrinated by my friend David Joffe [see chapter 3 on the evolution of neurofeedback]—who was the first to implement LORETA NFB, along with Marco Congedo, back in 2002 or 2003—to be very concerned about the vulnerability of LORETA NFB to artifact* and the dangers of training artifacts with such a powerful method. Joel Lubar deals with that via the filters he uses on sites and bands that are known to be artifact prone. What do you think?

MARTY: One thing I do is let clients see their live EEG as they are training, and I coach them about the artifact production. Another thing is Bob Thatcher's software is really good at not training artifact, it's uncanny at times. I haven't had the need to put in additional filters.

MICHAEL: As you gear up to train a lot of clinicians to do LZN, and you encounter relatively inexperienced practitioners who are not yet adept at reading the live raw EEG while working with a client, how do you help them perform competently?

MARTY: I think that is going to be essential, to impart these skills up front.

MICHAEL: Thanks to how Dr. Thatcher put the NeuroGuide NFB software together, LZN seems to be remarkably user-friendly, and even novice-friendly, but still, I would think relatively novice neurotherapists have to learn a lot of clinical or applied neurophysiology, to

---

*Because the LZN uses such vast amounts of critical data collected from nineteen sites through a "cap," it may be vulnerable to muscle movement, connection problems, and other variables extraneous to the EEG.

know how and when to override or modify the set of locations and bands and metrics you will be training at any one time.

MARTY: I think that it is crucial, essential, that the LZN user is well informed about the neurophysiology, where the symptoms are coming from, what are the likely networks to train or ignore, but at the same time, LZN requires knowledge about the whole psychodynamic impact of this work, so a solid command of clinical skills, diagnostics, patient management, psychotherapeutic issues even, is needed. LZN produces profound psychological shifts in clients, and not just people with chronic PTSD, or addicts. I am talking about people with head injuries, and with OCD, some ADHD adults, even people who have come in for gastrointestinal complaints or migraines, or neuroautomomic issues. The clinician must know how to recognize, manage, and even utilize these big psychological shifts as they come up. The psychological impact of LZN can be far greater than what we see in traditional neurofeedback (NFB).

MICHAEL: So, it seems that one of the requirements of a LZN training has to be that while you can be somewhat new to neurofeedback, you must be an experienced and resourceful clinician first.

MARTY: Absolutely . . . or, at a bare minimum, the clinician must have very ready access to expert supervision and mentoring around the psychodynamics and know when to call upon it. LZN really does change people's lives, and client awareness, and for the patient now to realize what he or she has been doing to cause or perpetuate self-destructive behaviors, or putting his or her family and friends through all these years, can often require fast and accurate intervention. At the same time, knowing how changes in the underlying client neurophysiology correlates with likely changes in client psychology is crucial. And frankly, this new science, neurotherapy, especially as it grows more powerful and impactful, requires a new school of thought that really isn't taught anywhere, or in any one set of courses. It evolves over years of mentoring with the best teacher/practitioners we have.

MICHAEL: Another focus: Does hardware matter in the use of NeuroGuide NFB?

MARTY: I don't know yet. I haven't compared amplifiers yet. I have heard from Joel and other people I trust that *Deymed* is superior to the BrainMaster *Discovery* and the *Mitsar* in the registration of the higher frequencies and distinguishing it from artifact, but LORETA is limited to the 1–30 Hz range, so it may not matter all that much for doing LZN. It's a wait-and-see sort of thing.

MICHAEL: If we could return one last time to the probable mechanics of LORETA NFB, what is the significance, in your mind, of training current source densities* with LZN vs. surface voltages as done in traditional neurofeedback that allows us to access and transform entire functional neural networks or symptom "systems" as Len Ochs and Barry Sterman have characterized it?

MARTY: I think it's because current source densities are roadblocks in the brain's information processing highways. If you clear out those roadblocks, accurately and completely, the brain quickly snaps back and works as intended. I know some of this happens with traditional neurofeedback, but I see a lot of LZN clients process traumatic memories and themes and make really profound connections as to what these memories have meant to them and their own "life story" or life narrative. We have everybody keep a journal as they go through this, and people come up with the most remarkable self-narratives as they start putting together the pieces of their lives in the most profound ways.

MICHAEL: I recently had a discussion with Joel Lubar on the topic of why it is so powerful to work with current source densities with LORETA vs. surface voltages, and he said, as I recall, that traditional NFB works with voltages, which are a measure of the electrical force or pressure that is detectable at the scalp. Thus, surface voltages are a measure of how the brain's electrophysiological activity comes together at certain gathering points. Electrical currents, on the other hand, are a measure of how fast electrons pass by a certain point, and as a result, it is a

---

*"Current source densities" (CSDs), simply stated, have to do with the probable sources or generators of the electrical current in the brain that will ultimately give rise to the EEG activity detected at the scalp or "surface."

sense of the *direction* of the source of the surface activity, and *that* is what gives us a sense of the network involved.

MARTY: That is what I believe is happening, and that is what I meant by the idea of detecting "key roadblocks" in specific neural networks. I will encourage Bob Thatcher to address this in his trainings. We haven't had a chance to discuss Bob's "phase reset"* NFB, which I have been using since he released it a few weeks ago, and which I use with LZN. I recently used it with an Alzheimers client and got some amazing changes that way in just ten sessions. Let me say, in closing, what a remarkable set of tools Bob Thatcher has given us, and just how big the impact of their skillful use could be.

The BrainAvatar System

While this book has been going through the editorial process, the gnomes of neurofeedback have been relentlessly innovating in their little cubicles. If LORETA neurofeedback is showing the extraordinary promise that Wuttke and Thatcher claim, resolving long-standing, serious problems in a single or a few sessions, releasing addictions, and bringing about major personality changes for the better, then the advocates of s-LORETA, a brand new system still being tested, may offer even more spectacular results. Leading this field is BrainMaster's Tom Collura.

Collura writes of his system: "BrainAvatar computes the s-LORETA projection instantaneously using high-speed time-domain methods, and accurately shows the momentary changes in EEG signals, in real time. The combination of BrainMaster's high-speed digital filters with our unique projection technology provides the ability to compute hundreds of whole-brain s-LORETA projections per second, and image and train on the data. Trained data can be from voxels or Regions of Interest (ROI's)" (along the Hagman hubs, default networks, or salience systems described in chapter 14).

Collura believes his system talks to be the brain so quickly that it

---

*"Phase" is one of the parameters measured in qEEG, and it is analyzed by the NeuroGuide database. It has to do with how the wave forms line up or "resonate" with each other.

forms an entirely new kind of brain/computer interface. It is certainly faster than the conventional neurofeedback that uses "fast Fourier transforms" or FFT's, which have to be calculated before the feedback signal is given; and he claims it is faster than the Thatcher system described above, delivering virtually instantaneous real-time feedback.

Collura believes that the BrainAvatar can interface with any of the existing protocols used in neurofeedback: "These include all of our Z-score protocols, including PZOK and Plus. You can do SMR, alpha, Infra-Slow, Slow-cortical potential, synchrony, or any other training along with the live sLORETA projector and analysis. You can use peripherals such as Heart Rate Variability, skin conductance, EMG, respiration, or others along with the s-LORETA as well. BrainAvatar pushes the mind-brain connection, to provide a mind-brain-body connection for research or biofeedback. You can evaluate a client sitting still, then visualize the changes as they read or do other tasks. Task-based EEG information is instantly available."

I wish I could include some of the amazing color plates and videos of the BrainAvatar in action, that were first unveiled in 2011 at the ISNR (International Society for Neurofeedback and Research), but alas, at this late date there is no more room in the book. These can easily be seen on line at: http://youtube/XCHzx3OP9bw, and more information at www .brainm.com/kb/entry/460/ and www.brainmaster.com/software/videos/ Brainmaster.wmv.

Collura said in a recent communication, "When Roberto Pasqual-Marquis, the inventor of the LORETA and s-LORETA recently saw our system, he said: The possibilities are endless" (Collura, private communication).

Conclusions

It is certain that in new, developing fields like neurofeedback there are going to be clinical mistakes, along with successes. I am eager for innovators and their trainees to train themselves, and then to hear honest feedback—from those around them—about how a particular new modality "feels." Especially with modalities that propose lasting changes in personality and functioning, the clinician should be a trained psychotherapist or mental health professional—just to be able to "field" some of the astonishing changes that may be brought about.

In my home office at Stone Mountain Center, in addition to regular professional training seminars, I encourage my clinicians to practice on themselves and people they know well, who are mostly robust and stable, and willing to give honest feedback on how they feel after treatments. In this way, clinicians are more equipped to help clients over bumpy places in treatment and achieve maximum outcomes. By treating each other, we also get to know each other better, and enhance workplace dynamics!

FOURTEEN

CONSCIOUSNESS

A NEUROFEEDBACK PERSPECTIVE

With Jay Gunkelman, QEEG, and
Juan Acosta-Urquidi, Ph.D., QEEG-T

I t is invisible, odorless, colorless; it takes on the shape of whatever is around us, but its absence can endanger our very existence. Freud and others frightened us by talking about its dark twin, which can undermine our intentions and expectations, leading to dreams we don't expect, slips of the tongue, and far worse disorders called *neuroses* and *psychoses,* where it is grotesquely distorted. Most people have it, at least we assume they do, and so do animals, in their several ways. At its best and brightest, it lights up our life. People who possess it in abundance seem to do well in living; those lacking in it, well—they cause a lot of problems for the rest of us!

What is it?

The word seems simple enough: *consciousness.*

But for all its vaunted accomplishments, modern science hasn't yet gotten a handle on it. Whole conferences of scholars from the East and from the West devote themselves to elucidating it. Should it best be explicated by biology, physics, chemistry, or psychology? (Or do all of them need to be included in the conversation?)

I think neurofeedback has a unique and wonderful contribution to make to the conversation and thus takes us a large step toward understanding this great mystery that is interwoven into our lives. Though we may never fully be able to wrap our minds around it, the attempt is perennially compelling.

For twenty-five years I taught a college psychology course called "The Psychology of Consciousness" that I hoped might be like what William James would have taught eighty years later, had he the tools and the knowledge we have now. The course touched on all of James's interests: altered states of consciousness, dreams, meditation, creativity, imagination, and on to the furthest reaches of human potential. Biofeedback was the piece that James would not have been privy to, but which he very much would have appreciated. Much to the surprise of the college administrators, who were used to average registrations for the basic psychology courses—General, Developmental, Social, or Abnormal, because they were required for various curricula—this course, which fit none of those "required" categories, was always full, and with a waiting list.

It would be easy to attribute the success to my pedagogical charisma, but I know better: *it was the subject of consciousness itself,* and the latitude I gave students to find out some interesting things about their own consciousness—*experientially.* The students leaped into self-study with a passion that usually belongs only to play or other forms of high pleasure. I gradually involved them more and more, as the course unfolded, in sharing with the other students what they had discovered in their own explorations. We observed how motivation causes awareness to fluctuate, how distraction occurs through shifts in internal states, how to evaluate the quality of one's own attention, both in school and outside; to learn to manipulate consciousness itself through meditation or qigong. Through EEG biofeedback, the students learned to identify the brain waves that accompany states of consciousness. Shall I review them once more for the reader, even as I did for my students?

Delta for deep sleep, injury, or metabolic dysfunction; theta for hypnosis or reverie—and connection with the creative unconscious; alpha for meditation or "empty mind" (anxiety when it's more frontal) and a gearshift to the other states; beta for concentration—or very high anxiety, as in high-beta. And gamma? Who knows, maybe supercon-sciousness, Zen mind, or "enlightenment," as some studies suggest. I admitted that we didn't have a *definition* of consciousness, but we could talk about its *transformations,* say in the circadian cycle (over the course of a day all of them appear, but at any given time, one, called the *dominant frequency,* predominates over the others). And does the brain get locked into a particular frequency or amplitude or pattern of coherence? Or can it change flexibly as the occasion warrants? (In *The Healing Power of Neurofeedback,* I identify flexibility as a sign of health.)

Modern psychology is still looking for a definition of what conscious-ness is and how it arises, but I believe that, as for my students, having a vocabulary for its states, and the changes between states, is extremely helpful. Let's start with some up-to-date human neurobiology, and one of the questions that has always plagued biologists who study the brain's use of energy (probably 25–30 percent of the body's entire use of glucose and oxygen).

The Salience and Default-Mode Networks

Diffusion tensor imaging, a type of functional MRI involving water molecules in the human brain, has helped reveal new things about the human brain in two conditions: at rest, or under task. These are called salience networks, and the functional analyses correspond quite nicely to anatomical features, giving the entire model an immediate probity and acceptance in neurobiological circles. White matter tracts (myelinated neuron bundles) interconnect five different (Hagman's model) or eight (VanDen Heuvel) core networks, humming away under our busy bonnets, even under passive conditions.

Probably the most important of these is the default mode network (DMN), which, along with the core network, plays a role in interoception and the maintenance of a sense of self. Exteroceptive, outside events or stimuli are neurologically effective only because they impinge upon this already dynamically activated thing usually called "the self." Connector hubs go down the "Z" line, the center of the brain, and also spread out centrally and parietally, through the corpus callosum and less so frontally. Scattered out from these hubs are "provincial hubs" that connect to each other but do not have the major linkages of the connector hubs. (Please see plates 12 and 13 of the color insert.)

We now know that the human brain at rest can be more active than under task. That is to say, consciousness without a task, and even without "content," still requires glucose and oxygen and the blood flow to deliver them. The default network is like the mainframe that's on whether or not you're stuffing awesome data-processing tasks into its maw.

Guess what, you lucky people? There's something going on in there all the time!

How do all these parts interrelate? I like the description from Newburg and d'Aquili:

> By working in concert, the two sides of the orientation associa-tion area are able to weave raw sensory data into the vivid, complex perception of a self and into a world in which that self can move. The fact that this "self" is a mental representation, and that it is assembled from bits of raw sensory data, does not mean, of course, that the physical body or the world does not exist. The point is that the only way the mind can know the self and experience the difference between the self and the rest of reality, is through the elaborate restless efforts of the brain. (Newburg and d'Aquili 2001, 28)

If you think about it, there is something miraculous going on here, in a polyrhythmical dance of brain waves between the two (parietal) hemispheres, that supports the idea of a self in a world: "What kind of a world is this?" (right hemisphere) and "What kind of creature am I in it?" (left hemisphere). As mentioned in chapter 5 on attachment disorders, these two areas may be heated up white-hot, so to speak, under adverse circumstances—a cruel foster placement, a cold and rigid orphanage, trapped in a locked cage (for an Australian shepherd). In a sense, the one implies the other. We know that crazy environments help fashion crazy people, and the reverse is true as well, as Hitler showed the world half a century ago.*

Generic neurobiology has recognized since the time of Wilder Penfield that the sensory and motor representations (homunculi) of the body are arrayed along the Rolandic fissure, on both sides of the "sensorimotor strip," and are connected to the contralateral side of the body (they are interconnected with U-shaped fibers that allow almost instantaneous communication, say in an athlete or a musician who requires immediate sensory feedback on the effects of a behavior). Common knowledge also recognizes the role of the frontal lobes in planning, sequencing, and organizing behaviors (the so-called executive functions). To talk to each other, each of the homologous sites must send messages through the slender bridges, the corpus callosum or the anterior commisure. How do billions of neurons talk through telephone lines made up of mere millions (1/1000 of the total number of voices clamoring from each hemisphere)?

The answer involves something beyond structure, namely, rhythm, resonance, and that strange thing called "emergent properties." But we are getting ahead of the game. First we must go down the central axis of the brain.

The Deep Grottoes of the Brain: The Insula and the Cingulate Gyrus

Our quest for the mainsprings of human consciousness now takes us deeper into the brain, into areas that control these networks, and involve how self-awareness and our idea of past and present selves help us plan behaviors and understand the emotional texture of our lives. The recent neuroimaging experiments cited reveal an area of which Penfield and his generation knew little, because it was generally inaccessible to probes, which concentrated on the cortical surface made available only during

---

*Alice Miller has speculated on the rigid German family and upbringing in producing Hitler. See Alice Miller on "How could a Monster Succeed in Blinding a Nation," www.naturalchild.org/alice_miller/adolf_hitler.html.

open-brain procedures. Interestingly, for what they reveal about our inner ideas of ourselves and our experience, these newly charted areas lie deep in the shadowed fold between the hemispheres, where they join, and along the grottoed folds of the interior of the cortex.

With a midway position between the "old brain" (the limbic system and brainstem) and the "new brain" (the neocortex), lies the insular cortex, or "insula." The front part of this region (the anterior insular cortex or AIC) is definitely connected to "gut feelings." It registers nonpainful distention of the digestive tract, hence satiation; awareness of temperature, pleasurable voices, faces, music, and sexual arousal; and awareness of changes in one's own heartbeat (not an unimportant somatic variable). With its intimate connection to the amygdala, it feels the "approach-avoidance" and "fight-or-flight" emotions. It is also adjacent to the hippocampus, which registers and stores memories largely based on their emotional salience. As one study shows, when unpleasant faces were paired with gastrointestinal sensations, there was a synergistic effect, hinting that James and Lange were just right about our guts commenting on our outer experience (Craig 2009, 59). The AIC responds to music, rhythm, happy faces, self-recognition (as in seeing your picture or yourself in a mirror), time perception, the feeling of knowing something, awareness of the present moment, as in now, attention, boredom (which sabotages attention), and perceptually based decision-making.

Impairments of the AIC are involved in strange distortions in awareness called *alexithymia* (inability to communicate about one's own emotions)—attributed mainly to Vulcans (like Mr. Spock) on *Star Trek*, autistics, or "wooden" politicians. Even more interesting is *anosognosia*. Do you remember the point in the movie *Young Frankenstein* in which Dr. Frankenstein, played by Gene Wilder, calls Igor's attention to the hunchback's all-too-apparent hump? Igor (played brilliantly by Marty Feldman) smiles ghoulishly and asks, "What hump?" Anosognosia is the denial that one possesses some obvious (to others) physical defect, such as poststroke paralysis in half the body, or a repetitive tic. (Impossible, you might think, but true! Think of *The Man Who Mistook His Wife for a Hat*!—Oliver Sachs' famous study.) More subtly, the insula weaves somatic and emotional memory into "now," allowing us to match or mismatch feelings or to notice things that don't fit or seem disjunctive ("All right, I don't get it! What the heck is going on around here?").

The reader may have encountered the old saw that time is stretchable according to psychological experience: "Three hours of tender conversation with a lover can seem to pass in ten minutes. Ten seconds sitting on a hot stove can seem like three hours." The anterior insula is intimately involved with timing. It is the part of you that notices the sound track is not synched to the movement of the movie actor's lips.

Then there is something both wondrous and strange. The insula contains large, spindle-shaped neurons called VENs.* VENs seem to be implicated in what truly separates us from (lower) animals. They seem to yield both self-consciousness and self-awareness (more on the differences between these two later). These notable neurons are found among the familiar (also large) and ubiquitous pyramidal neurons that are positioned vertically through the six cortical layers. VENs are lacking in dogs and cats (and rodents and reptiles of all sorts) and macaques. They seem to appear, albeit sparsely, among gorillas, chimps, and bonobos. But they are found among all sorts of cetaceans (whales), bottlenose and Risso's dolphins, and Asian and African elephants. Giant neurons for giant creatures!

Animals who have a certain abundance of VENs—and they are found not only in the AIC, but the anterior cingulate cortex (ACC) and the dorsolateral prefrontal cortex (DL-PFC)—pass the mirror test. That is to say, they recognize themselves in a mirror, an elemental and immediate form of feedback. This is known to happen among elephants, where stringent tests have revealed that the great pachyderm can notice an X painted on its face by seeing it in a mirror. Your dog or your cat, intelligent and socialized as it may seem, probably cannot pass the mirror test—maybe with the exception of very talented individuals. Elephants, on the other hand, not only seem able to form a self-image, their ability to perform music with other elephants shows an ability to access that self in relation to others, clearly an advanced neurological trait.

---

*VEN stands for von Economo neurons, named after an early-twentieth-century neuroscientist, Constantin von Economo (1876–1931), who first identified them.

An experienced horse trainer has told us of an incident in which she walked in front of a mirror with Kitwell, an Arabian-cross (very intelligent) that she was training. (For the most part, horses, like dogs and cats, do not recognize themselves in mirrors—in fact, they have been known to attack "the other horse" or try to jump through the mirror into the other room that seems to be there.) On this occasion, the trainer touched herself, then the mirror, then Kitwell and the mirror. "All of a sudden, he got it. He was almost jumping up and down with excitement." He touched her sleeve while looking in the mirror, then touched the mirror with his nose. "He was vocalizing, nickering, and kept touching my sleeve and touching the mirror—it was very moving," she said, and the only experience like it that she ever had, but thereafter Kitwell responded to mirrors. (Thanks to Carla Adinaro for this story.) My wife, Robin, a horsewoman, hearing this story, reminded me that horses and elephants indeed are relatives, and that horses vary greatly in their sensitivity and ability to socialize with their handlers. In any case, Kitwell may have had rudimentary VENs.

In human beings, the abundance of VENs follows aging; adult human beings have many more of these neurons than youth or infants. Note that these are not the same as the "mirror neurons" discovered by Rizzolatti and the Parma Group during the 1990s. (Mirror neurons, found in macaques, are all about "monkey see, monkey do" imitation rather than self-reflection. Mirror neurons, found in the inferior frontal gyrus, and also in the parietal area, show a similar pattern of response whether it is oneself or another having an experience or engaging in a behavior.)

The mechanism of connection between the two types of neurons has not been studied extensively, but it is tempting to speculate that mirror neurons and VENs are involved in social role-play and the ability to put oneself in the other's place. Thus we have the rudiments of a theory of the neural substrate of empathy, and perhaps even a moral conscience: "Do unto others as you would have them do unto you!" These insights stand fairly high on the scale of psychological development and may be involved in something as non-Darwinian, and gratuitously selfless, as *altruism*. There are stories of (VEN-possessing) dolphins engaging in extraordinary acts of saving humans drowning at sea, not infrequently human children, as if they understood their predicament—and their helplessness.

Defects in the AIC, as well as the aforementioned *alexithymia* and *anosognosia,* include *aphasia* (loss of basic kinds of linguistic abilities), *amusia* (cannot hold or repeat a simple tune), *ageusia* (loss of taste discrimination), anxiety, drug craving, eating disorder, conduct disorders, panic disorder, mood disorders, and schizophrenia (Craig 2009, 66).

"No other region of the brain," writes Bud Craig in an academic paper, "is activated in all of these tasks, and the only feature that is common to all of these tasks is that they engage the awareness of the subject. Thus, in my opinion, the accumulated evidence compels the hypothesis that the AIC engenders human awareness" (Craig 2009, 65).

Craig further goes on to define what he means by awareness: "Knowing that one exists (the feeling that 'I am')." He says, even more poignantly, "An organism must be able to experience its own existence as a sentient being before it can experience the existence and salience of anything else in the environment" (Craig 2009, 65).

Craig thus puts Socrates' *Gnothi seauton,* "Know thyself," before Jesus's "Do unto others as you would have them do unto you" in the moral sequence. (You have to have self-awareness before the actual reality of the *other* comes into salience.) Such high ethics are missing in frontotemporal dementia and sociopathy, where the person with a disturbed insula, or dorsolateral prefrontal cortex, has no ability to empathize with the other. Is the ability to be aware of oneself prior to being aware of, and able to value, "the neighbor"? When one is aware of oneself with all one's own emotional fragility and vulnerability (the fear of the criticism of others directed at oneself is in part localized in the AIC), can one then empathize with another self over there, not me but "very like me," who may be in trouble or suffering?

If the AIC *perceives,* the ACC (anterior cingulate cortex) *behaves* (agency). The ACC also has VENs, as does the dorsolateral prefrontal cortex (DL-PFC). Impairments of both these regions of interest (ROIs) can cause impairments of ability to inhibit behavior—impulsivity and potential violence being the consequences. Attachment problems (chapter 5) adversely affect these areas, as well as the orbital prefrontal cortex. It is probably through this kind of impairment that the future criminal sociopaths, demagogues, and dictators are hatched. (See also Miller 1971.)

Here also is obsessive-compulsive disorder, OCD (chapter 9). Amen and others, using SPECT scans, have shown anterior cingulate problems generally present in OCD. Anxiety (and my early toilet-training problems) tell me I am hopelessly "soiled" (AIC). I have an almost irresistible urge to wash my hands—and then I do! (ACC). I feel a little better for a short while, and then the thoughts recur (AIC), followed by the behavior (ACC), completing the vicious cycle of *obsessive* then *compulsive* disorder: disturbing intrusive thought followed by irresistible ritualized behavior. Also involved is a limbic organ called the *caudate nucleus,* one of the basal ganglia. ("Nucleus" means many neurons come together in a densely innervated area, like a little brain.) The caudate is part of the *striatum* and closely interconnected with the *putamen* and the *globus pallidus.* The caudate interconnects with dopamine neurons, and thus it is extremely activating. In OCD, the question then becomes, what turns the caudate off? Adjacent to the thalamus and the brainstem, including the *reticular activating system* (RAS), the caudate is definitely a kind of "gas pedal."

Talk therapy is usually ineffective in OCD; medication avails somewhat (Anafranil and SSRIs are customary), but as we have seen from Dr. Hammond's chapter, neurofeedback, skillfully applied, is quite efficacious. How could it do this? I am speculating here, but I think it may work first by breaking up established dysfunctional patterns (hypercoherences). Then the energy of the neurofeedback treatment enters and offers, at least, the possibility of redirection, another pathway, and maybe other thoughts and behaviors. Further, the caudate nucleus is known to be a center of *feedback* in the brain. *Feedback? What kind?*

The answer is "all kinds." We need feedback to know if things are too hot, too cold, too heavy, too light, what it feels like when I do this and when I do that. How does the consequence of what I do affect me? *Feedback is so intrinsic, not only to the human, but to all organisms, that it is a wonder that until now the principle hasn't been used or exploited at every level of biophysical self-regulation.*

It is also tempting to speculate here on how neurofeedback can sometimes (as Freud bragged about psychoanalysis) "speed up the process of maturation." This would include childhood and adult developmental models, such as, for example, Kohlberg's or Maslow's, in which higher stages of development transcend earlier, more concrete, autistic, or self-preoccupied stages in the interest of "universal ethical principles" or "self-actualization." In these later stages, one's own well-being is seen to be intimately connected to the welfare of others, and even the entire human race. Universal ethical principles may even go further in addressing the concerns of deep ecology or the welfare of all (interrelated) life forms.

Neurofeedback may grease wheels that are already there; the neural machinery (structure) is in place. There they are, lined up like good little soldiers: the insula, the cingulate gyrus, the dorsolateral prefrontal and orbital prefrontal cortices, the caudate nucleus, and the other basal ganglia. They just have to be tweaked, and maybe time-synchronized, to work. And when they work and coordinate together, ultimately, we are told, the self-aware and simultaneously socially-aware human being flowers: altruistic and socially contributive behaviors carry their own intrinsic rewards.

When people are preoccupied with dysfunctional and uncomfortable problems such as anxiety, OCD, or even primary narcissism, they cannot possibly function at their own built-in potential. They are conscious of their own problems (and the complexities attached) rather than other people, or humanity's endless need for socially contributive individuals. Again and again, I have seen people, as they conquer their (pathological) self-preoccupation and isolation, become nicer, kinder, and more creative humans. Freed from the habitual dysfunctional loops, energy becomes available, and using it constructively carries its own intrinsic rewards.

Human consciousness, possibly the most awesome mystery in the world, is vulnerable to its own (neurological) traps, and yet it can also participate in its own rescue. As Bud Craig puts it: "The key to the cortical (that is, mental) representation of the sentient self is the integration of salience across all relevant conditions at each moment. . . . In this view, the neural basis for awareness is the neural representation of the physiological condition of the body, and the homeostatic neural construct for a feeling from the body is the foundation for the encoding of all feelings" (Craig 2009, 66).

Here's another way of thinking of the motto from Juvenal, the Roman often cited in college classics courses: "Mens sana in corpore sano," "A sound mind in a healthy body." That is to say, that body, according to this sophisticated view, is *always involved in our perception*—and in the background of our awareness. The anterior insula helps us select from among many sources of input, interoceptive as well as exteroceptive, the salient one that deserves our attention at that moment. The choice will be clearer, and probably more sensible, if those (proprioceptive) images are relatively clear and stable, rather than riding on choppy waves of anxiety or the lugubrious groundswells of depression. In other words, working on oneself fairly frequently and systematically, especially through neurofeedback, breathing regulation, or meditation, is the best way to have a firm and reliable inner platform for responding to stimuli—or initiating action from within, based on balanced and considered criteria.

On Meditation and Self-Regulation

It is to be prayed that the mind be sound in a sound body.
Ask for a brave soul that lacks the fear of death,
which places the length of life last among nature's
*   blessings,*
which is able to bear whatever kind of sufferings,
does not know anger, lusts for nothing and believes
the hardships and savage labors of Hercules better than
the satisfactions, feasts, and feather bed of an Eastern
*   king.*
I will reveal what you are able to give yourself;
For certain, the one footpath of a tranquil life lies through
*   virtue.*

JUVENAL, *SATIRES*, BOOK IV, SATIRE X

In meditation, if it is successful, as Davidson's work has underlined, there is a quieting all over the cortex, but especially in the right parietal region (and by definition, the left too, since they are homologous). Sitting with half-lidded eyes in a Zen ashram day after day, interrupted by walking *kinhin* with a measured gait, has neurological consequences—as anybody who has given it a committed try has found out. Contrast such an immersion into existential quiet with, say, the state you might be in as a citizen in postwar Baghdad—waiting for some horrendous "other shoe" to drop in the form of an explosion, a mine going off, or a sniper cutting down pedestrians. In the latter condition, the sense of self and the sense of the world in reciprocity are laced with fearful, high-frequency (high-beta) brain waves. Nothing is safe, calm, reliable. I think we would say that if, under those circumstances, you could achieve brain waves that match those of a guy in an ashram—under these circumstances—you are pretty advanced and should start teaching others immediately.

The above is not at all impossible, as some adepts have proved, just very difficult. As the hundred-year-old penniless renunciate Joseph Campbell met in India, said: "Anxiety doesn't eat me. I eat anxiety!" (For lunch and dinner, we presume, since as a mendicant, he may not get any regular food at all, and he never knows where he's going to sleep.) Here the idea of spiritual practices takes on new significance. That is to say, the initiate, or the adept, cultivates the wisdom of molding his own environment through practices. (The Tantric yogi meditates in the burial ground while sitting upon an actual corpse.)

Will, which the aforementioned researchers usually localize in the frontal and prefrontal areas, is accompanied by redundancy; it's what allows you to read a book in a noisy restaurant. (While in graduate school at Columbia and living on the Lower East Side, I had an almost hour-long commute by noisy New York City subways. I remember getting some of my most intense studying done during those times. I'm sure a terrorist attack would have gotten my attention—I wasn't that lost to the world—but the ordinary subway noise and bustle simply strengthened the concentration.)

In the next section of this chapter, we see that there are many ways of conceiving of "the will."

Then there is "the mind that minds itself." How does this miracle arise, which we call self-awareness? Certainly there are rudiments of this ability in the animal mind, as horses and dogs can learn to critique their own performance and seem almost to strive to do better or please their master.

My colleague Lester Fehmi believes that it happens through "whole brain synchrony" and beyond—that is to say, a part of the brain, characterized by either different frequency or out of synchrony with the rest of the brain, stands aside and critiques the performance of the rest of the Faustian organ. That is to say, we can be self-critical as well as critical of others. In fact, people who are unable to criticize or stand-apart from their own behavior exhibit pathologies we call narcissistic, autistic, or sociopathic. And yet, as Fehmi shows, it is the whole synchronous entrainment of the disparate parts that constitutes healthy—and even self-transcendent—self-awareness.

In my consciousness course, I would help students differentiate between "self-consciousness"—generally not a good thing in its conventional meaning, because our sense of self is laced with anxiety, and self-criticism usually makes us stumble and falter—and "self-awareness." Self-awareness is preferable because if we eliminate anxiety and a self-punitive approach, we may learn something about ourselves. This is also called "metacognition," or, alternatively, "mindfulness." Biofeedback, as well as the spiritual disciplines, are bound by the rules of feedback. Feedback of the self without judgment seems to be an extremely powerful self-transformation tool. Why? Because the "witness," or the self-observing self, extends an exercised, "soft" awareness that is quite large and quite impartial—it watches long enough to learn something and refrains from leaping into judgment—which, after all, is just another mechanical form of behavior.

To use Fehmi's paradoxical term, it is an "open focus," a term that intrigues us because of its contradictory nature. Can we practice broadening our experience so that it includes everything and anything potentially present? Fehmi's work (Fehmi and Robbins 2007) suggests that it is so. The will may be exerted independent of any content; we can will to be empty and receptive as well as highly focused on a reading or math problem. Newburg and D'Aquili in *Why God Won't Go Away* point out the curious symmetry between hyperarousal that leads to quiescence—as in frenzied trance dance that leads to ecstatic contemplation, and the attaining of such intense quiescence that there is suddenly a surge of activation—as in the various forms of *samadhi* or *satori*. And Barry Sterman (1996 and 1999) has pointed out the synchronous alpha spindles that follow a complex and difficult act, such as landing a fighter plane (even in simulation). He has suggested that this may even be the brain's way of self-rewarding for a job well done—a little *mini-satori*, if you will.

Consciousness and the EEG

We have now looked at the structure and the locations of what we call consciousness, or awareness. The dynamics of the EEG provide an entirely different way of looking at what goes on in our unfolding miracle. We have talked about rhythms all the way along, and we have seen that consciousness follows frequency (and to a certain extent amplitude) in its dynamic. From delta (0.5–4 Hz) all the way to gamma (28–70 Hz), we find a certain logical congruence: slow waves equal slow thinking or sleep itself. Fast waves imply quick processing of data and lightning insights—or reflexes. We also have seen how patterns of frequency go together (coherence), talk to each other, or dance together (comodulation). We have also discussed brain synchrony versus asynchrony and the part that each plays.

It is quite clear that consciousness studies and neuroscience are trying to have a conversation. But none of the sophisticated modern imaging techniques, with the possible exception of the fMRI, have such an intimate and immediate relationship to each other as the EEG and consciousness. In the very early days of biofeedback and neurofeedback, people were measuring the EEGs of yogis and Zen masters to see if they were different from normal folk (mostly they *are* different—Kasamatsu and Hirai, 1963). In response to outside stimuli, some meditating yogis have very slow responses (P-300 waves), and some, as in Zen meditation, are very quick. In the 1960s the great neurofeedback pioneer Elmer Green was attaching

EEG electrodes to swamis as they sat on beds of nails. He and his wife, Alyce, and later daughter Pat Norris and her husband, Steve Fahrion, joined the team. This is also when Jim Hardt was left alone for three hours in Joe Kamiya's lab and emerged, he said, "a totally different being" (www .biocybernaut.com/about/discovery/part1.htm#nav1top).

Learning from Jay Gunkelman

A lot of people are teaching that classical orthodoxy at universities is "the gospel according to neuroscience." I am here to teach you the heresy.

JAY GUNKELMAN, QEEG

Whenever there is a neurofeedback conference, I look for my friend Jay Gunkelman, whom I have known for years. He does not have a lot of letters after his name, but top world professionals look to him for his expertise in the EEG. The founder of q-Metrx, he may have evaluated more quantitative EEGs than anyone in the world.

Twenty-some years ago, Jay was diagnosed with a rare tumor of the pituitary gland. When the surgeons went deep into his brain to see what they could do (I will spare the reader the details of how they get in there), the gland itself exploded, leaving Jay with no pituitary at all, and a lifetime of dependency upon steroid hormones. Always energetic and full of creativity, Jay used his condition, which allows him only about three hours of sleep a night, to become one of the world's foremost brain researchers.

Even as a neurofeedback professional, to hear Jay lecture is an extraordinary experience, because of the amount of material he presents—very solid conventional research and literature—along with truly radical ways of thinking about it. I was lucky enough to catch Jay just after his lecture at the AAPB national meeting in San Diego in 2010, for a couple of hours of intense discussion. Fortunately I had my recorder.

Stephen Larsen Interviews Jay Gunkleman, QEEG

STEPHEN: How does cutting-edge brain science help us unravel this perennial question of defining consciousness?

JAY: Consciousness is an exchange between two media, the glial environment, with its slow cortical potentials [SCP], which are DC [direct current], and the AC [alternating current] oscillatory *environment* of the brain waves, which arises from the familiar *action potentials* of the neurons. Consciousness is an *emergent property* of the two dimensions interacting—and with millisecond resolution.

STEPHEN: And what of the will? What directs intention?

JAY: *Intention is a DC phenomenon.* Intend something, and you can see the DC area light up with electronegative charge, then not intend, it turns electropositive, then intend again, electronegative. Every single one of those covert intentions shows up. *Attention* is simply the *intention* to perceive. I have data on this. When you intend to feel something in the hand, the hand area of the brain lights up with DC energy. The perceptual "set" to experience something is a DC phenomenon. Intention and attention: these covert states form the mind. This isn't restricted to the head. The acupuncture points are also DC-negative hot spots.

STEPHEN: Is this the same thing as *qi,* or *prana* in the Eastern systems? It doesn't matter whether it moves through channels in the brain or body? And these systems say our essential body is made up of energy.

JAY: I think it is. Intending seems to be covert, unless you look at DC field potentials. When you intend to see something in the left hemifield, the right side of the brain lights up.

The system exists within and around the early development of the human body; the radially symmetrical egg can be shown to have a charge, and in a sense we are built around our energy body, not the other way round. The embryo will grow into a blastula ball with a neural tube and finally make a little critter. The electromagnetic field has a front, back, bottom, top. The flesh fills it out.

Which came first, the chicken or the egg? I think the DC field potentials came before the brain. The mind existed as a developed entity before the brain. In acupuncture, for example, you can see if analgesia has been established in the hand before pricking it. With

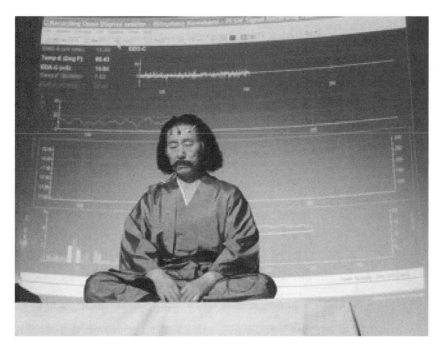

*Fig. 14.1. Mitsumasa Kawakami connects to the powerful
Thought Technology BioGraph Infiniti System.*

hypnosis you can nerve-block a pain signal. If it's electropositive, you're not feeling anything. The mind is controlling the brain's neural networks. The FDA has approved a device that utilizes the SCPs and gamma. The little machine tells the anesthesiologist whether the patient is too deep or too shallow. Doctors use this little device because it improves outcomes from surgery.

STEPHEN: I think we both were there at the AAPB annual meeting, in Las Vegas, in 2001 or '02, when that amazing Japanese yogi, Kawakami, did his feats while hooked up to biofeedback devices. Eric Peper was moderating.

JAY: I was indeed there. I've been with him, and measured him, a number of times. He was hooked up to everything: EMGs, temperature trainers, GSR [electrodermal]. I was asked to place the EEGs myself. The other measures didn't show much, as he inserted the skewers through his cheeks, his tongue, his neck.

But the EEG told the tale of how he did it. He shifts the somato-sensory strip in his brain to electropositive to turn it off. The AC EEG quits dancing along the strip. He's not there. He does the stick, finishes, and presto: it turns electronegative; up comes the AC EEG. Kawakami has done a very nice demonstration of the mind's ability to control the brain. The yogi intentionally modulates the sensory strip of his brain.

STEPHEN: Some people have called it dissociation or something like that.

JAY: I would call it something else. "Dissociation" has a pathological ring to it, and it's usually involuntary; whereas this guy is showing what could seem like superpowers to the rest of us, and he's completely conscious.

STEPHEN: I think of Jack Schwartz, who did similar things. He was captured during the war, and he knew the Nazis were probably going to kill him. I remember him saying that, "with nothing left to lose," he went into a definite altered state; he talked to them in a certain persuasive way, and they let him out.

JAY: Jack went on to found the Eleuthera Institute and teach lots of people how to use their minds to control their bodies. Kawakami did it through Kundalini Yoga.

STEPHEN: I heard you say something in your lecture about a "BS detector." I found it fascinating. Doesn't everybody have, or want, a BS detector?

JAY: I have a slide of a person who has been exposed to a semantic non-sequitur: "I can't get no satisfaction" [the one that makes English teachers cringe]. You could call it a "semantic–non sequitur detector," or, if you prefer, "a BS detector." At 100 ms (milliseconds), it hits my sensory cortex; at 200 ms, it hits the front of my head; at about 300 ms, I can differentiate that sensory input from what it expected. It takes another full cycle to be consciously aware of what you just saw. At about 400 ms, the frontal area locks in to see what the BS is, about 50 ms before you encode this information in memory.

The perceptual areas are locked out. "Don't give me any more BS until I figure out what this other stuff is!" The areas at front of the head lock together, and the areas at the back are locked out. This is, in fact, "binding." . . . It is instantaneous, can't be the thalamus, because the alpha is diffuse. What you see here is that when alpha is time-synchronized, when it hits the front of the head, it is out of phase with the back of the head, because of the different transit time; it's a different circuit. (We are talking here about the neurology of how the brain detects incongruities or something out of place, whether "BS" or "non sequitur"—this is neurologically measurable; this is why so many neuroscientists think something like an EEG-based "lie detector" is a possibility.)

When you hear people say that there is "phase locking," I say, "Is that a theory too good to be true?" In reality the diffuse projections from the thalamus don't have phase lock. You can see this in real EEG data. Phase lock gamma comes in 45 ms after a cognitive task. Gamma is a resonance within the neural network. It's produced everywhere, *it is an emergent property of a bound network being bound.* Being bound, the network will "ring" with gamma. [Note: There are technical discussions about something called the "binding rhythm" that ties all separate neurological events in the brain together. Rodolfo Llinas has proposed gamma—40Hz and above—as a candidate, but Gunkelman here says even gamma is too slow; only a DC "field potential" moving at the speed of light is fast enough. —Editor]

STEPHEN: Rodolfo Llinas and his colleagues at NYU speculate that gamma (40 Hz and higher) is the "binding rhythm" of consciousness, because it is found all over the brain. Do you agree?

JAY: I do not. A lot of people are teaching that classical orthodoxy at universities is "the gospel according to neuroscience." I am here to teach you the heresy.

E. Roy John showed that in 2005. DC fields can synchronize neural networks, they can initiate rhythmicity within a millisecond. Can it be in different locations at the same time? Hell, yeah, it's a field distribution. It travels at the speed of light. We're looking at something that can bind fields in a millisecond, the DC cortical

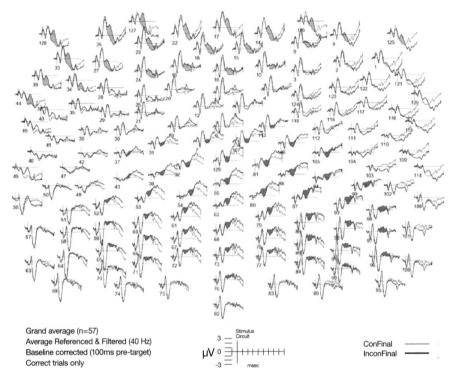

Grand average (n=57)
Average Referenced & Filtered (40 Hz)
Baseline corrected (100ms pre-target)
Correct trials only

Stimulus
Circuit

μV

ConFinal
InconFinal

msec

Fig. 14.2. D. Tucker 1994: An "Unexpected Semantic Difference"
elicits changes with a 400 ms latency

potentials. This system, the slow cortical potentials, runs the brain; *the mind controls the brain!*

A lot of people are speculating about this topic in the field. What are the mechanisms? Are distant parts of the brain tied together by the thalamus? If so, they would have to get the messages at exactly the same time, but they don't. The EEG says that doesn't happen. Gamma can't be the binding rhythm; it occurs 45 milliseconds after a relevant stimulus. That's a little late if it's going to be a binding agent; if it's going to bind, it has to be immediate, not a propagated rhythm. I know this was the big theory during the 1990s; there were "position papers" on it. But the gamma is just fast AC. Even gamma doesn't have the speed to explain some of the phenomena in the brain that emerge from DC field potentials, which are instantaneous (the speed of light, not of neurons).

STEPHEN: I know you presented some stuff on ADD. That it's not so much the area of the brain that's involved in separating ADD from normals but the way the brain runs more globally or systemically.

JAY: ADD guys aren't using a different *area* of the brain; they use the same areas, only the effect is weaker depending on how impaired they are. They're just not very good at attention. Edelman says, "Consciousness is the remembered present." It takes two events to create an experience. The first is the perceived reality; then there is accessing the memory trace for comparison. It takes two ERP [event-related potential] cycles for consciousness about an event to occur. The DC field resonance and phase locking of EEG rhythms yields consciousness when they're *nested*.

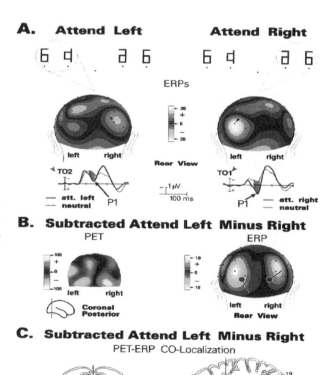

Fig. 14.3.
Shifting attention
volitionally shifts
the ERP's cortical
distribution

You remember my image of nested rhythms. The limbic system generates theta [4–8 Hz, crucial for certain hippocampal memory functions], but there are little 100 Hz nests within a theta waveform. [*How many gamma wavelets can nest within a theta wave?*]

STEPHEN: Did you say that has something to do with our short-term or sensory memory?

JAY: That's our digit span: typically 7 units nest within there [the vaunted magic #7 + or -2]. (This was explored by Bell Labs cognitive psychologists over fifty years ago, that's why we have 7- digit phone numbers—it's about all that the average human can hold in working memory at once—unless you group the individual units in a familiar area code or an "acronym.") This nesting ends up being an important thing. The entire EEG is a "base nest." Remember when it's DC-negative it's on, DC-positive, it's off. DC nests any brain wave. But in memory you have the idea of DC nesting theta and theta nesting gamma; they're all nesting!

I'm going to show you a slide I presented on the high- and low-functioning ADD compared to normals. It's called "nesting" in clinical practice.

In the normal, here is where a stimulus happened. And one second after that, six packets of gamma nested in theta. They're big and strong. In the high-functioning ADD they're still there, but weak. In the low-functioning ADD there are some nests missing. Aware, healthy, or you could say, conscious, functioning requires nested gamma. When it starts to uncouple, it says the person is not really awake. Can't keep a vigilant focus. Gamma drops out. [Gamma training for ADD?] Gamma not being around puts them in stage one sleep. They're "zoned out."

STEPHEN: Would that be like driving down the freeway and zoning out, so you forget the last ten minutes? You can be miles further than you last remember?

JAY: It's the same thing. ADD kids look like people in stage one sleep. They're not really controlling conscious awareness. Consciousness is

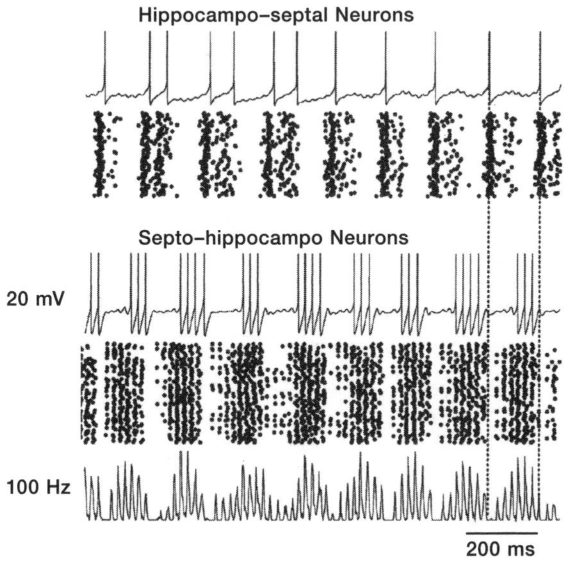

Hippocampo–septal Neurons

Fig. 14.4. The resonant DC fields and phase-locked EEG rhythms yield consciousness from within their "nested rhythms"

20 mv

Septo–hippocampo Neurons

100 Hz

200 ms

a cross-spectral interaction between DC fields and the EEG rhythms. You have to find out which of the many types of ADD or ADHD people have, then you can implement a careful program of neurotherapy to help them rectify it.

STEPHEN: The part in your lecture that really fascinated me had to do with healing. I'm interested in the kinds of resonance that go on between healers and healees.

JAY: You could ruin your career going into some of this stuff. Grad students are made to shy away from these topics. To really investigate the healing process with the EEG, you have to have the healer and the healee each hooked to a computer. Then how do you lock the computers together within a millisecond of synchrony? Well, you can reset the clocks so they are identical, and so that you can superimpose the two EEG recordings on top of each other. Phase synchrony would look like an amplification of the EEG. It is something that tests the resonant properties of a system. Let's talk about this model.

Suppose the healer and healee are like tunable bells, could go up and down in frequency. If we're in an environment with a resonant frequency, if things are in resonance, they sound louder, but they're not. It would be putting out the same amount of volume, but the resonance would sound louder when you hit the resonant frequency. The bell next to me is going to start to ring at that frequency, and in phase, because of the *standing potentials*. If you could see this phenomenon happening in a room full of water, you would see standing potentials, as if the wave were standing still. If you were swimming in it, you would sink into a trough, because gravity will pull you to the point of least resistance The second bell is going to ring, but weaker, then stronger when it gets into phase; as soon as the phase synchronizes, it looks like it's amplified.

STEPHEN: Would the Schumann resonances* be such a standing wave?

JAY: Exactly. This gets into really weird stuff. Imagine you're traveling at the speed of light, with all the other little electrons. How many times do you go around Earth in a second? Answer: 7.83 cycles per second. This is what happens when lightning hits; it rings the Schumann resonance of Earth. The small fluctuations in this resonance, say 7.81–7.85, are tracked by the U.S. Geological Services. They predict important things like earthquakes. The ionosphere is a resonant plane, and the ground is another conductive plate. In between is the atmosphere, a nonconductive resonant chamber. Then we think of the harmonics. Double the first resonance and then double that. When you get out to the fifth or sixth harmonic, then you have gamma. Starts slow, but gets faster.

STEPHEN: It is such a fascinating thing that Earth resonates in Hertz, or cycles per second; and that is also how the human brain resonates. We know that early astronauts got really disoriented; their circadian cycles went off, until they introduced an artificial Schumann resonance into the spacecraft or satellites. Then their daily cycles regulated themselves.

---

*Schumann resonances are the basic electromagnetic rhythms of Earth; they range from 7.81–7.85 cycles per second and average out at 7.83.

JAY: So I'm coming back to the healers. We were flown into Arizona by a gentleman named Luke Hendrickson, who was interested in gathering scientific data on healing. One of the healers was a Dr. Bankson [who had been studied at the Princeton Engineering Anomalies Lab, known as the PEAR Lab, because he was able to heal skin cancer in mice in a controlled study]. Leslie and Rebecca Sherlin did the pasting on of electrodes [for qEEG], and *Mitsar* [the Russian qEEG company] provided the instruments. [Leslie Sherlin was a past president of the ISNR and participant in many EEG research projects.]

But after all the expenses were paid, there wasn't enough money left to pay for analyzing the data. So I told Luke Hendrickson to go ahead and do it himself. He said, "But I don't know anything about the EEG!"

I said, "Just look over the raw data till you find something." What he found was resonance between the healer and healee all at around 7.81 and its harmonics. You see the phase of the healer going down, then a second later, two little chirps, and they're in phase, then it amplifies.

Now this is scientifically interesting stuff, along the lines of a double-blind study. Get someone who knows little or nothing of the EEG to just notice outstanding features in the two EEGs, and he comes up with a resonance that compares with the Schumann resonance. That blows my mind, and should blow a few others!

STEPHEN: My colleague, Juan Acosta-Urquidi, has been recording qEEGs on shamans and healers for several years. I think he has lots of data. He sees alpha suddenly increase, and perhaps that is the moment of resonance. He has done about twenty-five or thirty individual case studies; and there are commonalities.

JAY: I've seen it and find it very impressive. I've been speaking to the neurofeedback community about Juan's work and think this is tremendously important. I said: "The hard scientist in you needs to be related to this subtle energy world. If it's there, I think it can be measured. And when we're looking at these relationships, it can be really fun data. If you think the subtle energies are so subtle that they can't be measured, well, I think you're wrong. If its real you can study it and publish about it!"

STEPHEN: I think I'll do that! To get back to your main point, we who are psychotherapists as well as clinical biofeedback providers know this instinctively. When you have a good resonance, a good relationship, with your patient, he or she is likely get better. Jerome Frank proved this in his Hopkins study, which studied the different psychotherapy systems for efficacy. Frank found it was not the theory, whether psychoanalysis, Ericksonian, Jungian, or Rogerian therapy that mattered, no matter how dearly attached the therapist to his or her system, but the resonance and empathy between the client and the therapist.

JAY: I want the EEG division of AAPB and the ISNR to talk to ISSSEEM [the International Society for the Study of Subtle Energies and Energy Medicine, which originally came out of the work of Elmer and Alyce Green at the Menninger Foundation], because we have a common substrate in energy and neurobiology. Our tools are their tools. I say to neurofeedback researchers: "Our tools are getting so sophisticated now. We need to talk to the energy specialists, the ones who study shamans and healers. You could do a better job together. Your tools— even concepts—might do things theirs can't, and vice versa." I am a spokesman for integration, or reintegration.

STEPHEN: I love that about you, Jay. Your heart always outdistances even your—rather formidable—head. I thank you so much for this interview.

Neurofeedback Terms and Concepts Presented
in the Gunkelman Interview

Binding rhythm: Several facts have fueled the search for a "binding rhythm" in the EEG, among them the extremely quick, almost instantaneous nature of thought; how frequencies and amplitudes "sweep" through the brain; the fact that the traditional frequency ranges from delta to beta sometimes seem to morph in and out of each other, so that a decrease in one range shows an increase in another. Perhaps most importantly, consciousness itself is not dependent upon any brain state but seems to persist through all of them, even sleep itself. Rodolfo Llinas, formerly of NYU, along with many others in the neuroscience community, have a daring but plausible hypothesis: that gamma, the highest EEG range to be graced with a name (some say 28–100 Hz, some 40 Hz and up), is the only wave fast enough to explain all the phenomena described, plus ERPs or event-related potentials, such as the P-300 wave (300 milliseconds).

Gunkelman here is marshaling evidence for another mechanism entirely, in a sense two dimensions of energy, one manifesting as the traditional EEG, an alternating current, changing from positive to negative with each sinusoidal wave. We know that the "hidden brain," as it is sometimes called, moves through a different, nonneuronal network, the microtubules of the glial cells, which outnumber the neurons 10:1 and previously were thought to be a mere "scaffolding" holding the neurons in place. But modern neuroscience accords them roles of a much higher order of complexity: nourishment, repair of neurons, moderating the neurotransmitter environment, dendritic growth, and last but not least neural plasticity, as brains grow new neurons (along with the help of BDNF, or brain-derived neurotrophic factor).

DC field potentials: According to James Oschman, the connective tissue of the entire body is permeated by electromagnetic field potentials. That is why we experience emotions almost instantaneously throughout the body. In athletics and the martial arts, this "second nervous system" is much faster and more accurate, and it has nothing to do with conscious thought; in fact, it works at its best in the absence of conscious or intentional thought.

According to Gunkelman (and Oschman's theory is comparable), the term *binding rhythm* might be misleading, as the energy moves in the connective tissue (including the glia) at literally the speed of light (far faster than even the fast myelinated neuron-bundles, conducting impulses at maybe 18'/second). The term *rhythm* added to *binding* might be misleading, Gunkelman says, as it is not faster frequencies that carry the familiar EEG frequencies but something more like a slow-moving *tsunami* of energy, similar to the qi of acupuncture or the prana of yoga, which Gunkelman also equates with will, attention, and intention.

Now you might be saying, "Why slow?" when he says the effect is almost instantaneous. The measured current indeed flows slowly between the poles. In neurofeedback its frequency is referred to as slow cortical potentials and infralow frequencies (see chapter 13), but the field potentials are what is quick.

The Schumann resonance: Many people get worked up just thinking about the Schumann resonance and try to get a lot of metaphysical mileage out of it. But perhaps a very brief history will show just how remarkable Gunkelman's observation—made by a "blinded" researcher—really is.

The existence of a "resonant frequency" of Earth itself was first proposed by Nikola Tesla after he made "artificial lightning" in Colorado Springs around the turn of the century. Tesla was a man ahead of his time in many ways. It was not until half a century later that Professor W. O. Schumann asked his students to find the frequency for what he postulated must be a standing wave, formed in the cavity between Earth's surface, a conductor, and the ionosphere, also a conductor. The two spherical layers were separated by a non-conducting medium, the atmosphere, which thus would be charged with electricity.

His students came pretty close: 10 Hz, they said. In 1954, Schumann and Konig came up with a more exact measurement: 7.83 plus or minus about 0.02 Hz. It is predicated on the number of lightning strikes happening worldwide—about 300 simultaneously, the summarized electromagnetic bursts measurable in Hz. Of course in human physiology, 10 Hz, mid-alpha, is "neutral" on the EEG gearshift, with delta and theta below and beta and gamma above.

By EEG convention, 7.83 would be just below the alpha range, in high theta, or close to that legendary "crossover" that alpha-theta neurofeedback therapists try to induce to help people recover traumatic memories more gently (theta opens the doorway to the unconscious, alpha soothes the recall, the theory goes). The correspondence between the geomagnetic frequency, in the ELF or extremely low frequency range, and the human brain rhythm was noted by a German physician, Dr. Ankermüller, to Schumann. Schumann assigned his star graduate assistant, Herbert Konig, to the task. Konig's finding is displayed in plate 17 of the color insert.

The same rhythm is found in many mammals, including a hippocampal rhythm in rats of 7.7. Further strengthening the relatedness of the frequencies is that studies conducted at the Max Planck Institute showed that people electromagnetically shielded from the Schumann resonance became chronologically disorganized, as did experimental subjects (cited by Wolfgang Ludwig) deprived of only part of the wave. The relationship was brought home when astronauts, sailing blissfully above the ionosphere and thus shielded from the resonance, became disorganized. Only when an electromagnetic pulse based on the Schumann was introduced into the satellite did the circadian (daily) rhythm reestablish itself.

Increased EEG Alpha Spectral Power During Energy Healing

Abstract ISSSEEM 2010

JUAN ACOSTA-URQUIDI, PH.D., QEEG-T

This study provides objective scientific data that energy healers can shift brain states when engaged in healing. A broad sample of practitioners from many traditions were voluntarily recruited for this study, including Reiki, Pranic, Johrei, faith healing, shamanic, Vedic, and Quantum Touch. A partial report has been previously communicated (Acosta-Urquidi 2010). Most qEEG data was recorded using *Mitsar* 201 amplifier (St.

Petersburg, Russia), nineteen-channel electrocap, referential linked ears, impedances ca. 5K Ohms; Lexicor NRS-24 was also employed in some early studies. Data from N=14 healers (6 male, 8 female) was analyzed using NeuroGuide software (www.appliedneuroscience.com). Peak absolute FFT spectral power values (uV2) were compared before (baseline resting eyes closed) and during healing state. Data was statistically analyzed (paired correlated samples t-test).

Healers were observed to shift brain states in several frequency bands: theta (4–8 Hz), delta/beta, and alpha (8–12 Hz). However, the most consistent and reproducible result, found in 96 percent of the healers studied, was a change in the alpha band. A robust increase in global alpha spectral power was measured. The peak alpha power values were compared for EC condition: mean 116.06 vs. HS condition: mean 208.85; t-2.82, P<0.014 (two-tailed). The mean percent increase in alpha power was 80 percent.

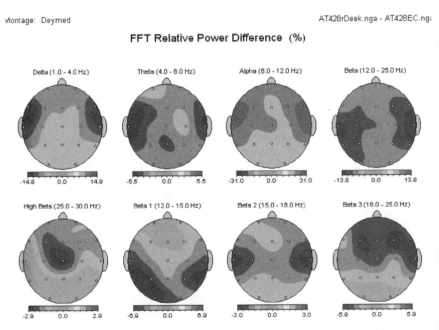

Fig. 14.5. Difference topographic brain maps showing that alpha relative power is selectively increased in a Deeksha healer. Copyright Juan Acosta-Urquidi, Ph.D., QEEG-T. (See plate 16 for a color version.)

Healers were recorded in two conditions: with the client in the room (some healers preferred light touching of client) and distant healing. In three cases, the clients receiving the healing were qEEG recorded, and all three produced a robust increase in alpha spectral power (average 170 percent increase). It is emphasized that these studies measured shifts in EEG brain states; no claims as to the efficacy of the healing were investigated.

The unexpected finding that different healing traditions all share a common increase in alpha power during HS may be explained by a recent

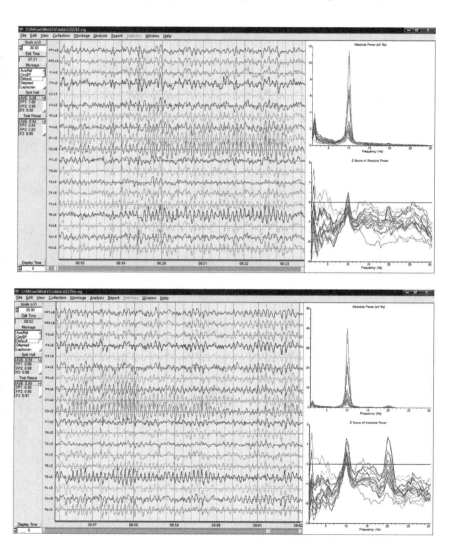

Fig. 14.6. Subject JJ receiving healing from spiritual healer KJ

qEEG study of a Buddhist meditator by the author. A robust increase in alpha power (143 percent increase) was revealed only during a powerful visualization task, suggesting the healers similarly focus on visualizing the specific target to receive the healing energy.

Recently, simultaneous qEEG recordings of both healer and client have reported a cross-spectra correlation at 8 Hz during HS condition, and it was suggested that Earth's Schumann resonance frequency may act as a connectivity mechanism underlying healing.

Brain Waves and Heart Waves: Psychophysiological Studies of Healers, Mystics, and Shamans

JUAN ACOSTA-URQUIDI, PH.D., QEEG-T

Objective: To explore the psychophysiology of the energetic transaction between healer and client using qEEG and HRV analysis.

Materials and methods: qEEG was performed using *Lexicor* NRS-24 and *Mitsar* 201 equipment with standard *Electrocap 19* channel 10–20 hookup, referential linked ears montage, bandwidth, 0–40 Hz (up to 60 Hz in some cases). Data analysis software used: Neurolex, NREP, WinEEG, and NeuroGuide. Statistical analysis consisted of correlated samples paired t-tests.

HRV analysis performed with the Heart Rhythm Scanner 1500 ECG unit, BioCom Technologies, Poulsbo, Washington. The qEEG protocol consisted of an initial 10 minute baseline resting eyes closed, recorded from healer, followed by a 15–20 minute healing session. In some cases, the client receiving the healing was recorded.

For HRV analysis, a 5–10 minute baseline was recorded from the client, followed by a 10–20 minute healing session, during which HRV was continuously monitored. A session consisted of the healer doing energy work directed at the client without any body or hand contact; healer-client separation ranged from 0.5 to 10 feet. In some cases, HRV analysis of the healers was also included in the session. Healers and clients voluntarily participated in this study. Healing modalities included: Vedic, Reiki, Pranic, Heart-spiritual, Falun-gong, shamanic.

Results of qEEG study: The most consistent finding was a robust increase in EEG alpha power (range: 50–150 percent) for the healer during the healing session. The client's alpha power was also significantly increased (50–100 percent, when monitored in some experiments). Power in the other EEG bands (delta, theta, and beta) was also shifted during healing, reflecting the diverse sample of healers' baseline profiles.

Changes in assymetry, phase, and coherence were also noted.

Results of HRV study: All healing sessions (N=12) produced significant shifts in baseline HRV values. Two types of responses were recorded, depending on the initial HRV signature and the emotional experience: increased SDNN* (average 48 percent, N=4) and decreased SDNN (29 percent, N=8). LF/HF ratios also changed: increased (average 155 percent, N=6); decreased (186 percent, N=6).

Of interest was the observation that power-frequency spectral peaks often shifted to the very low frequency VLF region (increased sympathetic drive) in healers and clients without a significant rise in mean heart rate.

Conclusions

This study demonstrates that robust EEG changes are associated with the "healing state." The increased alpha power is the common finding that holds true for the diverse healing traditions studied.

HRV analysis is a sensitive tool capable of detecting energetic transactions between two subjects, physically separated but in close proximity (0.5 to 10 feet). Further tests are underway to examine the mechanisms underlying this spiritual, physioemotional energetic interaction.

Summary: Dr. Acosta has presented evidence here that has never before been assembled, specifically, that there are resonances measurable, particularly power (amplitude squared) in the alpha frequency range (8–10Hz) between healers and healees. It does not seem to matter which "school" or tradition of healing the healers belong to—from Reiki to qigong to shamanic—the energy dynamics are similar. This is similar to Prof.

---

*SDNN is a straightforward and useful metric of HRV and represents the standard deviation of all normal RR intervals (those measured between consecutive sinus beats).

Jerome Frank's work in the 1960s and '70s that showed that irrespective of the specific belief system of the therapist, it was the resonant dynamics between therapist and client that determined the efficacy of the psychotherapy. This is landmark science!

Neurofeedback, Subtle Energy, and Mindfulness Disciplines

From the early days of biofeedback, there has been, it seems, a natural resonance between spiritual disciplines, psychophysiological control, and the scientific zeal to take these things out of the murky world (for some) of "mere mysticism" and into the world of science. Can yogis really stop their hearts and allow themselves to be buried alive for days in states of suspended animation? Can they sleep on beds of nails, pierce their skins with skewers (or resist piercing, as in the qigong Iron Shirt technique)? Can they walk on fire? Can they defy gravity and levitate, or fly?

There is a whole population of scientists these days poised between belief and disbelief (where any good scientist must be poised, "Let's see, now . . ."). Many of these scientists, over the years, have been my mentors and friends.

One of my most amusing memories of this interface was a science documentary from the 1970s involving *gtum-mo*, the Tibetan practice of "psychic heat," that I used in my Psychology of Consciousness course. Harvard's Herbert Benson and a team of investigators set out to explore the scientific parameters of the yogis who sat outside naked on subfreezing nights and dried wet sheets with the heat of their bodies.

Benson was always a conservative, meticulous researcher who allowed himself at times to be pulled further and further into the Twilight Zone of the very unusual. But he was always careful to record everything. He was on a field research trip to the Himalayas and had just fitted out a gtum-mo yogi with all manner of sensors and electrodes.

The yogi did everything he was supposed to, sat outside naked on a subfreezing night beneath the blazing Himalayan stars. The wet sheets were put on him, and he did his practice. (Yogis have described an inner visualization, repeated each day for many months, of a tiny spark of fire in the belly that, with breath control, waxes into a glowing ball in the belly, an inner furnace. You have to be under rural circumstances in Tibet, in winter, to realize how useful a skill this might be.)

The yogi showed no apparent discomfort with the cold, but something else was bothering him. He didn't meet his own previous performance standards and seemed genuinely discomfited about something. Since he spoke only Tibetan, communication had to go through a translator, but with some awkward body language and hesitant translation, the yogi finally told what was wrong. It was the *rectal temperature probe* Benson's team had inserted before his meditation that had "ruffled his wa" and impaired his concentration. He was trying to be polite, and he was sure the scientists meant well, but, well, he had never done such a thing before—it was quite apparent that, for some reason, he found the event humiliating (www.drikung.org).

"Ah," I said to the lecture hall. "East meets West!"

After the laughter in the room subsided, we had a very interesting discussion about how culture-bound our systems of knowledge really are.

From the early days of biofeedback, Elmer Green was examining yogis and Zen masters. Biofeedback helped show that there were interesting differences between yogis' inwardly directed attention and the samurais' outwardly directed attention. In recent times, no one more than Richard Davidson at the University of Wisconsin has investigated the EEG of meditating Tibetan (Nyingmapa and Kagyupa) monks (Davidson et al. 2003).

Davidson said that the results unambiguously showed that meditation activated the trained minds of the monks in significantly different ways from those of the volunteers. Most important, the electrodes picked up much greater activation of fast-moving and unusually powerful gamma waves in the monks, and found that the movement of the waves through the brain was far better organized and coordinated than in the students. The meditation novices showed only a slight increase in gamma wave activity while meditating, but some of the monks produced gamma wave activity more powerful than any previously reported in a healthy person.

The monks who had spent the most years meditating had the

highest levels of gamma waves, he added. This "dose response"—where higher levels of a drug or activity have greater effect than lower levels— is what researchers look for to assess cause and effect.

In previous studies, mental activities such as focus, memory, learning, and consciousness were associated with the kind of enhanced neural coordination found in the monks. The intense gamma waves found in the monks have also been associated with knitting together disparate brain circuits, and so they are connected to higher mental activity and heightened awareness as well.

Davidson's research is consistent with his earlier work that pinpointed the left prefrontal cortex as a brain region associated with happiness and positive thoughts and emotions. Using functional magnetic resonance imagining (fMRI) on the meditating monks, Davidson found that their brain activity was especially high in this area.

Davidson concludes from the research that meditation not only changes the workings of the brain in the short term, but it also quite possibly produces permanent changes. That finding, he said, is based on the fact that the monks had considerably more gamma-wave activity than the control group even before they started meditating. A researcher at the University of Massachusetts, Jon Kabat-Zinn, came to a similar conclusion several years ago.

Resonance with Earth's magnetic field; resonance between healer and healee; tuning the discharges in the brain to lightning flashes in the atmosphere; permanent changes in the chemistry and dynamics of the brain through meditation; the use of the EEG to change consciousness and to heal the brain; mindfulness practices and the cultivation of universal human ethical principles: these are the modern equivalents of disciplines—and the insights gained from them—that have preoccupied thoughtful and adventuresome human minds for millennia. What we know now deepens and widens the knowledge of the past and its ancient wisdom traditions. Can the new technologies of the mind, led by neurofeedback, point the way to new stages of human evolution and technologies of consciousness not even yet dreamed of?

Twentieth-century psychology began with two different approaches to consciousness. Sigmund Freud said that consciousness was merely "the tip of the iceberg," only 10 percent above water, while 90 percent, *der Unbewisst,* the unconscious, floated invisibly—and ominously—below the surface. William James (James 1902/1997), the innovative American psychologist, said something a little different and a little more hopeful than Freud's pessimistic view of human nature in his famous paragraph from *The Varieties of Religious Experience*:

> Our ordinary waking consciousness, rational consciousness as we sometimes call it, is but one form of consciousness, whilst all about it, parted from it by the filmiest of screens, there lie potential forms of consciousness entirely different. We may go through life without suspecting their existence, but apply the requisite stimulus, and they are there in all their completeness, definite forms of mentality which probably have somewhere their field of application and adaptation. No account of the universe in its totality can be complete that leaves these other forms of consciousness quite disregarded.

And so it continues today. The world runs on waking, rational consciousness, while people slip into fantasies, daydreams, and night dreams, or can't wait to get home at the end of the day to imbibe or smoke some chemical "requisite stimulus," so that the world and ourselves become altered from the grinding routine of the workplace, the marketplace, or the political forum. Whether legal, illegal, or prescription (stimulants, tranquilizers, painkillers, or drugs for antianxiety, depression, or psychosis), people seem to need to see the all-too-familiar from another perspective and somehow break through the habitual conscious conditioning of the ordinary.

This book shows us that there are many more ways of exploring consciousness and its modifications than the chemical, pharmaceutical route. Neuerofeedback, energy medicine, and energy psychology give us access to the same alternative ways of experiencing without the hangover or the side-effects. Many people who have experienced the clarity of a neurofeedback session, whether the LENS, alpha-theta, SMR or beta training, Z-scores, ILF, or HEG training, say they would never swap that clarity for the chemical cloud that comes with alcohol, pot, or psychedelics. With the chemical, once ingested, you are in the thrall, the biochemical field of that substance, until it leaves the system—and that could be hours or even days.

James himself tried peyote (the mescaline-containing cactus) and nitrous oxide, and while enthralled by what he found, he felt there was something wrong or discontinuous about the transition between the chemically induced altered state and ordinary reality. Aldous Huxley was spellbound by the universe he saw on mescaline but disheartened by how down he felt when the psychedelic wore off. Having had personal experiences of LSD with Stanislav Grof himself, and *ayahuasca* in a variety of religious and shamanic ceremonies, including the jungles of the Amazon, I have come to feel similarly. While something unmistakably magical and visionary may be bestowed by the "medicine" (sometimes called an "entheogen," or a "glimpse of God"), I have to live my everyday life in some version of ordinary consciousness, and I like my altered states to be continuous rather than discontinuous with it.

Because of this, I tend to rely upon (and teach my clients, students, and trainees) techniques of yoga, breathing, and meditation, which can be immensely helpful aids to combating the boredom, anxiety, and depression that often plague ordinary consciousness in an alienated culture. But for me, neurofeedback has deepened and opened out still further everything offered by these traditional techniques: for example, exceptional clarity, optimal performance, the ability to dip into visionary or intuitive states and return quickly (because undrugged). And I love the ability to work on ordinary problems in nonordinary ways.

A few years ago I taught my old classic, the Psychology of Consciousness, to adult returning students for SUNY–New Paltz. The class was full, and the motivated students very appreciative of everything that I was able to bring to them. We discussed and practiced dreamwork, guided imagery, meditation, coherent breathing, and HeartMath. With or without the assistance of biofeedback equipment, we need to find graceful, intermediate ways between ordinary and altered consciousness. I entitled the course "Psychology as William James Would Have Taught It" if he had had the exquisite and sensitive little electronic robots (called "biofeedback machines") we now take for granted.

Just today, as I worked with clients suffering from depression, trauma, and TBI with just simple neurofeedback, breathing, and relaxation techniques, three different people said, "The world seems richer, brighter, more colorful." One said, "I feel so relaxed, I feel high, like I took something" (but they hadn't). It was very affirming and very bonding to realize that we were both standing and smiling in a miracle—the miracle of everyday life!

CHANGING THE WORLD, NEURON BY NEURON

A s I consider the range of topics covered in this book, I have a sensa-tion close to what is called in Yiddish *nachas*. It is loosely trans-lated as "pride of offspring."

Don't get me wrong: Books are not my only "babies"! My wife, Robin, and I have two healthy, capable adult children of whom we are enormously proud. They are off in the world, and my son, Merlin, has children of his own, so we are grandparents. (Recently at a biofeedback training seminar, someone referred to me as some kind of "grandpa"— since I started my first college biofeedback program in 1970, and I realize that is now forty-one years ago.) That was a different era, and so much has changed: the world, technology, and our understandings of the brain and body and how they function.

And yet, so much is the same: human suffering and neurosis. There is still more, not less, PTSD in the world, although when I first started practicing biofeedback, the Vietnam War had just finished leaving its hor-rific legacy on a generation. According to epidemiological studies, there is more autism, more ADD, more outright terrorism. The events of 9/11 are a mere decade behind us, and global warming seems to be releasing ever more violent weather: hurricanes, tornadoes, people struck by lightning in the fierce storms that accompany the climate change in which we now find ourselves. The returnees from the Gulf War, Iraq, and Afghanistan are among us, with their nightmares, their emotional disquiet, their addictions, and their failures in marriage and family. Every now and then someone "goes postal," showing how fragile our adaptation and security really is.

Then there are the little everyday vexations: robots that ring our phones, merciless bill collectors, technology that is almost, but not quite, there—and doesn't work right when we need it the most. According to many psychologists, there is an "information overload" that makes us feel like we are swimming in turgid sea of knowledge, some of which is useless, and a lot of which is scary. How do we lead meaningful lives in the midst of so much meaningless chaos? Someone recently sent me a nostalgic e-mail: "I long for the days when *people* robbed *banks*" (not the other way 'round). The financial stresses of rising fuel prices, dwindling resources, the very quest for clean air and water, leave most of the human species frazzled—if not desperate.

How could something as puny as the biofeedback/neurofeedback I practice every day do anything at all in the midst of such chaotic tribulation?

Thoughtful people have tried to analyze the problem in its broad outlines: Our "paradigm" is twisted or corrupted, our *weltanschauung,* our very way of conceiving of the world, is wrong somehow. We think our resources are inexhaustible, our country eclipses all others in spiritual and moral "righeousness," our religions, our economy are "better"! My old mentor Joseph Campbell would say we have introduced an error, an inflation, in our mythology. We have gotten to a place the Greeks called *hubris* and the depth psychologists call "inflation." One of my clients dreamed twice of a great, destructive *tsunami* in the week before the 2011 Japanese earthquake. When it actually happened, she said she felt relieved; the awful anticipation of something dreadful was over.

So back to my original question: What difference could something as puny as biofeedback or neurofeedback make in the midst of such massive problems?

First of all, it uses no resources to achieve its results. It pollutes no rivers, as we are finding the tons of tranquilizers and other pharmaceuticals have done. (Rejected by the bodies of the patients for whom they have been prescribed, they enter the ecology as a new kind of toxic waste.)

The amount of energy neurofeedback uses is minimal, along the lines of computers and cell phones, which are already manufactured and utilized for other purposes. Biofeedback, in fact, relies on the same technology that is driving us crazy with the robots that spy on us and ring our phones when we are trying to relax on weekends. Its sophistication is the same Silicon Valley technology that puts satellites in orbit or tracks terrorists. (The perverse biofeedback healers, though, think the technology can be adapted to their own purposes—love, not war, if you will.)

The "little robots" of biofeedback do not have their own agenda, and they unflinchingly speak the truth—about our high blood pressure, our over-revved brains and hearts, our insomnias, and our obsessions. Unlike the really high-end medical technologies, the MRI and PET and SPECT scans, though, they are not in the hands of the health-care elite. They are available to what I call "Mom and Pop" shops: the Othmers, Ochslabs, BrainMaster, the Fehmis—dear, heartful, concerned folks who have our best interests in mind, who truly want us to get better and are not concerned with making themselves billionaires. *The essential myth, the basic paradigm of biofeedback, is to empower people, to give them a role in their own healing, to put wellness back in their own hands.*

Every day clients sit in our offices and tell us how much it means to be listened to as deeply as we do, to know we respond to the nuances of their daily struggles and the vicissitudes of their journey, to get counsel in how to calm themselves in the midst of authoritarian or corporate rejection or heartless foreclosure. One intelligent woman client, fed up with impersonal institutional care, said: "You don't know how careful and caring you really are!" (It was a heartfelt and affirming moment.)

In a crazy society, people do crazy things—to themselves and to each other: they drink too much, take drugs, drive too fast, take chances—either an outright expression of the stress they labor under, or the arrogance of entitlement, usually a misplaced compensation for helplessness.

I love to head disaster off at the pass. For example, one young business owner confessed to me that, well, he was drinking a bit too much during his business lunches and in fact had started an affair with his "hot" gal Friday. He was getting home later and later; the kids were long in bed so he couldn't say goodnight, and—whoops—he had just been charged with driving while intoxicated.

This is the point at which the therapist, be he or she psychotherapist or neurotherapist, says: "You have some choices here. Lots of people make the same mistakes. (Read the newspapers if you think I'm putting you on.) It's only a matter of time; your excesses are coping mechanisms for the enormous stress you feel you are under. Take a look down the pike! You definitely need some tools for stress reduction. Which will they be? Does the stress of providing for your family mean you deprive them of your company and degrade the family's quality of life?"

In this man's case, neurofeedback, HRV training, and psychotherapy worked together to save a marriage and a family. But the cultural landscape is littered with sand traps. "Of course you are under stress; now how do you want to deal with it?" One route prescribes intoxication and the ultimate dismemberment of your family, yourself, or both! The other is less adrenalized but a lot more satisfying and ultimately deeper: the method of assuming control over your own life. Which will it be?

Cultural dismemberment incites personal dismemberment, and vice versa. Are we the victims of a pathological culture, or does our individual pathology produce a sick culture? (Or do we participate in a type of feedback loop?) Whichever it is, personal responsibility can play an influential role in our lives, both personal and social. Political process, the media, families, and individuals, all need honest feedback, feedback that does not lie. That is why I am a fan of NPR, C-Span, the BBC (for the most part), and faithful reporting wherever it is done, not of things as we wish they were—or certain factions would like us to believe they were—but of things *as they are*. Look all over the world, and where you see interventions and distortions in the feedback process, you will see pathology.

In these pages, you have learned that some people put personal responsibility and honesty above opportunism and pious profiteering. They set their own lives aside to help loved ones, or to contribute something to the greater good of our communities and our lives. Using tiny amounts of energy—but more importantly, knowledge and skill—new, humanistically oriented technology has declared itself. It is not unimportant, because its target is nothing less than "command central": the human brain. It is where all our hopes and dreams cluster, and where they are fulfilled, die a slow death of ennui, or explode in a fast death of risk-taking and anxiety.

When we suffer in large ways, it gets our attention, and in turn it is brought to the attention of caring—and hopefully skilled—professionals. The outcome is the vision of optimal performance for us all, whether we are scientists, athletes, students, artists, business people, or tradespeople. By helping those among us with the most glaring problems, we help ourselves with our multitude of small impairments. So neurofeedback can help people with big problems such as stroke, brain trauma, and PTSD; it can help children who have been grievously neglected (attachment disorder) or for some reason (still unknown) are autistic, or attention compromised. But it can also help those of us who labor under mild depression, fatigue—or good ol' laziness—or who have temporary setbacks like Lyme disease or economic woes.

Whenever a parent with a child at risk (seizures, autism, TBI, ADHD) comes in, I listen to him or her with empathy, and then I say, "And you? Is there anything we can do to make your job a little easier and give you a sense of relief?" I will often do a pro-bono treatment or two—which sometimes swings the balance—or suggest some other resources: an adaptogen like Rosavin for more energy; the daily practice of coherent breathing or qigong.

In this way, little by little, maybe even neuron by neuron, we change the world!

RESOURCES

Ameriden International

(808) 405-3336

http://Ameriden.com

One of the major distributors of Rosavin (*Rhodiola rosea*), a Russian-discovered adaptogen, which can help with a variety of fatigue syndromes, Lyme disease, depression, and other problems. Ameriden carries other excellent products for allergy relief, energy for physical performance, and natural treatments for illnesses.

Art of Living, International

www.artofliving.org

A yoga society following the teachings and practices of H.H. Sri Sri Ravi Shankar. The practices are also called Sudarshan Kriya Yoga (SKY). Seminars are taught in many countries around the world and most major cities in the United States.

Association for Applied Psychophysiology and Biofeedback (AAPB)

(303) 422-8436

www.aapb.org

A membership body that represents professional practitioners (as does the AMA for medicine, and the APA for psychology or psychiatry). Coordinates regional membership groups such as the Northeastern Biofeedback Society, puts on annual and other conferences. Has lists of providers and contact information.

American Institute of Biofeedback Technologies (AIBT)

drmaryjo@sabosystems.com or www.therippleeffect.org.

A training and certifying body directed by Dr. Mary Jo Sabo at Biofeedback Consultants in Suffern, New York.

Biofeedback Certification International Alliance (formerly the Biofeedback Certification Institute of America)

(303) 420-2902

www.bcia.org

A professional nationwide certifying body for practitioners. Maintains lists of certified practitioners and manages "blueprint" for certification requirements.

HeartMath Institute

(800) 450-9111

www.heartmath.com

Offers training programs, education, literature, research, and licensure in HeartMath as a one-on-one provider.

Interactive Metronome

www.interactivemetronome.com

Interactive Metronome has its own program for training professionals in IM methods and also has machines used for therapy or training.

International Society for Neurofeedback and Research (ISNR)

(800) 847-4986

www.isnr.org

A professional body for practitioners of neurofeedback as a subspecialty of biofeedback. Puts on annual and other conferences, coordinates research, raises funds, and gives grants for research.

J & J Engineering

(360) 779-3853

J & Jengineering.com

Manufacturer of finely calibrated EEG processors and generic bio-feedback machines that can be used for the LENS. (For the LENS, however, these must be combined with OchsLabs proprietary software.) Best to buy from Dr. Len Ochs at ochslabs.com.

LENS Practitioner Listings

(707) 823-6266

(707) 823-6225 (fax)

www.ochslabs.com

OchsLabs maintains a list of practitioners currently working in the United States and in Australia, Germany, and Singapore. It is available on this website. The list is maintained by Dr. Len Ochs and includes practitioners' credentials and contact information. Also see Biofeedback Certification International Alliance (BCIA).

Life Extension Foundation

(800) 544-4440

www.lef.org

Provider of high-quality nutritional supplements.

OchsLabs

(707) 823-6225

ochslabs.com; cathywills@ochslabs.com

OchsLabs is where Dr. Len Ochs conducts his practice of the LENS. The center treats patients with traumatic or acquired brain injuries (including those in a coma), autism, chronic fatigue, mood problems from depression to bipolar (manic-depression I and II), post-traumatic stress disorders, and ADD and ADHD.

Open Focus Training

(609) 924-0782

www.princetonbiofeedback.com

Open Focus training is offered by Dr. Les Fehmi at the Princeton Biofeedback Center. Programs are available for professionals in both Dr. Fehmi's alpha-synchrony neurofeedback training and the accompanying attentional technique called Open Focus.

Stone Mountain Center, PC

(845) 658-8083

http://stonemountaincenter.com

Stone Mountain Center, in the Hudson River Valley of New York, is where Stephen Larsen conducts his practice of the LENS, HeartMath, psychotherapy, Interactive Metronome, and Open Focus. Contact the center to arrange for a screening or intake interview. Dr. Larsen also coordinates professional training programs around the country and biannually at Stone Mountain Center.

Glossary of Neurofeedback Terms and Acronyms

AAPB: The Association for Applied Psychophysiology and Biofeedback is a national organization representing biofeedback providers. See AAPB.org.

ABA (study): A research design in which subjects are exposed to condition A (the independent variable, for example), then B (nothing done, for example), then A (the independent variable) again, to observe the effect of the different conditions on the dependent variable—effect or result.

ACC: The anterior cingulate cortex is a central region corresponding to Fz on 10–20 maps, often indicating OCD problems according to psychiatrist Daniel Amen.

AchE: Acetylcholinesterase is an enzyme that digests (erases) the neurotransmitter acetylcholine.

ADD: Attention deficit disorder is a generic term that includes a variety of attentional problems.

ADHD: Attention deficit hyperactive disorder is a disorder in which there is restlessness and impulsive behavior in addition to distraction.

AIC: Anterior insular cortex is a frontal internal region associated with self and social perception.

ALS: Amyotrophic lateral sclerosis (also known as Lou Gehrig's disease) is a degenerative disease characterized by loss of muscle control and fatigue; it affects the nervous system.

ANS: The autonomic nervous system consists of two branches: the sympathetic and the parasympathetic. Found external to the CNS (inside the skull and spinal column) in chains of ganglia and plexi throughout the body, it regulates "automatically" involuntary functions.

APA: Two professional organizations share this acronym: the American Psychiatric Association, a division of the AMA, whose members usually have the M.D. degree as well as a psychiatric residency, and the APA, the American Psychological Association, whose members are professional psychologists, and usually have an M.A. or Ph.D. degree.

ATP: Adenosine triphosphate is the "fuel" of the mitochondria, related to energy throughout the whole body.

AVS: Audio-visual stimulation; it uses rhythmical sound and lights to entrain certain rhythms in the brain.

BCIA: The Biofeedback Certification International Alliance, a professional nationwide certifying body for practitioners (see resources).

BDNF: A brain-derived neurotrophic factor, a neurohormone that stimulates the growth of brain cells, improving brain function.

C2 I-330: A biofeedback instrument made by J & J Engineering, the C2 I-330 was first made available during the 1990s and has undergone several developmental changes since then. It can measure parameters such as EMG, GSR, and temperature, as well as EEG.

CAM: Complementary and alternative medical approaches, generally using natural or noninvasive methods.

CES: Cranioelectrical stimulation (a form of "microcurrent stimulation," as in the alpha-stim machine) is used when there is physical pain or a blockage. Can also help with anxiety and addictive problems when used cranially.

CHADD: Children with ADD is a parents' organization for ADD children generally supported by the manufacturers of stimulant medications, who are sometimes hostile to neurofeedback.

CNS: The central nervous system is the part of the nervous system enclosed by the skull and spinal cord.

CNSQ: The central nervous system questionnaire designed by Dr. Len Ochs to screen for a variety of central nervous system problems.

COSMODIC: A type of electrical stimulator in the SCENAR line, manufactured in Russia, used for RSD, neuropathies, and pain complexes.

CP: Cerebral palsy is a severe developmental disability usually occurring perinatally and characterized by one or more sensorimotor and cognitive handicaps.

CRPS: Chronic regional pain syndrome, also called reflex sympathetic dystrophy (RSD), is a chronic progressive disease characterized by severe pain, swelling, and changes in the skin.

CT or CAT: Computer-assisted tomography (or computed axial tomography) is a body and brain-scanning ionizing technology similar to X-rays.

CTE: Chronic traumatic encephalopathy, a possible alternative diagnosis for the wasting disease that afflicted baseball great Lou Gehrig (from multiple concussions—Gehrig was a "battering-ram" halfback at Columbia before he went into baseball).

DHA: Docosahexanoic acid is an Omega-3 fatty acid found in fish oils and known to cross the blood-brain barrier as an antioxidant.

DHEA: Dehydroepiandosterone is a vitality-enhancing corticoid made in the body by the adrenals, or taken supplementarily. Measurable improvements in DHEA are observed with HeartMath training.

DID: Dissociative identity disorder, formerly "multiple personality disorder," is a severe form of dissociation, a mental process, which produces a lack of connection in a person's thoughts, memories, feelings, actions, or sense of identity.

DL-PFC: The dorsolateral prefontal cortex, involved in emotional regulation, empathy, and higher order cognition.

DMN: Default mode network is a core system in the brain that is always active, even if no voluntary or reactive behavior is going on.

DSM IV-r: *The Diagnostic and Statistical Manual of Mental Disorders— Revised* is currently under revision, having passed through many prior versions. It is used by all mental health professionals to diagnose or label conditions. *DSM IV-r* diagnoses are also used to determine eligibility for third-party reimbursements.

DTI: Diffusion tensor imaging is a sophisticated, recent method of tracking pathways through the brain using water molecules.

ECT: Electroconvulsive therapy, also called "shock treatment," is a commonly used psychiatric (medical) treatment for depression, which must be administered by medical doctors or under medical supervision.

EDF: EEG disentrainment feedback is an early name for what is now called the LENS.

EDS: EEG-driven stimulation is another early name for the LENS.

EEF: EEG feedback is another early name for the LENS.

EEG: Electroencephalograph is the brain wave-reading machine invented and named by Hans Berger in 1924.

ELF: Extremely low frequencies in the electromagnetic spectrum (3–300 Hz).

EMDR: Eye movement desensitization and reprocessing was discovered by Francine Shapiro and is used for therapeutic amelioration of traumas and painful memories.

EMF: Electromagnetic fields are areas of energy that surround electrical devices. Power lines, electrical wiring, and appliances produce EMFs.

EMG: An electromyograph is a machine that measures and displays muscle tension. It is either administered medically (in a subcutaneous fashion using needles) or on the surface—a much less invasive technique used in biofeedback.

ERP: Event-related potential is a measurable brain wave reading subsequent to a known stimulus.

FFT: Fast Fourier transform is a mathematical method of analyzing raw brain waves into the familiar ranges of delta-gamma.

fMRI: The functional MRI is a generation beyond the traditional MRI, or magnetic resonance imaging device. The fMRI is able to catch dynamic processes in the brain or the body as they are unfolding.

FNS: The Flexyx Neurotherapy System is an early version of the LENS.

GABA: An amino acid that acts as a neurotransmitter in the central nervous system. It inhibits nerve transmission in the brain, calming nervous activity.

GSR: The skin galvanometer is a machine that shows a readout of changes in the skin's conduction of electrical stimuli. It is a way of measuring stress, a determinent in the classical "lie detector."

HANDLE (approach): The Holistic Approach to Neurodevelopmental

Disorders and Learning Efficiency, developed by Judith Bluestone.

HBOT: Hyperbaric oxygen therapy; known to help with traumatic brain injury and conditions caused by ischemia and brain anoxia.

HE (High Efficency): The usual LENS treatment is administered with the stimulation signal embedded on a "carrier wave" of 15–150 megahertz. To maximize delivery of the signal for more sensitive patients, and to go "deeper" in the physiology, Len Ochs developed HE treatments in which the signal is on a much narrower band of kilohertz. Unfortunately this has been only available on the software for the older generation of J & J machines and is not available on the newer Atlantis (Brainmaster) machines as of this publication.

HEG: Hemoencephalography is a measure of cortical blood flow to the pre-frontal cortex; it was pioneered by Dr. Hershel Toomim (nirHEG) and Dr. Jeffrey Carmen (pirHEG).

HPAA: The hypothalamic-pituitary-adrenal axis is a central regulation system involving brain and endocrine functioning.

HRV: Heart-rate variability is a measure of cardiac health reflecting moment-by-moment changes in the heart rate, generally indicating cardiac health and responsiveness in biofeedback protocols.

I-400: An earlier generation biofeedback instrument made by J & J.

ILF: Infra-low frequency training is a recent development in neurofeedback pioneered by Dr. Siegfried Othmer, his wife Susan, and Mark Smith.

ILT: Interactive light therapy is an early version of the LENS.

IM: Interactive metronome is a biofeedback device invented by musician James Cassily to help musicians with their tempo; it is now used for ADD and a variety of other CNS problems.

IRB: Institutional review board is a body that independently oversees clinical and research activities at many centers or facilities, to verify that the studies are conducted ethically and reliably.

ISNR: The International Society for Neurofeedback and Research is a professional body for neurofeedback. It conducts annual meetings (see www.ISNR.org).

ISSSEEM: The International Society for the Study of Subtle Energies and Energy Medicine is an outgrowth of the Council Grove conferences usually held annually near Denver, Colorado.

ITP: Ideopathic thrombocytopenic purpura is the condition of having an abnormally low blood platelet count, for no known reason.

LD: Learning disabled; the disability can be verbal or nonverbal in nature.

LED: Light-emitting diode; used in visual stimulation or in photoelectric applications such as "photonic stimulation."

LENS: Low energy neurofeedback system is the latest, and hopefully final, name for the neurofeedback system developed by Dr. Len Ochs (earlier versions were called ILF, EDF, EDS, FNS).

LORETA: Low-resolution EEG-based tomography, which uses a mathematical equation called "the inverse solution" to move from surface electroencephalography to reveal deeper brain problems.

LS: Least stim is a kind of LENS map that delivers the least possible RF stimulation.

LZN: Live Z-score neurofeedback using instantaneous comparisons of the subject's brain waves to a normative database.

MEG: Magnetoencephalography, which uses magnetic sensors, not electrodes, to measure EEG activity.

MMPI: The Minnesota Multiphasic Personality Inventory is a questionnaire-based psychological test or "inventory" with established reliability and validity.

MRI: Magnetic resonance imaging is a physiological imaging technology involving powerful magnets to reveal structural anomalies.

MS: Multiple sclerosis is a degenerative disease affecting the myelin sheath of the nervous system, causing severe impairments in motor control and many aspects of functioning.

MTBI: Mild traumatic brain injury is usually the result of a concussion or other injury that is not life-threatening or leading to major impairment. However, the suffering may still be quite significant, with symptoms of many kinds including disturbances of mood, cognition, sleep, or endocrine imbalance. The index (MTBI) was developed by Dr. Robert W. Thatcher to score the severity of mild TBI.

NIMH: National Institute of Mental Health is a branch of the U.S. government–run National Institutes of Health (NIH).

nirHEG: A type of near-infrared hemoencephalography developed by Hershel Toomim.

NLP: Neuro-Linguistic Programming is a hypnotic and therapeutic system developed by Grinder and Bandler from the work of hypnotist Dr. Milton Erickson.

NxLink: A database of EEG recordings originally developed at NYU.

OCD: Obsessive-compulsive disorder is a disorder characterized by an obsession with primarily repetitive thoughts and/or a compulsive urge to enact rituals or other behaviors.

ORF: Optimal reward frequency is a metric developed by the Othmers and also used by Mark Smith, to determine the best treatment levels in ILF or NFB.

PANDAS: Pediatric autoimmune neuropsychiatric disorders are often mistaken for other diagnostic categories such as ADD or OCD. (See also Pediatrics and Developmental Neuropsychiatry Branch, Intramural Research Program, National Institute of Mental Health, Bethesda, Maryland 20892. swedos@mail.nih.gov.)

PCS: Postconcussive syndrome occurs after a loss of consciousness and can be a symptom of a sports injury.

PDD: Pervasive developmental disorder is a disorder characterized by a failure to achieve normal sequences of developmental milestones.

PET: Positron-emission tomography; a neuroimaging technique

pirHEG: Passive infrared hemoencephalography, developed by Dr. Jeffrey Carmen.

PNS: Peripheral nervous system, nerves outside the bony enclosure of the skull and spinal cord (CNS).

PTSD: Post-traumatic stress disorder is a disorder resulting from the psychoneurological aftereffects of severe, tragic, or violent experiences.

qEEG: Quantitative EEG.

QRIBb: A test for Lyme disease.

RAD: Reactive attachment disorder.

RAS: The reticular activating system is a deeper, older part of the brain involving sleep, waking, and activation cycles.

RF: A part of the electromagnetic spectrum from 3 kilohertz to 300 gegahertz, used for many communicational devices from radios to televisions, usually propogated by an antenna and received by a "receiver." Also used in very weak form for the "carrier waves" for the LENS type of neurofeedback.

RFI: Radio-frequency interference filters; used on some LENS processors to diminish radio-frequency emissions.

ROI: Region of interest is an area of intense or clustered brain wave activity, internal or external to the "hubs" discovered through diffusion tensor imaging.

RSD: Reflex sympathetic dystrophy, also called "complex regional pain syndrome."

RTB, RTS Protocols: Rocking the Brain, and Rocking the Spectrum are "advanced" protocols developed by Dr. Nick Dogris for the LENS software. They usually use a succession of increased "stim" feedbacks at different "offsets" (RTB) or at different frequency ranges (RTS). Renamed as "ramping protocols" after being acquired by Ochslabs.

rTMS: Repetitive transcranial magnetic stimulation is a form of bio-electromagnetic medicine developed by Dr. Alvaro Pascual-Leone, which uses repeated magnetic stimulation to the brain to alleviate depression—often done at major medical centers.

RVS: The reactivity-vitality-suppression questionnaire was developed by Dr. Len Ochs to assess neurological sensitivity.

s-LORETA: Standardized low-resolution EEG tomography that, like LORETA, uses the "inverse solution" to generate activity in deeper brain structures from surface electroencephalography (EEG). S-LORETA is said to be capable of accurate, zero-error localization.

SAD: The standard American diet usually referred to (disparagingly) as the diet available in American convenience stores and fast-food restaurants, with empty calories, dyes, preservatives, and poor nutrition.

SCENAR: A Russian energy healing device that is used in healing pain syndromes.

SCP: Slow cortical potentials are at the bottom end of the AC spectrum (too low in frequency to be measured by most AC processors) and regarded as DC or direct current fluctuations.

SD: Standard deviation is a statistical measure of variability from the norm. In LENS it is used to indicate energy in a site by a blue bar on top of the black bar in a histogram.

SDNN: A measure of heart-rate variablility calculated over longer periods.

sEMG: Surface electromyography is the use of electromyographs from the surface of muscles, a noninvasive method employing skin electrodes, compared to needle electromyographs, which people often find painfully invasive.

SMR: Sensorimotor rhythm is a range of brain waves just above "alpha," originally discovered by Dr. Barry Sterman in cats, to have an inhibitory effect on seizures.

SPECT: Single-photon emission tomography, a diagnostic technology, is a type of nuclear imaging test that measures how blood flows to tissues and organs (it is the diagnostic specialty of Dr. Daniel Amen). Reports vary on its diagnostic utility and efficacy from "wonderful" to "not very useful." An adverse opinion is found at www.quackwatch .com/06ResearchProjects/amen.html.

SQUID: Superconducting quantum interferometric device magnetometers, which monitor the electrical activity of the brain.

SSRI: Selective serotonin reuptake inhibitor is a drug, such as Prozac or Zoloft, that seeks to help depressed patients by preventing the "reuptake" of serotonin, an activating, "feel-good" neurotransmitter.

SSRS: The subjective symptom rating scale is a numerical scale developed by Dr. Stephen Larsen to monitor patient symptoms on a session-by-session basis.

TBI: Traumatic brain injury; can be structural (long axonal shearing) or functional (involving blockades of certain brain areas because of the brain's own neuroprotective mechanisms).

TCM: Traditional Chinese medicine is an ancient 3000+-year-old form of "energy medicine" based on the flow of "chi" or "qi" energy through the meridians of the body; these meridians correspond to specific organs or organ systems. TCM is the basis of such disciplines as qigong and acupuncture.

TENS: Transcutaneous electrical nerve stimulation is a form of bioelectrical stimulation used by physical therapists or chiropractors to relax muscles.

TMJ: Temporomandibular joint disorder is a disorder characterized by a tense jaw and/or teeth-grinding.

TMS: Transcranial magnetic stimulation is also called rTMS (repetitive transcranial magnetic stimulation). It is identified as a noninvasive energy medicine, a polarizing magnetic impulse that has been tested as a treatment tool for various neurological and psychiatric disorders including migraines, strokes, Parkinson's disease, dystonia, tinnitus, depression, and auditory hallucinations.

TOVA: Test of the variables of attention is a computer-administered test for attentional problems that registers errors of commission as well as omission (compulsivity verus inattention). The TOVA is regarded as fairly reliable and valid.

ULF: Ultra-low frequency range (usually electromagnetic), 300 Hz–3000Hz (or 3KHz).

VENS: Von Economo neurons are special, large neurons identified in some advanced primates and humans (but not "lower" animals); these neurons are involved in both self-perception and awareness of others.

VLF: Very low frequency range, 3 Khz–30KHz.

VNS: Vagal nerve stimulation is a form of bioelectromagnetic medicine in which an implant is attached to the vagus nerve (one of the ten cranial nerves) to control some of the side effects of Parkinson's disease and other problems.

Y-BOCS: Yale-Brown Obsessive Compulsive Scale measures, developed by Dr. Wayne Goodman, is a questionnaire-type instrument that measures obsessive-compulsive thinking. The scale is measured from 0 (no symptoms) to 40 (extreme symptoms).

Bibliography

Ackerman, D. L., and S. Greenland. "Multivariate meta-analysis of controlled drug studies for OCD." *Journal of Clinical Psychopharmacology* 22, no. 3 (2002): 309–17.

Acosta-Urquidi, J. "Increased EEG Alpha Spectral Power During Energy Healing." *International Society for the Study of Subtle Energies and Energy Medicine* (2010).

Aina, Y., M.D., and J. Susman, M.D. "Understanding Comorbidity With Depression and Anxiety Disorders." *Journal of the American Osteopathic Association* (2006): S9–S14.

Barlow, D. H., ed. *Clinical Handbook of Psychological Disorders: A Step-by-step Treatment Manual* [4th edition]. New York: The Guilford Press, 2008.

Baxter, L., et al. "Caudate Glucose Metabolic Rate Changes with Both Drug and Behavior Therapy for Obsessive-Compulsive Disorder." *Archives of General Psychiatry* 49 (1992): 681–88.

Berger, H. "Uber das Elektrenkephalogramm des Menschen Vierzehnte Mitteilung (On the Electroencephalogram of Man, Archives of Psychiatry and Neurology)." *Archiv fur Psychiatrie und Nervenkrankheiten* 108 (1938): 407–31.

Birbaumer et al. "Slow Potentials of the Cerebral Cortex and Behavior." *Physiological Reviews* 70 (1990): 1–41.

———. "Area-Specific Self-regulation of Slow Cortical Potentials on the Sagittal Midline and Its Effects on Behavior." *Electroencephalography and Clinical Neurophysiology* 84 (1992): 353–61.

Bowlby, J. *Attachment and Loss.* 2nd ed. New York: Basic Books Classics, 1982. (Original work published 1969.)

———. *Loss: Sadness and Depression.* New York: Basic Books Classics, 1982.

Bowlby, J., and S. A. Mitchell. *Separation: Anxiety and Anger.* New York: Basic Books Classics, 1976.

Brody, A. L., et al. "FDG-PET Predictors of Response to Behavioral Therapy and Pharmacotherapy in Obsessive Compulsive Disorder." *Psychiatry Research* 84 (1998): 1–6.

Brown, B. B. *New Mind, New Body.* New York: Harper & Row, 1974.

———. *Stress and the Art of Biofeedback.* New York: HarperCollins, 1977.

Brown, R. M., M.D., and P. L. Gerbarg, M.D. *The Rhodiola Revolution: Transform Your Health with the Herbal Breakthrough of the 21st Century.* New York: The Rodale Press, 2004.

Brown, R. M., M.D., P. L. Gerbarg, M.D., and P. R. Muskin, M.D. *How to Use Herbs, Nutrients, and Yoga in Mental Health Care.* New York: W. W. Norton & Company, Inc., 2009.

Brown, R. M., M. D., T. Bottiglieri, and C. Colman. *Stop Depression Now: SAM-e, the Amazing New Treatment.* New York: Berkley Books, 1999.

Bruner, J. S. *On Knowing: Essays for the Left Hand.* Cambridge: Belknap Press of Harvard University Press, 1962.

———. *Actual Minds, Possible Worlds.* Cambridge, Mass.: Harvard University Press, 1986.

Budzynski, T. "The New Frontier." *Megabrain: The Journal of Mind Technology* 2, no. 4: 1994.

Campbell, J. *The Flight of the Wild Gander: Explorations in the Mythological Dimension.* New York: The Viking Press, 1951.

———. *Myths to Live By.* New York: The Viking Press, 1972.

Campbell, J., and Bill Moyers. *The Power of Myth.* New York: Doubleday Anchor, 1988.

Carmichael, Mary. "Who Says Stress Is Bad For You?" *Newsweek,* Feb 13, 2009. www.thedailybeast.com/newsweek/2009/02/13 (accessed October 2011, search on title).

Childre, D. L., H. Martin, and with Donna Beech. *The HeartMath® Solution.* San Francisco: Harper/SanFrancisco, 1999.

Coban, R., and J. R. Evans. *Neurofeedback and Neuromeditation Techniques and Applications.* Atlanta, Ga.: Elsevier Press, 2010.

Coben et al. "Feedback of Slow Cortical Potentials: Basics, Application, and Evidence." Neurofeedback and Neuromodulation Techniques and Applications (2011): 214.

Cowan, J. "Alpha-Theta Brainwave Biofeedback: The Many Possible Theoretical Reasons for Its Success." *Megabrain Report* 2, no. 4 (1994): 29–35.

Craig, B. "How Do You Feel—Now? The Anterior Insula and Human Awareness." *Nature Reviews (Neuroscience)* (2009): 59, 66.

Crane, A., and R. Soutar. *Mind Fitness Training.* San Jose, Calif., and New York: Writers Club Press, 2000.

Davidson, R. J. "Cerebral Asymmetry, Emotion and Affective Style." In *Brain Asymmetry.* Cambridge, Mass.: Bradford Books, MIT Press, 1995.

Davidson, R., et al. "Alterations in Brain and Immune Function Produced by Mindfulness Meditation." *Psychosomatic Medicine* 65 (2003): 564–570.

Demos, J. N. *Getting Started with Neurofeedback.* New York: W. W. Norton & Company, 2005.

Dogris, Nicholas. "The LENS and Autism: A Case Study of JJ." *NeuroConnections* (July 2007).

Doidge, N. *The Brain That Changes Itself.* New York and London: Viking Penguin, 2007.

Dolan, R. "On the Neurology of Morals." *Nature Neuroscience* 2 (1999): 927–29.

Donaldson, C. C. S., G. E. Sella, and H. H. Mueller. "Fibromyalgia: A Retrospective Study of 252 Consecutive Referrals." *Canadian Journal of Clinical Medicine* 5, no. 6 (1998): 116–27.

———. "QEEG Patterns, Psychological Status and Pain Reports of Fibromyalgia Sufferers." *American Journal of Pain Management* 13, no. 2 (April 2003).

Dougherty, D. D., et al. "Prospective Long-term Follow-up of 44 Patients Who Received Cingulotomy for Treatment-refractory Obsessive-compulsive Disorder." *American Journal of Psychiatry* 159, no. 2 (2002): 269–75.

Erikson, E. H. *Childhood and Society.* New York: W. W. Norton, 1950.

———. *Identity: Youth and Crisis.* New York: W. W. Norton, 1968.

Esty, M. L., Ph.D. "Traumatic Brain Injury and Its Treatment with FNS." In *The Healing Power of Neurofeedback.* Rochester, Vt.: Healing Arts Press, 2006: 103–13.

Fehmi, L. G., Ph.D. "The Megabrain Interview." *Megabrain Report: The Journal of Mind Technology* 2, no. 4 (1994): 30–39.

Fehmi, L. G., Ph.D., and G. Fritz, Ed.D. "The Attentional Foundation of Health and Well-being." *Science* (Spring 1980).

Fehmi, L. G., Ph.D., and J. McKnight, Ph.D. "Attention and Neurofeedback Synchrony Training: Clinical Results and Their Significance." *Journal of Neurotherapy* 5, nos. 1/2 (2001): 45–61.

Fehmi, L., Ph.D, and J. Robbins. *The Open-Focus Brain: Harnessing the Power of Attention to Heal Mind and Body*. Boston and London: Trumpeter, an Imprint of Shambhala Publications, 2007.

Foa, E. B., G. S. Steketee, and B. J. Ozarow. "Behavior Therapy with Obsessive-Compulsives: From Theory to Treatment." In *Obsessive-Compulsive Disorder*, New York: Plenum, 1985: 49–149.

Foa, E. B., and M. E. Franklin. "Obsessive-compulsive Disorder." In *Clinical Handbook of Psychological Disorders: A Step by Step Manual*, 209–63. New York: Guilford, 2001.

Fontenelle, L. F., et al. "Low-resolution Electromagnetic Tomography and Treatment Response in Obsessive-compulsive Disorder." *International Journal for Neuropsychopharmacology* 9 (2006): 89–94.

Frank, J. D., and J. B. Frank. *Persuasion and Healing: A Comparative Study of Psychotherapy*. Baltimore, Md.: The Johns Hopkins University Press, 1991. (Original work published 1973.)

Freud, A. *Psychoanalysis: For Teachers and Parents*. Translated by B. Low. Boston: Beacon Press, 1960.

Gazzaniga, M. S. "The Split Brain in Man." *Scientific American* (1967): 24–29.

———. "The Split Brain Revisited." *Scientific American* (July 1998).

Gazzaniga, M. S., and R. W. Sperry. "Language After Section of the Cerebral Commissures." *Brain* 90, no. 1 (1967).

Gibbs, F., and J. Knott. "Growth of the Electrical Activity of the Cortex." *Electroencephalography and clinical neurophysiology* I (1949): 223–29.

Goodman, W. K., C. J. McDougle, and L. H. Price. "Pharmacotherapy of Obsessive Compulsive Disorder. *Journal of Clinical Psychiatry* 53, supplement (1992): 29–37.

Gould, E. "Stress, Deprivation, and Adult Neurogenesis." In *The Cognitive Neurosciences*. Boston: MIT Press, 2004.

———. "How Widespread Is Adult Neurogenesis in Mammals?" *Nature Reviews Neuroscience* 8: 481–88.

Gould, E., et al. "Hippocampal Neurogenesis in Adult Old World Primates." *Proceedings of the National Academy of Sciences* USA 96 (1999): 5263–7.

———. "Neurogenesis in Adulthood: A Possible Role in Learning." *Trends in Cognitive Science* 3 (1999): 186–92.

———. "Neurogenesis in the Neocortex of Adult Primates." *Science* 286 (1999): 548–52.

Green, E., A. Green, and D. Walters. "Voluntary Control of Internal States: Psychological and Physiological." *Journal of Transpersonal Psychology* 11 (1970): 1–26.

Green, E., and A. Green. "Biofeedback and States of Consciousness." In *Handbook of States of Consciousness*. New York: Van Nostrand Reinhold, 1986.

Greist, J. H. "Treatment of Obsessive Compulsive Disorder: Psychotherapies, Drugs, and Other Somatic Treatment." *Journal of Clinical Psychiatry* 51, no. 8 (1990).

Gross, C. G. *A Hole in the Head: More Tales in the History of Neuroscience.* Cambridge, Mass.: The MIT Press, 2009.

Grove, William M. "The Reliability of Psychiatric Diagnosis." In *Issues in Diagnostic Research*. Edited by C. G. Last and M. Hersen. New York: Plenum, 1987.

Gruzelier, J. "A Theory of Alpha/Theta Neurofeedback, Creative Performance Enhancement, Long Distance Functional Connectivity and Psychological Integration." *Cognitive Processing* 10, supplement 1: S101–9.

Gunkelman, J. "Depression: Neurofeedback and QEEG." *Futurehealth Proceedings* (Winter Brain Conference, Miami) (February 2001).

Gunkelman, J., et al. "EEG Phenotypes Predict Treatment Outcome to Stimulants in Children with ADHD." *Journal of Integrative Neuroscience* 7, no. 3 (2008): 421–38 [qeegsupport.com; novatech.com].

Gunkelman, J., et al. "The Healing Connection: EEG Harmonics, Entrainment, and Schumann's Resonances," *Journal of Statistics Education* 24, no. 6 (Winter 2010).

Hammond, D. C. "QEEG-guided Neurofeedback in the Treatment of Obsessive-compulsive Disorder. *Journal of Neurotherapy* 7, no. 2 (2003): 25–52.

———. "Treatment of the Obsessional Subtype of Obsessive Compulsive Disorder with Neurofeedback." *Biofeedback* 32 (2004): 9–12.

———. "Hypnosis, Placebos, and Systematic Research Bias in Biological Psychiatry." *American Journal of Clinical Hypnosis* 50, no. 1 (2007a): 37–47.

———. *LENS: The Low Energy Neurofeedback System.* New York: Haworth Press, 2007(b).

———. "QEEG Evaluation of the LENS Treatment of TBI." *Journal of Neurotheraphy* 14 (2010a): 70–77.

———. "The Need for Individualization in Neurofeedback: Heterogeneity in QEEG Patterns Associated with Diagnoses and Symptoms." *Applied Psychophysiology & Biofeedback* 35 no. 1 (2010b).

———. "Placebo and Neurofeedback: A Case for Facilitating and Maximizing

Placebo Response in Neurofeedback Treatments." *Journal of Neurotherapy* 15, no. 2 (2011): 94–114.

Hammond, D. C., and L. Kirk. "First, Do No Harm: Adverse Effects and the Need for Practice Standards in Neurofeedback." *Journal of Neurotherapy* 12, no. 1 (2008): 79–88.

Harlow, H. F. *Learning to Love.* New York: Aronson, 1974.

Harmony, T. "Neurometric Assessment of Brain Dysfunction in Neurological Patients." *Functional Neuroscience,* vol. 3 (1984).

Hollon, M. F. "Direct-to-consumer Advertising: A Haphazard Approach to Health Promotion." *Journal of the American Medical Association* 293, no. 16 (2005): 2030–33.

Holzapfel, et al. "Behavioral Psychophysiological Intervention in a Mentally Retarded Epileptic Patient with Brain Lesion." *Applied Psychophysiology and Biofeedback* 23, no. 3 (September 1998): 189–202.

http://cns-wellness.com/brain-based-intervention/photonic-stimulator/69-neurofield. Accessed Jan 2011.

http://dreamhawk.com/inner-life/animal-children. Accessed Dec 2010.

http://moregehrig.tripod.com/id29.html. Accessed Oct 2011.

http://sportsillustrated.cnn.com/vault/article/magazine/MGG11; search on Ann McKee. Accessed Oct 2011.

James, W. *The Principles of Psychology: The Famous Long Course Complete and Unabridged.* Cambridge, Mass.: Harvard University Press, 1983. (Original work published 1890.)

———. *Varieties of Religious Experience.* New York: Touchstone, 1997. (Original work published 1902.)

Janov, A., M.D. *Primal Scream.* New York: Doubleday, 1970.

Jenike, M. A., et al. "Cingulotomy for Refractory Obsessive-Compulsive Disorder: A Long-term Follow-up of 33 Patients." *Archives of General Psychiatry* 48 (1991): 548–55.

John, E. R. "Principles of Neurometrics." *American Journal of EEG Technology* 30 (1990): 251–66.

Kamiya, J. "Conscious Control of Brainwaves." *Psychology Today* 1 (1968): 57–60.

———. "Autoregulation of the EEG Alpha Rhythm: A Program for the Study of Consciousness." In *Mind Body Integration: Essential Readings in Biofeedback,* 289–98. New York: Plenum Press, 1979.

Kasamatsu, A., and T. Hirai. "Science of Zazen." *Psychologia* 6 (1963): 86–91.

Keune, P. M., et al., "Frontal Alpha-Asymmetry in Adults with Attention Deficit Hyperactivity Disorder: Replication and Specification." *Biological Psychology* 87, no. 2 (May 2011): 306–10.

Khan, A., S. Khan, and W. A. Brown, "Are Placebo Controls Necessary to Test New Antidepressants and Anxiolytics?" *International Journal of Neuropsychopharmacology* 5 (2002): 193–97.

King, P. "Concussions: The Hits That Are Changing Football." *Sports Illustrated.* SI Vault (2010).

Kirk, Stuart A., and Herb Kutchins. "The Myth of the Reliability of DSM." *Journal of Mind and Behavior* 15, nos. 1 and 2 (1994): 71–86; www .academyanalyticarts.org/kirk&kutchins.htm (accessed August 2011).

Kirsch, I. *The Emperor's New Drugs: Exploding the Antidepressant Myth.* New York: Basic Books, 2010.

Kirsch, I., et al. "Initial Severity and Antidepressant Benefits: A Meta-analysis of Data Submitted to the Food and Drug Administration." *PLOS Medicine* 5, no. 2 (2008): 260–68.

Klein, M. *The Psychoanalysis of Children (The Writings of Melanie Klein).* Edited by H. Thorner. Translated by A. Strachey. New York: The Free Press, 1984. (Original work published 1932.)

Kohut, H. "The Analysis of the Self: A Systematic Approach to the Psychoanalytic Treatment of Narcissistic Personality Disorders." *The Psychoanalytic Study of the Child,* no. 4. New York: International Universities Press, 1971.

Larsen, Stephen, Ph.D. *The Mythic Imagination: Your Quest for Meaning Through Personal Mythology.* New York: Bantam Books, 1990.

———. *The Healing Power of Neurofeedback: The Revolutionary LENS Technique for Restoring Optimal Brain Function.* Rochester, Vt.: Healing Arts Press, 2006.

———. *The Fundamentalist Mind: How Polarized Thinking Imperils Us All.* Evanston, Ill.: Quest Books, 2007.

———. "Turning on the Lights: How Neurofeedback Helped a Cultural Genius Do Soul Retrieval" (preliminary version, audio/visual presentations), National LENS Conference. Los Gatos, Calif.: 2009.

Larsen, Stephen, Ph.D., K. Harrington, and S. Hicks. "The LENS (Low Energy Neurofeedback System): A Clinical Outcomes Study on One Hundred Patients at Stone Mountain Center, New York." *Journal of Neurotherapy* 10, nos. 2/3 (2006): 69–78.

Larsen, Stephen, Ph.D., et al. "The LENS Neurofeedback with Animals." *Journal of Neurotherapy* 10, nos. 2/3 (2006): 89–104.

Larsen, Stephen, Ph.D., and V. Zelek. "Turning on the Lights: How Neuro-feedback Helped a Cultural Genius Do Soul Retrieval." (Audio/visual presentation) International Society for Research and Neurofeedback (ISNR) Annual Meeting. Denver, Colo.: 2010.

Lehrer, Jonah. "The Reinvention of the Self." *Brain and Behavior* (2008); *Seed Magazine* August 22, 2010.

Lehrer, P. M., R. L. Woolfolk, and W. E. Sime, eds. *Principles and Practice of Stress Management.* New York: The Guilford Press, 2007.

Lorenz, K. *Studies in Animal and Human Behavior,* vol. 1. Translated by R. Martin. Cambridge, Mass.: Harvard University Press, 1970.

———. *Studies in Animal and Human Behavior,* vol. 2. Translated by R. Martin. Cambridge, Mass.: Harvard University Press, 1971.

Lubar, J. F., et al. "Quantitative EEG and Auditory Event-related Potentials in the Evaluation of Attention Deficit/Hyperactivity Disorder: Effects of Methylphenidate and Implications for Neurofeedback Training. *Journal of Psychoeducational Assessment* (1995): 143–204.

Lubar, J. F., and J. O. Lubar. "Neurofeedback Assessment and Treatment for Attention Deficit/Hyperactivity Disorders (ADD/HD)." In *Introduction to Quantitative EEG and Neurotherapy* (1999): 103–43.

Maihofner, C., et al. "Effects of Repetitive Magnetic Stimulation in Depression: A Magnetoencephalographic Study." *NeuroReport* 16, no. 16 (2005): 1839–42.

Maihofner, C., et al. "Spontaneous Magnetoencephalographic Activity in Patients with Obsessive-Compulsive Disorder." *Brain Research* 1129 (2007): 200–205.

Maslow, A. H., ed. *New Knowledge in Human Values.* Foreword by P. A. Sorokin. Chicago: Henry Regnery, Gateway: 1959.

———. *Toward a Psychology of Being.* New York: D. Nostrand, Insight, 1968.

———. *Religions, Values, and Peak-experiences.* New York: Viking Press, 1970.

Mercer, J. *Understanding Attachment.* Westport, Conn.: Praeger Pubishing, 2006.

Miller, N. *Selected Papers on Learning, Motivation and Their Physiological Mechanisms.* Chicago: MW Books, Aldine, Atherton, 1971.

Monastra, V. J., et al. "Assessing Attention Deficit Hyperactivity Disorder via Quantitative Electroencephalography: An Initial Validation Study." *Neuropsychology* 13, no. 3 (1999): 424–33.

Monastra, V. J., J. F. Lubar, and M. K. Linden. "The Development of a QEEG-Scan for ADHD: Reliability and Validity Studies." *Neuropsychology* 2000.

Moncrieff, J. *The Myths of the Chemical Cure: A Critique of Psychiatric Drug Treatment.* New York: Palgrave Macmillan, 2009.

Morell, V., and V. J. Musi, "Minds of Their Own: Animals Are Smarter Than You Think" [Short film: *Birds and Bats*]. Interview with photographer Vincent Musi. *National Geographic,* March 2008.

Mueller, H. H., et al. "Treatment of Fibromyalgia Incorporating EEG-driven Stimulation: A Clinical Outcomes Study." *Journal of Clinical Psychology* 57, no. 7 (2001): 933–52.

Newburg, A., and E. d'Aquili. *Why God Won't Go Away.* New York: Ballantine Publishing, 2001.

Ochs, L. "EEG-driven Stimulation and Mild Head Injured Patients: Extended Observations." SSNR Meeting Paper (March 1994).

———. "The Low Energy Neurofeedback System (LENS): Theory, Background, and Introduction." *Journal of Neurotherapy* 10, nos. 2–3 (2006): 5–39.

Oschman, J. L. *Energy Medicine, The Scientific Basis.* Edinburgh: Churchill Livingstone, 2000.

———. *Energy Medicine in Therapeutics and Human Performance.* Philadelphia and New York: Butterworth and Heinemann (Elsevier Science), 2003.

Othmer, S., Ph.D. "EEG Biofeedback: An Approach to Personal Autonomy." *Megabrain Report: The Journal of Mind Technology* 2, no. 4 (1995): 22–29.

Othmer, S., and B. A. Othmer. "Post Traumatic Stress Disorder—The Neurofeedback Remedy." *Biofeedback Magazine* 37, no. 1 (2009): 24–31.

Othmer, S., and S. F. Othmer. "EEG Biofeedback for Attention Deficit Hyperactivity Disorder. *EEG Spectrum Publication* (1992).

———. "Introduction to Infra-Low Frequency Training." *NeuroConnections* 14 (Spring 2010).

Othmer, S., S. F. Othmer, and C. S. Marks. "EEG Biofeedback Training for ADD, Specific Learning Disabilities and Associated Conduct Problems." *Journal of the Biofeedback Society of California* (September 1992).

Othmer, S., S. F. Othmer, and D. A. Kaiser. "EEG Biofeedback Training for Attention Deficit Disorder: A Review of Recent Controlled Studies and Clinical Findings." *Journal of the BSC* (October 1995).

Othmer, Siegfried, S. F. Othmer, and Stella B. Legarda. "Clinical Neurofeedback: Training Brain Behavior." *Treatment Strategies, Pediatric Neurology and Psychiatry* (2010).

Othmer, Siegfried, S. F., et al. "Clinical Neurofeedback: Case Studies, Proposed Mechanism, and Implications for Pediatric Neurology Practice." *Journal Child Neurology* 26 (2011): 1045. (Original published online May 16, 2011.)

Pascual-Leone, A. "Transcranial Magnetic Stimulation and Neuroplasticity." *Neuropsychologia* 37 (1999): 307–17.

Pato, M., R. Zohar-Kadouch, and J. Zohar. "Return of Symptoms After Discontinuation of Clomipramine in Patients with Obsessive Compulsive Disorder." *American Journal of Psychiatry* 145 (1988): 1521–25.

Peniston, E. "EEG Alpha-theta Neurofeedback: Promising Clinical Approach for Future Psychotherapy and Medicine." *Megabrain Report: the Journal of Mind Technology* 2, no. 4 (1994): 40–43.

Peniston, E., and P. J. Kulkosky. "Alpha-theta Brainwave Training and Beta-endorphin Levels in Alcoholics." *Alcoholism: Clinical and Experimental Research* 13, no. 2 (March/April 1989): 125–33. Fort Lyon and Pueblo, Colo.: The Veterans Administration Medical Center, Fort Lyon and the Department of Psychology, University of Southern Colorado, Pueblo.

———. "Alpha-theta Brainwave Neuro-feedback for Vietnam Veterans with Combat-related Post-traumatic Stress Disorder." *Medical Psychotherapy: An International Journal* 4 (1991): 47–60.

Pigott, H. E., et al. "Efficacy and Effectiveness of Antidepressants: Current Status of Research." *Psychotherapy and Psychosomatics* 79, no. 5 (August 2010): 267–79.

Pribram, K. H. "The Neurophysiology of Remembering." *Scientific American* 220 (January 1969): 76–78.

———. *Brain and Perception: Holonomy and Structure in Figural Processing.* Stanford University and Radford University: Lawrence Erlbaum Associates, Publishers, 1991.

Prichep, L. S., et al. "Quantitative Electroencephalography (QEEG) Subtyping of Obsessive Compulsive Disorder." *Psychiatry Research* 50, no. 1 (1993): 25–32.

Ramachandran, V. S., M.D., and D. Rogers-Ramachandran, Ph.D. "Synaesthesia in Phantom Limbs Induced with Mirrors." *Proc. R. Soc. Lond.,* 263, no. 1369 (April 1996): 377–86.

———. "Phantom Limbs and Neural Plasticity." *Archives of Neurology* 57 (2000): 317–20.

Ramachandran, V., D. Rogers-Ramachandran, and S. Cobb. "Touching the Phantom Limb." *Nature* 377 (1995): 489–90.

Ramachandran, V. D., et al. "The Neural Basis of Religious Experience." *Abstract, Society of Neuroscience* 23 (1997).

Ramachandran, V., and W. Hirstein. "The Perception of Phantom Limbs. The D. O. Hebb Lecture." *Oxford Journals, Brain* 121, no. 9 (1998): 1603–30.

Ramón y Cajal, S. *Textura del sistema nerviosa del hombre y del los vertebrados*

("Histology of the nervous system of man and vertebrates"). N. Swanson and L. W. Swanson, translated from the French., D. L. Azoulay, translated from the original Spanish). *History of Neuroscience*, no. 6: 1995. (Original work published 1897–1899.)

Rauch, S. L. "Neuroimaging Research and the Neurobiology of Obsessive-Compulsive Disorder: Where Do We Go From Here?" *Biological Psychiatry* 47 (2000): 168–70.

Robbins, J. *A Symphony in the Brain: The Evolution of the New Brain Wave Biofeedback.* New York: Atlantic Monthly Press, 2000.

Ros, Thomas, et al. "Endogenous Control of Waking Brain Rhythms Induces Neuroplasticity in Humans." *European Journal of Neuroscience* 31 (2010): 770–78.

Sackett, D. L., M.D. et al. *Evidence-based Medicine: How to Practice and Teach EBM.* Edinburgh: Churchill Livingstone, 2000.

Sacks, O., M.D. *The Man Who Mistook His Wife for a Hat and Other Clinical Tales.* New York: Simon & Schuster, 1998.

———. *The Mind's Eye.* New York: Alfred A. Knopf, 2010.

Schacker, M., B. McKibben. *A Spring Without Bees: How Colony Collapse Disorder Has Endangered Our Food Supply.* Guilford, Conn.: The Lyons Press, 2008.

Schaffer, R. *Introducing Child Psychology.* Hoboken, N.J.: Blackwell Publishing, 2007.

Schoenberger, N. E., et al. "Flexyx Neurotherapy System in the Treatment of Traumatic Brain Injury: An Initial Evaluation." *Journal of Head Trauma Rehabilitation* 16, no. 3 (2001): 260–74.

Schoenberger, M., and J. Scott, eds. *The Little Black Book of Neuropsychology.* New York: Springer, 2011.

Schore, A. N. "Early Organization of the Nonlinear Right Brain and Development of a Predisposition to Psychiatric Disorders." *Development and Psychopathology* 9 (1997): 595–631.

———. "Attachment and the Regulation of the Right Brain" In *Attachment and Human Development,* vol. 2, 23–47. New York: Taylor and Francis, 2000.

———. *Affect Regulation and the Repair of the Self.* New York: W. W. Norton & Company, 2003.

———. *Affect Regulation and Disorders of the Self.* New York: W. W. Norton & Company, 2003.

Schwartz, J. M., et al. "Systematic Changes in Cerebral Glucose Metabolic Rate After Successful Behavior Modification Treatment of Obsessive-Compulsive Disorder." *Archives of General Psychiatry* 53 (1996): 109–13.

Skinner, B. F. *Walden Two.* New York: Macmillan, 1962.

———. *Beyond Freedom and Dignity*. New York: Alfred A. Knopf, 1971.

———. *About Behaviorism*. New York: Random House, Vintage, 1976.

Smith, Mark. "A Father Finds a Solution: Z-Score Training." *NeuroConnections* (April 2008): 22–25.

———. *A Training Manual for Professionals*. www.brainmaster.com/kb/28. 2010.

Soehner, E., et al. "High Anxiety, Deep Depression" In *The Healing Power of Neurofeedback*, 190–223. Rochester, Vt.: Healing Arts Press, 2006.

Sperry, R. W. "The Nobel Prize in Physiology or Medicine: Roger W. Sperry, David H. Hubel, Torsten N. Wiesel." (1981).

Spitz, R. A. *Emotional Deprivation in Infancy* [A Study by Rene A. Spitz, M.D. Seven-minute film]. 1952. The Psychoanalytic Research Project on Problems of Infancy. Retrieved from www.youtube.com/watch?v=VvdOe10vrs4.

Spitzer, R., J. Endicott, and E. Robins. "Research Diagnostic Criteria: Rationale and Reliability." *Archives of General Psychiatry* 35 (1978): 773–82.

Spitzer, R., and J. Fleiss. "A Re-analysis of the Reliability of Psychiatric Diagnosis." *British Journal of Psychiatry* 125 (1974): 341–47.

Sridharan, D., Ph.D. "The Neuroscience of Music Perception Explored through Functional Imaging and Computational Modeling." The Second Annual Stanford Symposium on Music, Rhythm, and the Brain. The Stanford Institute for Creativity and the Arts (May 13, 2007).

Sterman, M. B. "Studies of EEG Biofeedback Training in Man and Cats." In *Highlights of the 17th Annual Conference: VA Cooperative Studies in Mental Health and Behavioral Sciences* vol. PP. 5060. Veterans' Administration, 1972.

———. "Physiological Origins and Functional Correlates of EEG Rhythmic Activities; Implications for Self-regulation." *Biofeedback and Self-Regulation* 21 (1996): 3–33.

———. *Atlas of Topometric Clinical Displays: Functional Interpretations and Neurofeedback Strategies*. New Jersey: Sterman-Kaiser Imaging Laboratory, 1999.

———. "Basic Concepts and Clinical Findings in the Treatment of Seizure Disorders with Operant Conditioning." *Clinical Electroencephalography* 31, no. 1 (2000): 45–55.

Sterman, M. B., and L. Friar. "Suppression of Seizures in an Epileptic Following Sensorimotor EEG Feedback Training." *Electro-encephalography and Clinical Neurophysiology* 1 (1971): 57–86.

Surmeli, T., et al. "Obsessive Compulsive Disorder and the Efficacy of qEEG-guided Neurofeedback Treatment: A Case Series." *Clinical EEG and Neuroscience* 42, no. 3 (2011): 195–201.

Swingle, P. G., Ph.D. *Biofeedback for the Brain: How Neurotherapy Effectively Treats Depression, ADHD, Aautism, and More.* New Brunswick, N.J.: Rutgers University Press, 2010. (Original work published 2008.)

Taylor, J. B., Ph.D. *My Stroke of Insight.* New York: Viking, 2006.

Thatcher, R., Ph.D. "Validity and Reliability in Quantitative Electroencephalography." *The Journal of Neurotherapy* 14, no. 7) (April–June 2010).

Thatcher, R., Ph.D., and Duane M. North. "An EEG Severity Index of Traumatic Brain Injury." *Journal of Neuropsychiatry and Clinical Neurosciences* 13 (February 2001): 77–87.

Thatcher, R. W., and E. R. John, eds. "Foundations of Cognitive Processes." *Functional Neuroscience,* vol. 1. N.J.: Erlbaum Assoc., 1977.

———. "Neurometrics: Quantitative Electrophysiological Analyses." *Functional Neuroscience,* vol. 2. N.J.: Erlbaum Assoc., 1977.

Thompson, M., and L. Thompson. *The Neurofeedback Book: An Introduction to Basic Concepts in Applied Psychophysiology.* Wheat Ridge, Co.: The Association for Applied Psychophysiology and Biofeedback, 2003.

Urban, R. J., et al. "Serum IFG-1 Concentrations in a Sample of Patients with Traumatic Brain Injury as a Diagnostic Marker of Growth Hormone Secretory Response to Glucagon Stimulation Testing." *Clinical Endocrinology* 74, no. 3 (March 2011): 365–69.

www.appliedneuroscience.com.

www.biocybernaut.com/about/discovery/part1.htm#nav1top (accessed October 2011).

www.cdc.gov/concussion/headsup/high_school.html (accessed October 2011).

www.drikung.org (accessed October 2011).

www.ejnet.org/dioxin (accessed October 2011).

www.fda.gov/BiologicsBloodVaccines.

www.health4youonline.com/article_electro_magnetic_pollution.htm (accessed October 2011).

www.headinjury.com/sports.htm (accessed October 2011).

www.interactivemetronome.com (accessed October 2011).

www.med.nyu.edu/brl/aboutus (accessed October 2011).

www.naturalchild.org/alice_miller/adolf_hitler.html.

www.ncbinlm.nih.gov/sites/entrez?db=pubmed.

www.mrisafety.com/safety_article.asp?subject=170 (accessed November 2010).

www.scientificartsfoundation.org/page/page/3529693.htm.

www.vba.va/gov/bln/21/benefits/herbicide (accessed October 2011).

ABOUT THE
CONTRIBUTORS

Elsa Baehr, Ph.D., is the director of the NeuroQuest Ltd. clinic in Skokie, Illinois. In this position, she has helped more than one "fainting robin" to beat depression with treatment that also works for a wide variety of disorders and conditions, including Attention Deficit Hyperactivity Disorder (ADHD), hypertension, head injuries, and anxiety disorders. Using neurofeedback methods based on a protocol developed by J. Peter Rosenfeld, a psychology professor at Northwestern University, Baehr trains patients to alter their own moods by manipulating their brain waves much as a physical therapist helps people exercise and strengthen their muscles.

Mike Beasley, L.M.T., became interested in the world of science in 1979 when General Electric recruited him for research and development work, which led to him heading up their Silicon and Gallium Arsenide Device Labs. He later worked with foreign and domestic semiconductor research and development centers to develop the next generation protocols and reactors. In 2001 a violent crime involving his daughter refocused his efforts on the health care field. By 2003 his total orientation was on understanding chronic pain, tissue breakdown at implant/donor sites, biofilms, and researching alternative therapeutic methods to reduce chronic pain and PTSD. He founded a company called NeuroPaths in Austin, Texas, to research, understand, and use nondrug/noninvasive approaches to promote relaxation and enhance the body's own healing abilities.

Paul Botticelli, L.C.S.W., received his Bachelor of Science degree in Education from the State University of New York at Cortland, and two Masters degrees from the State University of New York at Stony Brook: one in liberal studies and one in social work. In addition, Paul has completed many courses of continuing education covering such diverse topics as ADD, ADHD, anxiety, alcoholism, autism, biofeedback, chemical dependency, child abuse, communication skills, domestic violence, eating disorders, EMDR, family therapy, financial counseling, gambling, neurofeedback, LENS, psychopharmacology, PTSD, and sexual abuse recovery.

Lynn Brayton, Psy.D., graduated from the Florida Institute of Technology in 1988 with a psychology doctorate. She completed her doctoral internship at the University of Alabama Training Consortium where she trained in Children's Hospital, adolescent medicine, blind rehabilitation, the VA Geriatric Program and Day Hospital. She has been in private practice in the New Orleans area since 1990, treating adolescents, families, and adults—working primarily with mood disorders, PTSD, adjustment problems, eating disorders, and psychological problems associated with physical illness. She utilizes neurofeedback, EMDR, strategic family therapy, and numerous other therapeutic modalities.

Jeffrey Carmen, Ph.D., obtained his doctorate at Syracuse University in psychology and education in 1978. He is currently a licensed psychologist who has maintained a practice in Manlius, New York, since 1979. For the past fifteen years he has specialized in the treatment of migraine headaches. He is also the inventor of the passive infrared hemoencephalography system, also known as pirHEG. This system was developed specifically for use with migraine headaches, but it has subsequently proven useful for almost any problem in which an individual responds too quickly and too strongly to benign stimuli.

Thomas Collura, Ph.D., is the founder and President of BrainMaster Technologies in Bedford, Ohio. He received undergraduate degrees in philosophy and biology from Brown University and a Ph.D. in biomedical engineering from Case Western Reserve University in Cleveland, Ohio. He has held staff and supervisory positions with AT&T Bell Laboratories and the Department of Neurology of the Cleveland Clinic. He has published numerous peer-reviewed articles and book chapters covering such topics as EEG, evoked potentials, brain mapping, and biofeedback. Dr. Collura is the past president of the neurofeedback division of the Association for Applied Psychophysiology and Biofeedback (AAPB) and of the International Society for Neurofeedback and Research (ISNR).

Nicholas Dogris, Ph.D., earned his doctorate from the California School of Professional Psychology in 1997, after receiving a masters degree in research psychology from Humboldt State University in 1990. He is currently a psychologist who practices in the Eastern Sierra Mountains of Bishop, California. He has been using neurofeedback for over seven years in his clinical practice, treating children, adolescents, and adults. Dr. Dogris has developed several innovations for the LENS and is committed to the research and development of the LENS technology. He is the inventor of the NeuroField, an energy replenishment and stress reduction device. NeuroField theory is based on the premise that the human brain emits a field of energy that extends outside the skull. This field of energy is theorized to be an interactive conduit that can travel to any region in the body. Dr. Dogris designed NeuroField after years of study and research.

Mary Lee Esty, Ph.D., L.C.S.W., and president of the Brain Wellness and Biofeedback Center in Bethesda, Maryland, conducted the first traumatic brain injury research using the flexyx neurotherapy system (FNS) with the Kessler Medical Rehabilitation Hospital in an NIH-funded study published in 2001. She was one of the first therapists using this new form of neurotherapy (now known as LENS) and is currently collaborating with USUHS, the military medical school, on another LENS/FNS study treating TBI and PTSD for Iraq and Afghanistan veterans. Since 1994 Dr. Esty has used LENS/FNS to treat over two thousand people diagnosed with various disorders including TBI, ADHD, depression, anxiety, Asperger's syndrome, pain, and other central nervous system problems.

Sebern Fisher, M.A., M.S.W., L.M.H., BCIA, practices psychodynamic psychotherapy and neurofeedback in Northampton, Massachusetts. She trains professionals nationally and internationally on neurofeedback, neurofeedback and attachment disorder, and the integration of neurofeedback with psychotherapy. Fisher was also the clinical director of a residential treatment center for ten years. She is presently consulting with the Sandhill Center in Los Lunas, New Mexico, on the integration of neurofeedback into their treatment milieu.

Michael Gismondi, L.M.H.C., received his masters in Clinical Psychology from Duquesne University in 1976 and did doctoral training in educational psychology and information science at the University of Pittsburgh, receiving his licensure in psychology in 1982. In the 1980s he consulted with Ford Aerospace and the U.S. Air Force on autonomous systems design for project MILSTAR. He has worked in the areas of medical artificial intelligence, business, and licensed psychotherapy. In 1995, he began his work in Neurofeedback, studying and working with many of the leaders of the neurofeedback and QEEG arena. His current interests center upon consultation and treatment delivery systems development, integrating many different models of NFB, QEEG, energy medicine, and so-called intelligent databases for progressive medical practices, with an emphasis upon the integration of EEG-guided stimulation with Z-scored LORETA, surface, and phase reset-based neurofeedback.

Jay Gunkelman, QEEG, is the Chief Science Officer of Brain Science International. Jay lectures on cognitive neuroscience topics worldwide, covering a full range of subject areas from the harder sciences (he authored the seminal paper on EEG endophenotypes) to the underlying physical mechanism of the principle of "connection" in distance healing. He is a former President of the International Society for Neurofeedback and Research (ISNR). In 1999 he officiated and spoke at the inaugural Australasian meeting, which was the predecessor of the Applied Neuroscience Society of Australasia (now ANSA).

D. Corydon Hammond, Ph.D., ECNS, QEEG, BCIA-EEG, is a psychologist and professor at the University of Utah School of Medicine in Salt Lake City, Utah. A past president of the International Society for Neurofeedback and Research (ISNR), he is currently the primary author of the ISNR's Standards of Practice. He has been doing neurofeedback for twenty years and is the author of more than one hundred professional publications. As a psychologist/MFT he uses neurofeedback training, biofeedback, clinical hypnosis, and/or counseling to work with a large variety of clinical conditions. He has practiced in University Hospital in Salt Lake City for over thirty years, is board certified in quantitative EEG brain mapping (EEG and Clinical Neuroscience Society), and is a diplomate of the Quantitative EEG Certification Board. He has also been board certified in neurofeedback by the Biofeedback Certification International Alliance.

Michelle Luster is a courageous survivor of head trauma; she had a very serious head injury early in her life but went on to raise a family and finish college. She feels that her final improvement was achieved using the LENS form of neurofeedback provided by Cambridge psychologist Dr. Harris McCarter.

Joel Lubar, Ph.D., BCIA-EEG, received his B.S. and Ph.D. from the Division of the Biological Sciences and Department of Biopsychology at the University of Chicago. He has published more than eighty-five papers, numerous book chapters, and eight books in the areas of neuroscience and applied psychophysiology. He is currently professor emeritus of psychology at the University of Tennessee, Knoxville. He is a former president of both the Association for Applied Psychophysiology and Biofeedback (AAPB) and the International Society for Neurofeedback and Research (ISNR). He is a senior fellow for the Biofeedback Certification International Alliance (BCIA) EEG division and a licensed clinical psychologist. With his wife Judith, a clinical social worker, he directs the Southeastern Biofeedback Institute. (See also www.eegfeedback.org/joelbio.html.)

Donald Magder, M.A., is an expressive-holistic therapist working in Southfield, Michigan. He also teaches psychology at Baker and Macomb Community Colleges. In his practice he uses gestalt and expressive therapy (bodywork) to clear old emotional patterns, and incorporates Jungian dream work, which allows his patients to connect more directly with spirit. For children he uses neurofeedback to help with ADD, ADHD, developmental delay, and autism. He is also a member of a metaphysical music troupe called Inner Mission, which emphasizes the unity of all religions.

Henry Mann, M.D., is a clinical psychiatrist from Stonington, Connecticut, who has worked in both public health and private clinics. He has personally tried and professionally applied many biofeedback techniques; his wife Carole practices neurofeedback almost exclusively. The Manns conduct many trainings for professionals at their commodious Connecticut residence, and "Hank" is known far and wide as a gourmet chef who loves to cook for his friends and colleagues.

Harris McCarter, Ph.D., is a psychologist in private practice in Cambridge, Massachussetts. He is the former director of Behavioral Medicine training at the Cambridge Hospital where he taught for eighteen years. He has authored two textbook chapters on anxiety disorders and has a special interest in learning problems and their impact on one's concept of self throughout the life span.

Victor McGregor, Ph.D., A.N.P., N.P.P., is a New York State Licensed Adult Health Nurse Practitioner (A.N.P) and an N.P. in Psychiatry (N.P.P.). He is National Board Certified (ANA) Nurse Practitioner in Psychiatry and Adult Health Mental Health (BCMHNP), and a consultant at the Northeast Center for Special Care in Lake Katine, New York. In addition, he has a private practice that specializes in neurofeedback, neurotherapy, and integrative psychiatry in Saugerties, New York.

Siegfried Othmer, Ph.D., received his doctorate in physics from Cornell University. He became interested in the EEG field while working on focal plane arrays at Hughes Aircraft. His son suffered from temporal lobe epilepsy and received much help for his condition from early EEG feedback treatments. Since 1985 Dr. Othmer has been engaged in the development of research-grade instrumentation for EEG feedback, and since 1987 he has been involved in the research of clinical applications utilizing that instrumentation. From 1987 to 2000 he was President of EEG Spectrum, and until 2002 he served as chief scientist of EEG Spectrum International. Currently he is chief scientist at the EEG Institute in Woodland Hills, California. Dr. Othmer provides training for professionals in EEG biofeedback and presents research findings in professional forums.

Barbara Dean Schacker, M.A., has worked in the field of speech and stroke recovery as a researcher, Sensory Trigger speech facilitator, and publisher for over thirty years. In 1973 she began to research the brain and language and, as a result of her work, found a way to get her "untreatable" global aphasic father to talk again nine years post-stroke. In 1984 she began research and work with speech pathologists to design a computer program for speech recovery. After three years of development and testing she developed the Sensory Trigger Method, a nonmedical way to make new pathways in the brain for speech recovery using the brain's own natural ability to learn through the sense of touch. She is the founder of Stroke Family.Org.

Mark Smith, L.C.S.W., is a clinical social worker with a background as an electrician and electronics innovator. He is regarded as a rising star in the neurofeedback community, having participated closely in the emergence of Z-score training, as well as infra-low frequency (ILF). He conducts trainings for Brainmaster Technologies and its affiliate, Stress Therapy Solutions.

Richard Smith, Ph.D., is a North Country clinical psychologist who has practiced for over thirty years in Plattsburgh, New York. Long familiar with biofeedback and consciousness studies, Richard feels his own treatment and training in the LENS with Dr. Stephen Larsen helped bring new life into his practice, and that his own clarity and focus in his mid-seventies is better than ever, due to the LENS.

J. Lawrence Thomas, Ph.D., Director of the Brain Clinic in New York City, has been a clinical psychologist and neuropsychologist specializing in diagnosing and treating adult ADD, LD, and mild head injuries for three decades. He has post doctorate certificates in group therapy, cognitive therapy, relationship therapy, and neuropsychology, and seven books to his credit. Dr. Larry Thomas has degrees from UC Berkeley, Yale, and CUNY, and has been on the faculty of NYU Medical Center for over twenty years. He is the past president of the Independent Practice Division and the Neuropsychology Divisions of the New York State Psychological Association (NYSPA), and is on the board of directors of the International Dyslexia Association and the New York Academy of Traumatic Brain Injury. He is board certified in EEG Biofeedback from the Biofeedback Certification International Alliance (BCIA-EEG). Dr. Larry Thomas was awarded the Distinguished Service Award by NYSPA in June of 2000, and in October 2001 he was elected as Distinguished Practitioner of Psychology in the National Academies of Practice, one of the highest honors in the field.

Hershel Toomim, Ph.D., together with his wife, Marjorie, were established innovators in the field of neurotherapy. Early in their professional history the Toomims' interest in advancing scientific inquiry in psychology and biofeedback led to their hosting monthly meetings of the Forum for Humanistic Psychology. In the early 1970s, the Toomims joined other scientists concerned with self-regulation at the first annual meeting for the Biofeedback Society of America. Later, as a logical extension of biofeedback, Dr. Toomim designed and built sets of biofeedback instruments—including temperature, muscle, skin, and brain wave feedback instruments. He then began building biofeedback instruments that were the first of their kind to use infrared light. He also developed the first calibrated biofeedback instruments to be used in dynamic psychotherapy, hence the inception of neurotherapy. His interest in neuroscience led, more recently, to the discovery of voluntary control of blood flow in the brain, hemoencepholography (HEG). A universally recognized giant in the field, he passed away on July 19, 2011.

Marty Wuttke, C.N.P., and director of the Southern Institute of Psychophysiology, has practiced and taught meditation, biofeedback, and neurofeedback for over thirty years. Known as "a trainer's trainer," he continues to integrate the best elements of applied neurophysiology, spiritual practices, and holistic medicine with the cutting edge technologies of neurofeedback. While he is perhaps best known for his work in the addictions field, in the last decade he has branched out to address neurodevelopmental and treatment-refractory conditions.

Victor Zelek, Ph.D., received his doctoral degree from Yeshiva University, Graduate School of Psychology in New York, majoring in clinical health psychology. He also holds a medical degree from Lithuania. Dr. Zelek completed his postdoctoral training at NYU Medical Center, Rusk Institute for Rehabilitation, where he worked as a supervising neuropsychologist for eight years. He is currently a licensed clinical psychologist and neuropsychologist who maintains a private practice in Rhinebeck, New York. Additionally, he is the director of the neuropsychology department at the Northeast Center for Special Care in Lake Katrine, New York. Dr. Zelek has been using neurofeedback since 1998. He is a diplomate of the National Registry of Neurofeedback Providers. Many patients with ADD, traumatic brain injury, stroke, Lyme disease, chronic fatigue syndrome, anxiety, depression, PTSD, addictions, sleep disorder, and headaches have benefited from this form of treatment in his practice. He has presented his neurofeedback research at many scientific conferences both nationally and internationally. Dr. Zelek is also a member of the scientific advisory board of the International Brain Research Foundation.

INDEX

Page numbers in *italics* indicate illustrations.

Books of Related Interest

The Healing Power of Neurofeedback
The Revolutionary LENS Technique for Restoring
Optimal Brain Function
by Stephen Larsen, Ph.D.

Joseph Campbell: A Fire in the Mind
The Authorized Biography
by Stephen Larsen, Ph.D., and Robin Larsen

The Mythic Imagination
The Quest for Meaning Through Personal Mythology
by Stephen Larsen, Ph.D.

The Shaman's Doorway
Opening Imagination to Power and Myth
by Stephen Larsen, Ph.D.

Zulu Shaman
Dreams, Prophecies, and Mysteries
by Vusamazulu Credo Mutwa
Edited by Stephen Larsen, Ph.D.

Where Does Mind End?
A Radical History of Consciousness and the Awakened Self
by Marc Seifer, Ph.D.

The Biology of Transcendence
A Blueprint of the Human Spirit
by Joseph Chilton Pearce

Walking Your Blues Away
How to Heal the Mind and Create Emotional Well-Being
by Thom Hartmann

INNER TRADITIONS • BEAR & COMPANY
P.O. Box 388
Rochester, VT 05767
1-800-246-8648
www.InnerTraditions.com

Or contact your local bookseller